Illuminations:
The Human Becoming
Theory in Practice
and Research

Illuminations: The Human Becoming Theory in Practice and Research

Edited by
Rosemarie Rizzo Parse, PhD, RN, FAAN

Professor and Niehoff Chair
Marcella Niehoff School of Nursing
Loyola University Chicago

Editor, *Nursing Science Quarterly*
President, Discovery International, Inc.
Pittsburgh, Pennsylvania

National League for Nursing Press • New York
Pub. No. 15-2670

ISBN 0-88737-637-1

The views expressed in this publication represent the views of the authors and do not necessarily reflect the official views of the National League for Nursing.

Library of Congress Cataloging-in-Publication Data

Illuminations : the human becoming theory in practice and research /
    edited by Rosemarie Rizzo Parse.
        p.   cm.
    Pub. no. 15-2670.
    Includes bibliographical references and index.
    ISBN 0-88737-637-1
    1. Nursing—Philosophy.   I. Parse, Rosemarie Rizzo.   II. Title:
Human becoming theory in practice and research.
    [DNLM: 1. Nursing Theory.   2. Philosophy, Nursing.   3. Nursing
Care.   4. Nursing Research—methods.   5. Human Development. WY 86
I29   1995]
RT84.5.I45   1995
610.73'01—dc20
DNLM/DLC
for Library of Congress   94-37463
                                                                            CIP

This book was set in Aster and Caledonia by Publications Development Company. The editor and designer was Nancy Jeffries. The cover was designed by Lauren Stevens.

Cover art created by Alj Mary.

Printed in the United States of America

The reader who is illuminated is, in a real sense, the poem.

—Henry Major Tomlinson

Contents

Preface

*N*ow that nursing is an identifiable body of scientific knowledge articulated through nursing frameworks and theories, nurse scholars are focusing on the development of unique research and practice methodologies to further enhance the discipline. It is essential that these methodologies be developed and utilized to strengthen the identity of nursing as a distinct discipline. Within nursing, there are two major paradigms, totality and simultaneity. These worldviews are different perspectives on the human-universe-health process, the central phenomenon of nursing. The totality paradigm holds that the human is a bio-psycho-social-spiritual organism who adapts to the environment and that health is a state of physical, mental, and social well-being. A number of frameworks and theories have philosophical assumptions rooted here. These include Orem's (1991) general self-care deficit theory, Roy's (Roy & Andrews, 1991) adaptation model, King's (1981) theory of goal attainment, and others. The simultaneity paradigm, initiated in 1970 with Rogers' science of unitary human beings, represents a different perspective. In this paradigm, focus is on the human as unitary, in mutual process with the environment, and on health as a value. Parse's human becoming theory arises from the assumptions of this paradigm and builds on tenets of existential-phenomenological thought. The Parse theory was created as an alternative to traditional natural science nursing when the author realized the limitations inherent in the totality perspective (Parse, 1981). These limitations were most visible in four major ways:

1. The value priorities of the person were subordinated to a set of norms defined by medical science.

2. The nurse rather than the person was considered the expert on health.
3. The meaning of lived experiences was not the focus of nursing; a human science approach had not yet been conceptualized.
4. The potential contributions of nursing as a unique discipline were obfuscated by the natural science approach to research and practice.

As an alternative to the traditional, the human becoming theory focuses on the experience of humans as freely choosing beings who cocreate health in mutual process with the universe. The person is respected as the expert on his or her own health, and the meaning of lived experiences is honored. This theory, then, rooted in the human sciences, clearly requires a different approach to research and practice.

The purpose of this work is to posit, with examples, the research and practice methodologies that evolved from the ontological base of Parse's nursing theory of human becoming (Parse, 1981, 1992, 1994). The practice methodology actually flows directly from the three principles of the theory. The central focus of practice is the meaning of lived experiences in the enhancement of quality of life for unitary human beings. The research methodology likewise flows directly from the theory and focuses on uncovering structures of universal lived experiences to expand understanding of the human-universe-health process.

This book clarifies the process of developing practice and research methodologies from a unique theory and illustrates how the human becoming theory is practiced and research conducted in a variety of settings. How nursing theory is translated into practice and research is a question that nurse scholars must respond to with ever greater awareness and precision. The book contains three major parts: theoretical conceptualizations, practice applications, and research reports. Each section contains an overview with a chapter by Parse and chapters by other nurse scholars.

This text will be very helpful for undergraduate students who are learning about nursing theory and how it guides practice, for graduate students and faculty who are studying the enhancement of nursing knowledge through practice and research, and for professional nurses who seek a model for nursing theory-based practice. The work is offered as a contribution to the evolution of nursing science.

REFERENCES

King, I. M. (1981). *A theory for nursing.* New York: Wiley.

Orem, D. E. (1991). *Nursing: Concepts of practice* (4th ed.). New York: McGraw-Hill.

Parse, R. R. (1981). *Man-living-health: A theory of nursing.* New York: Wiley.

Parse, R. R. (1992). Human becoming: Parse's theory of nursing. *Nursing Science Quarterly, 5,* 35–42.

Parse, R. R. (1994). *Human becoming: A theory of nursing.* Manuscript submitted for publication.

Rogers, M. E. (1970). *An introduction to the theoretical basis of nursing.* Philadelphia: Davis.

Roy, C., & Andrews, H. (1991). *The Roy adaptation model: The definitive statement.* Norwalk: Appleton-Lange.

Rosemarie Rizzo Parse, PhD, RN, FAAN
Professor and Niehoff Chair
Marcella Niehoff School of Nursing
Loyola University Chicago
Chicago, IL
Editor, *Nursing Science Quarterly*
President, Discovery International, Inc.
Pittsburgh, PA

Contributors

Barbara C. Banonis, MSN, RN
President, Peoplework Solutions
S. Charleston, WV

Kathleen Stentz Brinkman, MSN, RN
Nurse Specialist
Clermont County General Health District
Amelia, OH

William K. Cody, PhD, RN
Assistant Professor
The University of North Carolina at Charlotte
College of Nursing
Charlotte, NC

John Daly, PhD, RN
Associate Professor & Head
School of Nursing
Charles Sturt University
Wagga Wagga, NSW, Australia

Jacqueline Hatfield Hudepohl, MSN, RN
Assistant Professor
Northern Kentucky University
Melbourne, KY

Christine M. Jonas, MScN, RN
Clinical Nurse Specialist
The Queen Elizabeth Hospital
Toronto, Ontario, Canada

Lois S. Kelley, DEd, RN
Assistant Professor
Florida Atlantic University
College of Nursing
Boca Raton, FL

Gail J. Mitchell, PhD, RN
Chief Nursing Officer
Sunnybrook Health Science Center
Assistant Professor
University of Toronto
Toronto, Ontario, Canada

Rosemarie Rizzo Parse, PhD, RN, FAAN
Professor and Niehoff Chair
Marcella Niehoff School of Nursing
Loyola University Chicago
Chicago, IL
Editor, *Nursing Science Quarterly*
President, Discovery International, Inc.
Pittsburgh, PA

Diane L. Rasmusson, BAAN, RN
Addiction Counselor
St. Stephen's Community House
The Corner Drop-In
Toronto, Ontario, Canada

Marc D. A. Santopinto, MScN, RN
Nurse Specialist
London Psychiatric Hospital
London, Ontario, Canada

Marlaine C. Smith, PhD, RN
Assistant Professor
School of Nursing
University of Colorado Health Sciences Center
Denver, CO

Part I

Theoretical Conceptualizations Within the Human Becoming Theory

Rosemarie Rizzo Parse

*T*his section of the book contains five chapters, one on the human becoming theory, three on views of phenomena from the human becoming perspective, and one on a metaphor comparing the human becoming perspective with extant caring frameworks. The first chapter specifies the theory with its assumptions and principles. The human becoming theory (Parse, 1992, 1994), first created in 1981 as man-living-health, focuses on participative experience with the universe in cocreating becoming. This theory is rooted in the simultaneity paradigm (Parse, 1987). Each of the next three chapters includes a review of the general literature on a phenomenon with an elaboration of its meaning from the human becoming perspective. The three phenomena described are family, freedom, and suffering.

In chapter 2, on family, Cody embraces the notion that family includes close others, all those individuals (predecessors, contemporaries, and successors) closely connected with the person (Parse, 1981). In chapter 3, Mitchell describes freedom as a dimension of the paradoxical rhythm of restriction-freedom. Although one is free to choose in situations at explicit and tacit realms of the universe, choices are not always explicitly known or reflectively made. From this perspective, freedom is related to the nature of being human and does not depend on a standard of living or number of possessions. In chapter 4, Daly writes about suffering, a universal phenomenon lived uniquely by each person. It is a chosen way of living a moment—an all-at-once heaviness-lightness arising in the human-universe process. In chapter 5, Kelley offers a metaphoric interpretation of house-garden-wilderness, comparing the human becoming perspective with extant caring perspectives.

REFERENCES

Parse, R. R. (1981). *Man-living-health: A theory of nursing.* New York: Wiley.

Parse, R. R. (1987). *Nursing science: Major paradigms, theories, and critiques.* Philadelphia: Saunders.

Parse, R. R. (1992). Human becoming: Parse's theory of nursing. *Nursing Science Quarterly, 5,* 35–42.

Parse, R. R. (1994). *Human becoming: A theory of nursing.* Manuscript submitted for publication.

Chapter 1
The Human Becoming Theory

Rosemarie Rizzo Parse

Parse's human becoming (1981, 1992, 1994a), first created as man-living-health (1981), is a human science theory. The change in name was related to a change in the dictionary definition of the term *man,* from "mankind" to "male gender." The theory is grounded in the belief that humans coauthor their becoming in mutual process with the universe, cocreating distinguishable patterns which specify the uniqueness of both humans and the universe.

The human becoming theory is explained in detail in the book *Human Becoming: A Theory of Nursing* (Parse, 1994a) which is an update of *Man-Living-Health* (Parse, 1981). A historical perspective can be drawn from reading Parse (1981, 1990, 1992, 1994a, 1994b, 1994c). The assumptions and principles are set forth here, and the principles are discussed briefly.

The assumptions of the human becoming theory (Parse, 1992, p. 38), written at the philosophical level of discourse, are:

1. The human is coexisting while coconstituting rhythmical patterns with the universe.
2. The human is an open being, freely choosing meaning in situation, bearing responsibility for decisions.

3. The human is a living unity continuously coconstituting patterns of relating.
4. The human is transcending multidimensionally with the possibles.
5. Becoming is an open process, experienced by the human.
6. Becoming is a rhythmically coconstituting human-universe process.
7. Becoming is the human's pattern of relating value priorities.
8. Becoming is an intersubjective process of transcending with the possibles.
9. Becoming is human evolving.

Three assumptions about human becoming are:

- Human becoming is freely choosing personal meaning in situation in the intersubjective process of relating value priorities.
- Human becoming is cocreating rhythmical patterns of relating in open process with the universe.
- Human becoming is cotranscending multidimensionally with the emerging possibles. (Parse, 1992, p. 38)

The principles of the theory flow directly from the philosophical assumptions and are written at a theoretical level of discourse. The principles bring to light the notion of paradox as fundamental to human becoming. It is the only nursing theory that regards paradoxical processes as inherent in being human. The paradoxes are not considered problems to be solved or eliminated but, rather, natural rhythms of life.

Principle 1. *Structuring meaning multidimensionally is cocreating reality through the languaging of valuing and imaging* (Parse, 1981, p. 69).

This principle means that humans construct what is real for them from choices made at many realms of the universe. Humans are continuously languaging imaged values through speaking - being silent, and moving - being still. Valuing is the confirming - not confirming of what is cherished in the prereflective-reflective knowings of imaging. One cocreates meaning, and the meaning changes with experiences as new images arise, expanding possibilities. People live their treasured beliefs in the process of evolving.

Principle 2. *Cocreating rhythmical patterns of relating is living the paradoxical unity of revealing-concealing and enabling-limiting while connecting-separating* (Parse, 1981, p. 69).

This principle means that humans live in rhythm with the universe coconstituting patterns of relating. The patterns are paradoxical in nature—apparent opposites, but dimensions of one phenomenon. One reveals and conceals all-at-once the who that one is becoming, which incarnates the who one was and will be. But one cannot reveal all of who one is; there is always the mystery of being human. One is enabled and limited simultaneously by all choices, in that with each choice there are an infinite number of opportunities and limitations. No choice is without both. In moving together and apart all-at-once, one connects and separates with the universe in the rhythmical flow of cocreation. This connecting-separating is the mutual process humans live with the universe.

Principle 3. *Cotranscending with the possibles is powering unique ways of originating in the process of transforming* (Parse, 1981, p. 69).

This principle means that humans forge unique paths with shifting perspectives as a different light is cast on the familiar. The energizing force of forging ahead - holding back enlivens the ebb and flow of life as one lives conformity - non-conformity and certainty-uncertainty in moving the unfamiliar to the familiar. Humans seek to be unique and yet like others all-at-once as they live the inevitable ambiguity of creating different ways of becoming in transforming.

This theory posits that humans live at multidimensional realms of the universe all-at-once as they prereflectively and reflectively choose from options incarnating imaged value priorities. Through languaging, humans disclose and hide all-at-once the who that they are, while living the opportunities and limitations of being close to and apart from others. Humans change moment-to-moment as they actualize dreams and hopes through inventing new ways to propel beyond what is to what is not-yet.

The principles of the human becoming theory specify the view of the human-universe process as a rippling, risking flow weaving together the changing fabric of the now moment, incarnating the side waters of remembering and anticipating, while forging the present yet to be. Human becoming, then, is a cocreated process of evolving.

REFERENCES

Parse, R. R. (1981). *Man-living-health: A theory of nursing.* New York: Wiley.

Parse, R. R. (1990). Parse's research methodology with an illustration of the lived experience of hope. *Nursing Science Quarterly, 3,* 9–17.

Parse, R. R. (1992). Human becoming: Parse's theory of nursing. *Nursing Science Quarterly, 5,* 35–42.

Parse, R. R. (1994a). *Human becoming: A theory of nursing.* Manuscript submitted for publication.

Parse, R. R. (1994b). Laughing and health: A study using Parse's research method. *Nursing Science Quarterly, 7,* 55–64.

Parse, R. R. (1994c). Quality of life: Sciencing and living the art of human becoming. *Nursing Science Quarterly, 7,* 16–21.

Chapter 2

The View of Family Within the Human Becoming Theory

William K. Cody

*T*he purpose of this chapter is to elucidate the view of the family in Parse's (1981, 1992) human becoming theory. For Parse, the central phenomenon of nursing science is *the human-universe-health process*, which, for purposes of explication, may be thought of as the interrelationship of the human, the universe, and health (Parse, 1992). Health is viewed as the quality of life experienced by the person. This is the *lived experience* of health. Lived experiences of health inherently involve one's interrelationships with others in the universe. Family interrelating, then, is of crucial significance in Parse's theory.

The conceptualization of the human as a unique individual and free agent is a well-known and important attribute of Parse's theory. The strong belief in the uniqueness and freedom of the individual within the theory, however, does not delimit its scope in addressing family phenomena. Rather, this emphasis is intrinsic to the specific view of family in the theory. The assumptions, principles, and concepts of Parse's theory encompass a view of family that guides nurses in living the theory in any setting, with individuals, families, or groups. Parse originally presented the theory using family life situations as illustrations in her 1981 text, wherein she defined family as "the others with whom one is closely connected" (p. 81). This chapter is intended simply to adduce and explore the view of family already present in the theory.

NURSING AND FAMILIES

Practice with families has been integral to nursing since the time of Nightingale. The family is emphasized in most general nursing textbooks and has been given considerable attention at more advanced levels. Yet, there is a consensus within the profession that nursing is far from realizing its potential in family-centered practice (Gilliss, Highley, Roberts, & Martinson, 1989; Whall & Fawcett, 1991).

The notion has been advanced that to think about families and family health requires concepts and methods different from those through which personal health is studied (Feetham, 1991; Gilliss, 1983, 1989). If this assumption is made, the scientist then considers the family as a whole to be the unit of analysis, so that individual experiences are considered only in relation to what *the scientist* considers to be the family. Historically, this view is closely associated with a sociological perspective, and it reflects the beliefs embedded in structural-functionalist, systemic, and developmental family theories (Gilliss et al., 1989). It is not a view that is rooted in the discipline of nursing.

Nursing scholars have advocated borrowing family theory from other disciplines in order to advance nursing practice with families and nursing theory development in the area of family phenomena (Gilliss et al., 1989; Whall & Fawcett, 1991). There have been very few nursing theory-based, family-centered works in nursing. The literature exhibits strong tendencies to borrow intact family theories from other disciplines, to blend borrowed theory with nursing theory, and to adopt the sociological perspective of the family as "the unit of analysis" to arrive at a theory base for family-centered nursing practice (Gilliss et al., 1989; Whall & Fawcett, 1991). These tendencies reflect an assumption that the extant nursing theories are inadequate to guide practice with families. The smallest proportion of the nursing literature related to families is that which is rooted wholly in nursing's own theory base (Clements & Roberts, 1983).

If nursing is to be a full-fledged discipline with its own knowledge base, and if families are important to consider in nursing practice and scholarship, then nursing scholars must make explicit the views of family that are specific to the discipline of nursing. In light of nursing's heritage of working with families and its often-stated concern for the health of families, it is crucial for the development of nursing science to approach practice with families and family-centered studies from a perspective rooted in the discipline of nursing. There is a coherent theoretical perspective of family phenomena already present in Parse's theory, different from the theories from other disciplines that currently dominate family-related science. In order to appreciate this view, it is necessary to begin with the assumptions underpinning the theory.

PARSE'S ASSUMPTIONS IN RELATION TO FAMILIES

Parse (1981, 1992) uses the singular term "human" to refer to *homo sapiens* generically. The singular term "human" is an abstraction, as is appropriate for theory construction. The term does not refer to a particular man or woman, but to any human being. "Family" is a human universal, although families are configured and experienced with great diversity in different societies and life situations (Brown, 1990). The use of the singular noun at the abstract level does not indicate a restrictive focus on the individual. Rather, since the abstract term "human" includes all human phenomena, it encompasses family phenomena as inherent in being human.

Parse's theory is one of two major theoretical perspectives (the other being Rogers', 1970) in nursing's simultaneity paradigm. The fundamental beliefs of the simultaneity paradigm are that the human and the environment are mutually and simultaneously interrelating as a unity, that the human-universe-health process is more than and different from the sum of parts, and that health is an ever-changing process experienced by the human (Parse, 1987). From this view, clearly, the family, by any recognizable definition, could not *not* be significant in any human life.

To center on the family with Parse's theory, one has only to dwell with the notion of family while dialoguing with the theory. The very first assumption underpinning the theory is: "The human is coexisting while coconstituting rhythmical patterns with the universe" (Parse, 1992, p. 38). Thus, to be human is to coexist with others and to coparticipate in the creation of what is real. The second assumption is: "The human is an open being, freely choosing meaning in situation, bearing responsibility for decisions" (Parse, 1992, p. 38). To be human is to be open, mutually and simultaneously interrelating with the universe, assigning meaning to life experiences, and bearing responsibility for choices.

Already a view of family phenomena is evident: persons coconstitute families while coexisting with all humans; persons coexist with contemporaries, predecessors, and successors all-at-once (Parse, 1981). Persons assign meaning to experiences within the context of their lives, which includes the family, in whatever way it is configured. Persons freely choose meaning at many levels of the universe, and they bear responsibility for the choices. Families are coconstituted through this process. Family relationships are given meaning by the person through living a commitment with others. Living this commitment to family has consequences. Living with the consequences in a chosen way is bearing responsibility for the choices (Parse, 1981, 1992).

Further assumptions underpinning the theory posit the human as a living unity continuously coconstituting patterns of relating, transcending multidimensionally with the possibles (Parse, 1992, p. 38). Each person is a living unity with a unique, irreproducible interrelationship with the universe; each person experiences life in a personal way. What is experienced is coconstituted with others in the process of cocreating patterns of relating. This unitary process is simultaneously moving beyond what is to what is not yet. It is a

continuous process in which all humans and the universe coparticipate, a process of ever-evolving possibilities.

Health is viewed by Parse as the quality of life as experienced
by the human. Health is essentially synonymous with *becoming*,
which is an open, rhythmically coconstituting process of the
human-universe interrelationship (Parse, 1992, p. 38); health is
the human's pattern of relating value priorities (Parse, 1992,
p. 38). This assumption relates to the view that the human is a living unity freely choosing meaning in situation. Health is cocreated
with the universe and experienced uniquely by the human.

Parse further posits becoming as "an intersubjective process of
transcending with the possibles" and as "human unfolding" (Parse,
1992, p. 38). While one's life experience is uniquely one's own, it in-
terfaces multidimensionally with the experiences of others, as all
humans coexist and coconstitute patterns of relating with the universe in an ever-evolving process of emergence. The basic assumptions of the theory, then, affirm essentially that the family is
always with the person in multidimensional realms of becoming no
matter what the individual's circumstances may be. Parse's language itself strongly suggests that interrelating with close others is
a major focus of the theory with such terms as *coexisting, coconstituting, intersubjective process, cocreating,* and *cotranscending.* The
fundamental focus on human-to-human relating in the theory is
clear in the use of these words and in such phrases as "cocreating
rhythmical patterns of relating" (Parse, 1992, p. 38), a continuous
process of human becoming. With these assumptions, a philosophical perspective of the family is clearly articulated. There is no way
that each individual is not with family; this is of the very nature of
being human.

DISTINCTIONS FROM OTHER VIEWS OF FAMILY

Historically, family-oriented scientists have examined the social
circumstances of their time and have conceptualized the family in
terms of the prevailing norms, working on the assumption that the

business of family science is to predict and control family dynamics to promote the prevailing notion of normality in the science (Burr, Hill, Reiss, & Nye, 1979). Parse's basic assumptions about humans are very different; thus her view of family is very different. The view of the family in Parse's theory is unbounded by structural, functional, or systemic assumptions. There are and have been many diverse views of kinship and family in human history, and these views are continuously evolving. While all discourse is historically situated, Parse's view of the family, in relation to the predominant view, is radically open to possibilities and to diverse personal meanings and interpretations of family experiences. Parse does not propose a specific structure for the family or a particular dynamic that is designated as family health. Rather, family health is cocreated by persons as they live family process.

For Parse, as previously stated, health is the quality of life *from the person's perspective*. The relevance to health of any societal norm, then, is relative to the person's perspective. While personal values and beliefs, inasmuch as they are cocreated with others, do reflect (shared and unshared) sociocultural values and may even be related to some specific sociocultural norms, these values and beliefs are *personal* for the person who holds them. The goal of practice guided by Parse's theory is to participate in cocreating quality of life. This does not change when practice unfolds explicitly within a family context. The goal of nursing research guided by Parse's theory is to understand lived experiences of health. Neither does this goal change when the research is family-centered. Family-centered practice and research guided by Parse's theory are not intended to predict or control family dynamics, nor to promote normality. General sociocultural norms for families are irrelevant to practice and research guided by Parse's theory, except *as* they are actually valued by persons and families, and then it is only the living of the values that gives them significance.

Parse (1981) defines the family as "the others with whom one is closely connected" (p. 81). This definition underscores the *interrelational* and *perspectival* nature of the family. No two persons' experiences of family are precisely the same. To speak of the family as a whole (without reference to an individual) within this context, one could designate the family as *close others, from the perspectives of those involved.* But caution is warranted in speaking of "the family as a whole" at all. Different persons "in" a family have different beliefs about who is family and who is not. If one traces the multiple family relationships of each person in a given family constellation, unbounded by the conventional restrictions of birth, marriage, and adoption, one finds that the multidimensional family connections coexisting with any given circumscribed family constellation extend infinitely. This gives testimony to the interrelationship of all human beings. Parse's view of the human-universe-health process is unbounded by geographic space and calendar time. If the family must be construed as a "unit," it is a "unit" of *meaning*, for those involved. It is not a hypostatized structure or system with roles and functions but, rather, a flowing experiential process of interrelating.

Parse's assumptions clearly manifest a view that the human "is not alone in any dimension of becoming" (1981, p. 20). Yet, the human is also posited as "freely choosing personal meaning," an assumption that sets in strong relief the uniqueness of the individual as well. Differentiating self from others is inherent in "the intersubjective process of relating value priorities" (1992, p. 38). The human coexists with others, coconstitutes reality through interrelating with others intersubjectively, and differentiates self as a unique being through relating personal value priorities. Parse's view of the process of relating value priorities as an *intersubjective* one is similar to von Hildebrand's notion of the "paradox of subjectivity" (cited in Owens, 1970). Von Hildebrand held that both communality and individuality are intrinsic to being human; there is no degree of individuality that can eradicate communality as constitutive of being human and no degree of communality that can eradicate the uniqueness of the individual. Buber (1938/1965) expressed a similar view when he wrote, "The fundamental fact of human existence is neither the individual as such nor the aggregate as such . . . . The fundamental fact of human existence is man with man" (pp. 202–

203). Although the matrix of personal values through which one filters all that one experiences is uniquely one's own, relating personal value priorities connects one with others multidimensionally through the very awareness of options, the sharing and not sharing, the divulging and hiding, that are inherent in humanly lived experience.

The philosophical assumptions underpinning Parse's conceptualization of the family, then, are, broadly, those of the simultaneity paradigm related to human-environment simultaneity, the human as more than and different from the sum of parts, and health as an evolutionary process. The assumptions specific to the human becoming theory set forth a view in which the family is coconstituted through "choosing meaning . . . in the intersubjective process of relating value priorities," through "cocreating rhythmical patterns of relating," and through "cotranscending multidimensionally with the unfolding possibilities" (Parse, 1992, p. 38). This is a view of the family unrestricted by the hypostatized, objectivist, normative view of the family commonly found in conventional family science. Rather, the family is a chosen pattern of relating emerging multidimensionally with the unfolding possibilities, an intersubjective process of relating value priorities experienced by the human.

In the family science literature, evidence of a need to explore new ideas about family structure and family dynamics has been presented by Anderson and Goolishian (1990), de Shazer (1991), Fine and Turner (1991), Golann (1988), Hoffman (1985, 1990), Parry (1991), and others. Burton (1990), Lindsey (1981), Rapoport (1989), and Weston (1991) have explored a variety of family configurations that challenge the conventional conceptualization of family, reflecting the increasingly obvious fact that among families "diversity prevails" (Rapoport, 1989, p. 55). Family therapists like Parry (1991) advocate the elimination of "the gratuitous attempt to explain the meaning of a person's story with regard to a normative structure concerning what makes individuals, families, or systems in general tick" (p. 42). Hoffman (1990) describes a "postmodern" family therapy, wherein the "therapist comes into the family . . . without any set idea about what should or should not change. Together . . . interviewer and family may come up with some understandings or ideas for action that are different from those the family may originally have had in mind, and also different from those the therapist may originally have had in mind" (pp. 10–11). Fine and Turner (1991) posit the family therapist as one who "collaborate[s] with clients in coconstructing new realities" (p. 307). These perspectives reflect an opening up of family theory and a dimunition of the normative, judgmental view of family in family science. Parse's perspective of family is similar in some ways to these approaches, yet is distinct in that it is fully articulated with a theory base and practice method rooted in *nursing science*.

THE PRINCIPLES OF PARSE'S THEORY
IN RELATION TO FAMILIES

As mentioned earlier, Parse (1981, p. 81) defines family as "the others with whom one is closely connected." It is necessary to consider this definition of the family within the context of the theory as a whole to appreciate its meaning. The "others" referred to in the definition are continuously coexisting, cocreating, and cotranscending with others as well. Every human-to-human interrelationship is one wherein the individuals are continuously coconstituting reality, cocreating patterns of relating, and cotranscending with the possibles at many realms of the universe. The recognizable pattern that is family interrelating is encompassed by the principles of the theory. In this section, the view of the family that is implicit in each principle will be adduced for discussion. A basic familiarity with the definitions of the nine theoretical concepts in Parse's three principles is assumed (see Parse 1981, 1992).

Principle 1. *Structuring meaning multidimensionally is cocreating reality through the languaging of valuing and imaging* (Parse,

1981, p. 42). The principle of *structuring meaning multidimensionally* describes the view that family interrelationships cocreate values that are lived as persons coconstituting the family language their perspectives of life situations (Parse, 1981, p. 81). Values are relational and perspectival in that all options are cocreated with others yet always given personal meanings. Living a commitment to a family relationship expresses a valued image chosen from among infinite possibilities. Family relationships are not limited by geographic space or calendar time but extend multidimensionally and may include persons who are deceased and persons not yet born.

For example, young adult children often live value priorities that are different from those of their parents, while simultaneously sharing many of their parents' beliefs and cherishing close, meaningful family relationships. They often look at things differently and make choices that are different from those that their parents might wish them to make. They may choose to adopt a different religion, to adopt a different political view, or to become intimately involved with a person or persons of a different ethnic heritage or value orientation. Yet, all of these possibilities unfold within the context of the person's family life situation and are often synthesized with a continuing commitment to the family of origin as multiple patterns of personal living unfold. Deceased or absent persons may be highly significant family members, and persons are often deeply committed to their offspring and other successors years before they are actually born. The meaning of the family is structured for each person through expressing personal views of shared and unshared priorities, thus cocreating the reality of the family that is experienced.

Principle 2. *Cocreating rhythmical patterns of relating is living the paradoxical unity of revealing-concealing and enabling-limiting while connecting-separating* (Parse, 1981, p. 50). The principle of *cocreating rhythmical patterns of relating* expresses the view that family patterns of interrelating generate opportunities and limitations as persons coconstituting the family reveal and conceal aspects of self in rhythmic being-with-and-apart-from family and others (pp. 81–82). In living the connectedness of family, persons are simultaneously distancing themselves from others. This does not abrogate the fundamental coexistence of all humans but, rather, reflects the uniqueness of each individual within the context of coexistence. Each individual uniquely relates with certain others yet is open to a universe of relational possibilities. Involvement with others entails relative "noninvolvement" with (distancing from) others in some realms, while the basic commitment to the family relationship persists. Opportunities and limitations are manifest in family life situations as persons choose unique ways of living moment-to-moment and day-to-day, divulging and hiding aspects of self in the way they *are* with others. The way each person *is* for the self is different from the way the person *seems* to others (Parse, 1981, p. 52). Each person's choices cocreate the diverse and intricate rhythmical patterns of living with family and others.

For example, persons coming together to create a life partnership are simultaneously distancing themselves from other persons and other possibilities while each person's interrelationship with the universe continues to be unique. Living personal value priorities, which may be shared or unshared, creates opportunities and limitations in relation to the togetherness of the life partners. Presence with another is simultaneously divulging and hiding aspects of self. Sometimes what is shared with others seems more important in the moment than what is shared with one's partner, and sometimes one feels that only one's life partner truly understands. Persons in a committed relationship may decide to forego possibilities that would separate them, confirming their commitment to togetherness, or they may decide to pursue hopes and dreams they do not share. Presence with the cherished other in light of each individual's unique multidimensional interrelationship with the universe bears witness to the personal valuing of the relationship.

Principle 3. *Cotranscending with the possibles is powering unique ways of originating in the process of transforming* (Parse, 1981,

p. 41). The principle of *cotranscending with the possibles* specifies that, through choosing unique ways of living from among the many possibilities available in the ever-changing process of becoming, the family's interrelating energizes transforming with each family life situation (p. 82). As each individual becomes the who that he or she is, the self as actuality and potentiality all-at-once is not experienced in a vacuum but in continuous interrelationship with others. Affirming oneself in the flux of daily life is affirming one's view of reality and the way in which one relates with others. Unique ways of becoming are chosen from among an infinite variety of ways of being like and unlike others, while the outcomes of the choices are not known. Families evolve, cocreate diverse ever-changing situations, and move toward and away from various possibilities all-at-once as each person chooses unique ways of becoming. Patterns of relating, for the persons coconstituting the family and others, are reconfigured and given new meanings such that the fabric of life is continuously rewoven and new possibilities for relating emerge.

For example, the family is commonly viewed as those persons who aid and comfort one another in struggling through difficult times. What constitutes "difficult times," however, is relative and perspectival to the person experiencing them. For some persons, the birth of a baby or a promotion may be a joyous occasion entailing little or no difficulty. For others, such an occasion may be an extremely strife-filled event. Possibilities surfacing in each family life situation challenge the persons cocreating the family to choose their own unique ways of living with change. The examples of committing to parenting a child or embarking on a demanding new career are situations in which choosing a way of living with change evolves the family life situation while the outcomes of the choices are not fully known. Often the commitment to the family itself is strengthened through affirming such a choice; yet it is also possible that the ever-changing human-universe-health process may evolve toward different family configurations through the personal choices of those involved.

PARSE'S PRACTICE METHOD WITH FAMILIES

Living Parse's theory with families, the nurse coparticipates in *illuminating* the *meaning* of the family situation through explicating what is (Parse, 1987, p. 167). The nurse is present as the family relates the meaning of their situation. "In telling about the meaning, persons share thoughts and feelings with one another, which in itself changes the meaning of a situation by making it more explicit" (p. 168).

The nurse coparticipates in *synchronizing rhythms* through "dwelling with the pitch, yaw, and roll of the interhuman cadence" (Parse, 1987, p. 167). The nurse "does not try to calm these rhythms . . . but . . . goes with the rhythm set by the family" (p. 168). "The nurse focuses on the person's own meaning of that moment" (p. 169). The *personal* meanings of family life situations may (and often do) conflict. The nurse in true presence with the family bears witness to the reality of each person's interpretation of the family situation and makes no attempt to reconcile conflicts or achieve resolution. The persons with the family evolve their own meanings and cocreate their patterns of relating.

The nurse coparticipates in *mobilizing transcendence* through moving beyond the meaning moment to what is not yet (Parse, 1987, p. 167). The nurse is there with the family to focus on "dreaming of the possibles and planning to reach for the dreams" (p. 169). The shared and unshared priorities and the disclosed and undisclosed hopes and dreams of the persons living the family commitment cocreate the possibilities for the continuous evolution of the family. The focus of Parse's practice method is quality of life from the perspective of the persons with whom the nurse is present in practice. The nurse does not know what kind of family life would be comfortable or rewarding for the persons involved but recognizes that each person participates in cocreating ways of living as family that are meaningful for them. The nurse, in cocreating the quality of life with the family, is "there with" the persons of the family as they focus on the meaning of the family life situation, dwell with the ebb and flow of the family relationships, and reach beyond the now toward what is not-yet. Each person is the cocreation of self with closely connected others (family), other persons, ideas, and situations (the universe). So, even when the nurse is with one individual, the living family for that individual is always present.

PARSE'S RESEARCH METHOD WITH FAMILIES

The preponderance of family-centered research reflects deeply held assumptions about the structure and dynamics of "the family," what a "healthy" family is, and how it should and should not "function" (Burr et al., 1979; Gilliss et al., 1989; Whall & Fawcett, 1991). Family-centered research guided by Parse's theory is very different. Parse's (1987, 1990) original nursing research method may be used with families as participants (for example, see Cody's study in this volume, chapter 14). The processes of the method are essentially the same whether the research participants are invited to participate individually or as families.

In family-centered research with Parse's method, it is the participants' view of who is family that is important, not the researcher's. It should be made clear to prospective participants that the definition of family is open to their own interpretation. There is no need to attempt to recruit every member of a family into the research, since the view of family as a multidimensional experience involving contemporaries, predecessors, and successors all-at-once means that there will always be "absent presences" in the family discussion (see Cody's study, chapter 14).

Dialogical engagement with families occurs in essentially the same manner as with individuals. In dialoguing with families, however, the persons in the families also speak with one another. Family discussions unfold in diverse ways, with different ways of participating among the family members present. The researcher goes with the rhythm of the discussion and makes no attempt to iron out the unevenness of the discussion (for example, if one person speaks more than another). Rather, the researcher dwells with the sense of the whole experience.

In a family-centered research project, the process of extraction-synthesis (through which the researcher uncovers the structure of the phenomenon under investigation) involves attending to the various views arising in the discussion with the participant family. For each participant family, a multiplicity of views cocreates the reality of the family situation as lived by each person. Patterns of relating are brought into sharp relief when described from more than one viewpoint. The structure of the lived experience of interest that emerges from a family-centered study reflects the description of each *family* in the study. Through the participation of multiple family members in the research process, the cocreative processes of the family, the rhythmical patterns of family interrelating, and the family's coparticipation in moving beyond the now toward the not-yet are brought to the fore and made explicit. Parse's method surfaces the meaning of family experiences in a way that is specific to this nursing perspective and, therefore, contributes to knowledge of family life in a way that is unique to nursing.

SUMMARY OF PARSE'S PERSPECTIVE
OF THE FAMILY

The perspective of the family within Parse's theory may be described, in short, as "synergistic family becoming" (Parse, 1981, p. 129), reflecting Parse's assumptions regarding human coexistence and the coconstitution of reality. But, Parse also states, "One's perspective of health . . . can be known only through a personal description even though it is cocreated through interrelationships with others" (p. 81). This aspect of the theory is crucial to understanding Parse's focus on lived experience. "An experience of a situation," she writes, "while cocreated with others, belongs to one human being only" (p. 30). "Perspectives of self emerge in human encounters as individuals view themselves as well as view themselves being viewed by others" (p. 64). In the human experience of a life situation, both prereflective and reflective awareness of one's own and others' perspectives are present and are coconstitutive of the situation. The dynamic cocreation of life situations intrinsically involves one's close others and one's predecessors, contemporaries, and successors all-at-once (p. 26). The family cocreates each individual; thus, family health is the living of struggle and commitment, the experience of closeness and distance, opportunities and limitations, and the sharing of meanings and values—pushing-resisting and creating anew while moving with hopes and dreams (Parse, 1981, 1992).

Parse's theory offers a theoretical perspective to guide family-centered practice rooted in the discipline of nursing. It is a unique perspective of family, emerging from nursing's own heritage and scholarly genealogy, which offers new insights into family life as it is actually lived. Quality of life is enhanced in a unique way when nurses who practice with families are guided by Parse's theory.

REFERENCES

Anderson, H., & Goolishian, H. A. (1990). Beyond cybernetics: Comments on Atkinson and Heath's "Further thoughts on second-order family therapy." *Family Process, 29*, 157–163.

Brown, D. E. (1990). *Human universals*. Philadelphia: Temple University Press.

Buber, M. (1965). In M. Buber, *Between man and man* (pp. 118–205). New York: Macmillan. (Original work published 1938)

Burr, W. R., Hill, R., Reiss, I. L., & Nye, F. I. (1979). *Contemporary theories about the family* (2 vols.). New York: Free Press.

Burton, L. (1990). Teenage childrearing as an alternative life-course strategy in multigeneration black families. *Human Nature, 1*, 123–143.

Clements, I. W., & Roberts, F. B. (Eds.). (1983). *Family health: A theoretical approach to nursing care.* New York: Wiley.

de Shazer, S. (1991). Muddles, bewilderment, and practice theory. *Family Process, 30,* 453–458.

Feetham, S. L. (1991). Conceptual and methodological issues in research of families. In A. L. Whall & J. Fawcett (Eds.), *Family theory development in nursing: State of the science and art* (pp. 55–68). Philadelphia: Davis.

Fine, M., & Turner, J. (1991). Tyranny and freedom: Looking at ideas in the practice of family therapy. *Family Process, 30,* 307–320.

Gilliss, C. L. (1983). The family as the unit of analysis: Strategies for the nurse researcher. *Advances in Nursing Science, 5*(3), 50–59.

Gilliss, C. L. (1989). Family research in nursing. In C. L. Gilliss, B. L., Highley, B. M. Roberts, & I. M. Martinson (Eds.), *Toward a science of family nursing* (pp. 37–63). Menlo Park, CA: Addison Wesley.

Gilliss, C. L., Highley, B. L., Roberts, B. M., & Martinson, I. M. (Eds.). (1989). *Toward a science of family nursing.* Menlo Park, CA: Addison Wesley.

Golann, S. (1988). On second-order family therapy. *Family Process, 27,* 51–65.

Hoffman, L. (1985). Beyond power and control: Toward a "second order" family systems therapy. *Family Systems Medicine, 3,* 381–396.

Hoffman, L. (1990). Constructing realities: An art of lenses. *Family Process, 29,* 1–12.

Lindsey, K. (1981). *Friends as family.* Boston: Beacon.

Owens, T. J. (1970). *Phenomenology and intersubjectivity: Contemporary interpretations of the interpersonal situation.* The Hague: Nijhoff.

Parry, A. (1991). A universe of stories. *Family Process, 30,* 37–54.

Parse, R. R. (1981). *Man-living-health: A theory of nursing.* New York: Wiley.

Parse, R. R. (1987). Man-living-health theory of nursing. In R. R. Parse, *Nursing science: Major paradigms, theories, and critiques* (pp. 159–180). Philadelphia: Saunders.

Parse, R. R. (1990). Parse's research methodology with an illustration of the lived experience of hope. *Nursing Science Quarterly, 3,* 9–17.

Parse, R. R. (1992). Human becoming: Parse's theory of nursing. *Nursing Science Quarterly, 5,* 35–42.

Rapoport, R. (1989). Ideologies about family forms: Towards diversity. In K. Boh, M. Bak, C. Clason, M. Pankratova, J. Qvortrup, G. B. Sgritta, & K. Waerness (Eds.), *Changing patterns of European family life: A comparative analysis of 14 European countries* (pp. 53–69). London: Routledge.

Rogers, M. E. (1970). *An introduction to the theoretical basis of nursing.* Philadelphia: Davis.

Weston, K. (1991). *Families we choose: Lesbians, gays, kinship.* New York: Columbia University Press.

Whall, A. L., & Fawcett, J. (1991). *Family theory development in nursing: State of the science and art.* Philadelphia: Davis.

Chapter 3

The View of Freedom Within the Human Becoming Theory

Gail J. Mitchell

*H*uman freedom is an important notion for nurses who align their practice and research approaches with the human science tradition (Mitchell & Cody, 1992; Parse, 1981). The foremost authority on human science, Wilhelm Dilthey (1833–1911), heralded the human being's free will as "a given actuality that cannot be denied" (Dilthey, 1883/1988, p. 270). Scholars who view freedom as a given actuality of human existence equate freedom with self-determination and with a person's cocreation of life (Bauman, 1988; Gadow, 1979; May 1981; Parse, 1981, 1992, 1994; Sartre, 1965; Tillich, 1952). Parse (1992) refers to persons as co-authors of their human becoming, a process linked to unfolding, the relating of value priorities, meaning, and quality of life. Freedom is an expression of human becoming and thus of health, from Parse's view.

The seemingly obvious importance of freedom as a dimension of the human-health-nursing process has not been widely acknowledged in the nursing literature. Several authors have drawn attention to the unique opportunities available to nurses who practice in ways that respect the other's freedom (see, for example, Gadow, 1979; Gulino, 1982). Awareness of the value-laden nature of the theory-research-practice triad has helped to advance the view that whether human beings are conceptualized as having freedom, or not, is essentially a values choice. Literature over the past decade indicates a mounting commitment to create a nursing discipline that respects and honors human freedom (Allen, 1985; Carboni, 1991; Gadow, 1979; Gulino, 1982; Hall & Allan, 1986; Moccia, 1988; Parse, 1981; Polifroni & Packard, 1993; Winstead-Fry, 1980).

Regard for human freedom is clearly present in Parse's (1981, 1992, 1994) nursing theory, human becoming. Parse's regard for freedom is consistent with her alliance with the existential tenet, situated freedom. Situated freedom means that there are certain givens in any situation that coconstitute the opportunities and limitations defined by persons as they freely choose their own "self-project of personal becoming" (Parse, 1981, p. 19). It is proposed here that there are specific dimensions of freedom that, once explicated, will enhance scholarly understanding of lived experiences and human health. The purposes of this chapter are: (a) to briefly examine the nursing traditions that have restricted knowledge of human freedom; (b) to explicate the meaning of situated freedom, including several misinterpretations of the concept; and (c) to explore human freedom as viewed in the practice of traditional problem-based nursing and Parse's (1981, 1987, 1992) theory of human becoming.

TRANSCENDING RESTRICTIVE TRADITIONS

As stated above, the importance of human freedom, as a phenomenon of scientific concern, and as a dimension of the nurse-person relationship, has been overlooked by nurse scholars. The absence of nursing literature related to freedom surfaced speculation about why this phenomenon has been relatively ignored. One possible explanation contributing to the inattention is that the notion of human freedom stands in opposition to traditional nursing research and practice approaches, which for the most part, have promoted objectivity, reductionism, and determinism—concepts consistent with positivism.

The logical positivists, in particular British philosophers Hobbes, Locke, and Hume, attempted to eliminate the influence of personal values, purposes, and choices from scientific knowledge (Bronowski, 1956; Oldroyd, 1986). Bernstein (1983) calls this stance toward the world objectivism. He states that it reflects the "basic conviction that there is, or must be, some permanent, ahistorical framework to which we can ultimately appeal in determining the nature of rationality, knowledge, truth, reality, and goodness or rightness" (Bernstein, 1983, p. 8). According to the objectivist view, all scientific knowledge must be verifiable in the physical world (Oldroyd, 1986), and freedom is not verifiable. Rather, it is a value that is chosen and integrated into one's belief system, or not.

The positivist ontology is driven by deterministic goals that strive for prediction and control of human behavior. Some nurses promote these controls and suggest that prediction and control are the hallmarks of nursing practice (see, for example, Gortner & Schultz, 1988; Norbeck, 1987). Human choices based on individual values, and especially human freedoms, are just not compatible with deterministic beliefs. Riezler (1940) suggests, "A dehumanized science that dissolves a [person] into a compound of physical events should speak of determinism and indeterminism but never of compulsion or freedom" (p. 539).

Perhaps the most explicit disregard for human freedom can be found in Skinner's (1971) book, *Beyond Freedom and Dignity*. Skinner espouses a behaviorist view of human beings, and he refers to freedom as an evil notion propagated by the ignorant and prescientific thinkers of the world. Skinner proposes that "what people think are acts of freedom are merely forms of behavior that have proved useful in reducing threats" (p. 26). For Skinner, freedom is merely a learned reflex, and his behaviorist approach is structured to remove concepts like autonomy, dignity, and freedom from any explanation of human behavior. Although the behaviorism advocated by Skinner is not predominant in nursing today, both the positivist and behaviorist traditions bequeathed a legacy clearly evident in nursing practice and research activities.

The nursing process with its objectivist stance and subsequent diagnostic categorization prepares the traditional nurse to intervene with the intent of controlling the client-person or family in some direction toward "normal." The nursing process is structured for the purpose of comparing and judging data gathered in a systematic way according to the expert's frame of reference. Nursing research continues to be predominantly driven by the expert's desire to categorize, predict, and control human processes of health like grieving, suffering, and hoping. Traditional nurses who aspire to be engineers of human experience through prediction and control stand in opposition to human science nurses, as defined here, who aspire to explicate human experiences as they are lived and freely created by persons and families themselves. But, to fully understand the human science tradition one must first consider and study the existential concept of situated freedom.

SITUATED FREEDOM

Choosing one's self-project, one's path in life, is an inherent quality of being human (Parse, 1981). Persons exist with others in a universe that consists of many historical, cultural, and linguistic realities which are continuously changing and evolving. Parse (1981) refers to this situatedness as a person's "facticity." Heidegger (1962) wrote about being "thrown" into the world. Existing with a person's facticity or thrownness is the freedom to define one's direction.

Situated freedom is an essential dimension of the human being's unitary process with the universe, from Parse's view. Situated freedom is always honored as a truth about the person's unique becoming; it is an expression of the restriction-freedom paradox as it is lived by all human beings in their day-to-day relating. The intimate and ongoing expression of human-universe unity is the mutual process of situated freedom in Parse's theory.

Parse (1981, 1987, 1992, 1994) suggests that a person participates in projects by choosing value priorities, assigning meaning to situations, and assuming an attitude or point of view from which to consider one's position or relationship with the world. Fears and concerns, like hopes and dreams, are also created and are specific expressions of how persons co-author their lives. Even when one is born into incredible hardship, or when tragedies occur, the person is there in the midst of the situation. It is the person who makes choices about what daily happenings will mean, about how to be with others, and about what hopes and dreams are possible. As proposed by Parse (1981, 1987, 1992, 1994), the choices that form one's project or existence are made at multidimensional realms of the universe, and not all choices are reflective or explicitly knowable.

Situated freedom is different from views of freedom that limit and predefine the opportunities that persons might encounter in day-to-day life. The existential view of human freedom is misinterpreted by those who believe that persons labeled as poor, impaired, or disadvantaged cannot or do not make choices. The freedom of existentialism is not limited to the privileged of the world who can afford to choose their material possessions and places of domicile. To suggest that the poor and disadvantaged are not free to make choices is to delegate those persons to some status less than human. From an existentialist perspective, freedom has nothing to do with possessions and everything to do with being human, with passion, vitality, and sensitivity (de Beauvoir, 1991). Sartre (1966) said that freedom and being human are identical and that even choosing not to choose is freely choosing.

The existential view of freedom proposes that the essence of humanness, which is freedom, cannot be circumscribed or predefined in specific ways by cultural, physical, social, or economic circumstances. Anyone familiar with the book *City of Joy* (Lapierre, 1991) has encountered the meaning of situated freedom because this story expresses the ways that persons, despite incredible need and anguished suffering, cocreated their passion, joy, and transcendence in the slums of Calcutta. The story of those persons living in the slums, the complexity of their life meanings, and the depth of their love, etches the essence of humanness in time for all human beings.

Situated freedom is open to the mystery, transcendence, and creation of life (Heidegger, 1962; May, 1981; Parse, 1981; Sartre, 1965). This means that human beings co-author life, and what is not-yet is open to an infinite range of possibles. Human beings choose and unfold in ways that cannot be predetermined or predefined. The existential view of freedom does not limit and constrict what might be possible, because as Parse suggests, it is inherently human to create new projects, to surprise, and to move beyond the moment. And, to move beyond does not depend on a certain standard of wealth or health. Existential freedom is related to the disclosure of being itself—it is the way that the human story is shaped by every life, in situations of genuine living (de Beauvoir, 1991). Rollo May (1981) says that freedom is possibility and that "this gives freedom its great flexibility, its fascination, and its danger" (p. 10). Human life is full of risk, and the possibility of non-being is always there in day-to-day living. When experts propose that the poor and impaired cannot choose, they restrict views of human freedom and they restrict ways of knowing about how human beings create their self-projects.

Many nurses and other health care professionals have been influenced by the restrictive linear-hierarchial models about human possibles. Maslow's (1970) hierarchy of needs is one such model whose interpretation restricts views about human freedom and transcendent possibilities. It is suggested here that people do not progress up the hierarchy in step-like fashion as needs are met. Rather, persons choose and prioritize their needs according to personal values while living at levels of the hierarchy and beyond those levels, all-at-once. There are many examples in the literature and from practice that indicate that persons not only transcend Maslow's lower order needs—they choose to reject meeting some needs that "norm" experts might consider essential to well-being in order to live their personal value priorities.

For example, persons who are homeless described their choice to continue without shelter and food in order to keep their freedom on the street (Rasmusson, Jonas, & Mitchell, 1991). And, authors like Frankl (1959) have certainly shed light on the mystery of human transcendence in the midst of incredible adversity.

A second misinterpretation about the existential tenet of situated freedom relates to the belief that nurses who embrace this view somehow encourage suffering and pain in order to enhance transcendence. This belief is unfounded. What is believed by nurses endorsing existential tenets is that humans are inherently free and that life is inherently a struggle, an unpredictable journey that includes both suffering and joy, loss and discovery, peace of mind and anguished torment. All persons share in these universal experiences, and nurses who endorse the belief about the inherent freedom of human existence respect the universality of lived experiences, and their paradoxical nature. The nurse guided by Parse's theory recognizes that persons choose the meaning and the way to be with universal experiences in their own lives. The opposing beliefs of the traditional objectivist and behaviorist models are that life is, or should be, problem-free, predictable, controllable, smooth-functioning, steady, normal, un-lifelike.

Simone de Beauvoir (1991) posits that existentialism is the only philosophy that has an ethic. Existentialists believe that human beings choose to act or not act. This means that the nature of human existence is not predetermined or governed by natural laws; it is, rather, created by human beings who actively participate in the process (de Beauvoir, 1991; Heidegger, 1962; May, 1981). For those who believe that human actions are predictable responses to environmental or biochemical factors, there is little room for choice and thus little room for ethical or moral decision-making. "It is because there are real dangers and failures . . . that words like victory, wisdom, or joy have meaning" (de Beauvoir, 1991, p. 34). It is because human beings do choose how to act and what to say in situations that ethics can be considered a context-bound area of interest for nurses.

FREEDOM IN PRACTICE RELATIONSHIPS

Despite the relevance of human freedom in the process of health, there is very little in the nursing literature about freedom, especially from a nursing science perspective. May (1981) suggests that freedom is continuously recreating itself. This statement takes on added meaning when considered in light of the nurse-person relationship. Differences come to light when freedom is viewed from two different practice perspectives, the traditional nursing process and Parse's (1981, 1987, 1992) theory of human becoming.

Freedom and the Nursing Process

The inherently ethical nature of the nursing process with its diagnostic offshoot has been considered from a critical standpoint (Deegan, 1993; Mitchell, 1991). Essentially it is posited here that the nursing process does not afford recipients of care the opportunities for making their choices explicit or their self-projects known. Note that it is not possible to say that persons are denied freedom; individuals will choose their meanings, attitudes, value priorities, and concerns, whether nurses acknowledge them or not. But the ways freedom is lived and expressed are not enhanced or made explicit in traditional practice. Although existential freedom, or situated freedom, cannot be given or denied by others, there are certainly dimensions of freedom that surface and that present an opportunity for explication in nurse-person relationships.

Most nurses are familiar with the central role of nursing interventions aimed at securing compliance with expert directives in traditional problem-based approaches. For persons who choose to disregard expert directives there are various measures, from persuasion to restraint, in order to convince them otherwise. Problem-based practice aimed at fixing human beings creates discomfort for some nurses. Comfort levels with compliance-related issues flow from the values and beliefs of individual nurses and are related to their educational experiences and familiarity with other belief systems. Nurses guided by the traditional problem-based nursing process are not encouraged to explicate the ways human beings freely choose their life values and projects. Human freedom in traditional nursing practice is often kept hidden and restrained in order to facilitate the efficacy of the system and its experts.

Freedom and Parse's Theory of Human Becoming

For nurses who embrace the belief that persons are inherently free to choose their way of becoming, certain aspects of the nurse-person relationship take on new dimensions. Parse's (1987, 1992) practice dimensions and processes (illuminating meaning through explicating, synchronizing rhythms through dwelling with, and mobilizing transcendence through moving beyond) describe what happens when the nurse is truly present with others. Parse guides nurses to believe that others know their own way and that in the true presence of the nurse, the other's freely chosen way will manifest itself. In the nurse-person relationship, freedom is a living process that is witnessed and honored by the nurse.

Respect for the other's freedom means that the nurse guided by Parse's theory does not offer unsolicited information or give predefined directives. Parse's approach is obviously different from traditional biomedical nursing which does rely on predetermined teaching protocols and standardized care plans. In Parse's theory the person is not only free to choose from among options, but the person is also free to decide which options to consider, what possibles to define, and what meaning to assign to life situations.

There are infinite ways of viewing freedom in the nurse-person relationship. Whether or not nurses respect and honor freedom is shaped, at least partially, by the knowledge base used to guide practice. A practice example considered from the perspectives of the nursing process and Parse's theory may help to illuminate the distinct way of living values and beliefs in practice.

Mrs. P was recently diagnosed with diabetes. She had been started on insulin and was about to be discharged from the hospital. Prior to leaving the hospital Mrs. P indicated that she was planning to wean herself off insulin as soon as possible. The following forms of practice, with a focus on how freedom is viewed by the nurse, represent various ways nurses may be with Mrs. P.

The nurse guided by the traditional nursing process assessed a knowledge deficit in Mrs. P. The nurse notified the attending physician of the potential noncompliance and then arranged a teaching session to educate Mrs. P about the consequences of improper administration of insulin. Both the doctor and nurse explained to Mrs. P that she should take the insulin as directed. The question of Mrs. P's freedom to choose her own way of living with this situation does not surface for the traditional nurse or doctor. The logic of the objectivist perspective does not consider the human being as an active coparticipant in the situation. The nurse and doctor believe that if Mrs. P does not follow directives, she will suffer consequences and that alone is reason to eliminate the possibility of her freedom to participate.

The teaching intervention directed at increasing Mrs. P's knowledge is based on the assumption that if people are told what to do and given a rational explanation, they will do what is best according to the expert's belief system. For the traditional nurse an intervention will be considered successful if Mrs. P complies with physician orders and maintains an insulin regimen. Ultimately the traditional nurse acknowledges that Mrs. P is free to choose to ignore what the experts want, but then she would be noncompliant and in violation of what is viewed as an acceptable action. Punishment in some form typically follows for clients who disobey expert directives.

The nurse guided by Parse's theory does not act according to beliefs aimed at control, and therefore there is no attempt to give information in order to get Mrs. P to think and act in certain ways. The Parse nurse offers information when it is requested, and it is done under the person's direction. The nurse guided by Parse's theory focuses on bearing witness in true presence to Mrs. P's choice of self-project. Mrs. P knew she was supposed to take insulin, but she had decided she was not going to take it. She possessed the knowledge but did not value it.

The nurse listened to Mrs. P's plans without judging or appraising her views. Parse (1990) suggests that if nurses want to know what persons are going to do in situations, they should ask the person to speak about plans. Mrs. P started to speak about her diet and cutting down on sugar in order to get off the insulin. The nurse asked Mrs. P to talk some more about what it meant for her to be on insulin. Mrs. P said her father took insulin and it killed him. Mrs. P explained that if she stayed on insulin she might die, and she would not be satisfied if she didn't try other alternatives. The nurse asked Mrs. P what she saw as alternatives. As Mrs. P continued, she said she was not sure if she could get off the insulin, but she was not convinced she had to have it to live, and, therefore, would try alternatives. The Parse nurse continued to be with Mrs. P without judging her plans or trying to change her mind. The nurse asked Mrs. P how she would know whether or not she could go without insulin. Mrs. P said she was going to monitor her blood sugar and keep regular checks. She said she had to try to balance things. For the Parse nurse there was no knowledge deficit to correct for Mrs. P. She was freely choosing the meaning of her illness and how she wanted to be with it. The nurse's presence enhanced the woman's explication of her choices and possible consequences, and in this way she moved beyond the meaning moment.

Freedom is linked to valuing (May, 1981; Parse, 1981) and thus to health from Parse's perspective. Valuing is confirming cherished beliefs, a process of "choosing from imaged options and owning the choices" (Parse, 1981, p. 45). Values symbolize meaning, and giving meaning to multidimensional experiences is how persons cocreate their personal realities. Parse (1990) suggests that human beings are creative authors of their personal worlds. Health as a process of creative authorship is intimately linked to the person's chosen values. Indeed, Parse (1990) says health is "a synthesis of values" and "a personal responsibility that is chosen" (p. 137). From Parse's view the nurse cannot give health because it is freely created by persons themselves. And, the nurse cannot direct others about what choices are best because it is the person who has the unique vision of what might be. The nurse guided by Parse's theory listens and respects the vision, even when it is different from what others might choose. The Parse nurse celebrates the person's vision of freedom and seeks to know it so that others can enhance their understanding about human becoming.

THE CHALLENGES OF HONORING FREEDOM

It has been said that nurses live Parse's theory in practice, as opposed to applying it (Parse, 1992). To live the theory means to integrate the values and beliefs of the theory into day-to-day actions. Once integrated, the values consistently show themselves in the nurse-person relationship. To honor and respect others' freedom to choose their own way is one of the most challenging aspects of Parse's theory, perhaps the most challenging. To live respect for another's freedom requires an openness on behalf of the nurse to bear witness to the questioning, struggle, risk, and change inherent in moving beyond the now moment. It is not easy to respect the other's freedom to think things through in one's own way when the nurse knows other options that could be suggested. But, what must be recognized is that the very freedom to question means there are different possibles to invent and choose (May, 1981). From this perspective, the freedom to question is itself a leap into the future and thus a valued process (May, 1981).

It is not easy to respect the freedom of others when their views, from the nurse's perspective, are "limited." This is where other practice approaches diagnose knowledge deficits and give directives. And, this is where Parse's theory requires the nurse to respect that the person will define his or her own possibles in the open arena of true presence, an arena that nurtures human freedom. It has been this author's experience that, given the opportunity, persons do indeed ask questions regarding what they want to know. In a moment of silence people will indicate where they want to go and how they want to be. Quite often, the person's creations of meaning and possibles far surpass what the nurse might be able to offer. Traditional approaches in practice do not consider the person's co-authorship of life.

For instance, Mr. L, who had been admitted to acute care for depression after his wife of 64 years died, was discussing his pain and grief from being separated from his wife. Day after day Mr. L said he just could not get on with things, and he often spoke of wanting to die. He kept repeating, "I don't know what to do. I don't know what to do." A nurse guided by the traditional problem-based model attempted to move Mr. L through his grief process by pointing out all the reasons she could see that make life worth living. The nurse recommended to Mr. L that he join a support group and see a psychiatrist. This nurse also reminded Mr. L that it takes time to get over a loss, and she reassured Mr. L that things would eventually get better. These actions, though well-intentioned, did not facilitate Mr. L's disclosure of meaning and possibles. Further, the traditional approach did not respect Mr. L's freedom to question, search, and choose his own reasons for going on.

The nurse guided by Parse's theory believes the person knows the way, and when Mr. L spoke of not knowing what to do, the nurse stayed with his not knowing in the moment. By going with Mr. L's not knowing the nurse showed her willingness to bear witness to his pain and to the infinite possibilities that might surface in his searching for what might be. In the midst of open possibilities Mr. L engaged the opportunity to create choices and assign meanings. The nurse asked Mr. L what might help him to go on. After several moments, Mr. L said only one thing would help and that was for him to imagine that Mrs. L was still with him, still sitting at the breakfast table, still lying next to him at night. The Parse nurse went with Mr. L's imaging of the one thing that would help him to get through his pain. There was no judging or labeling Mr. L because of his way of being with the pain. Before the nurse left Mr. L he said that he knew his wife was dead and that he was going to have to face that, but for right now he had to pretend she was still by his side.

In the above example, Mr. L's freedom goes far beyond selection from predefined options to freely creating ways of connecting and separating from the pain. Nursing practice based on the traditional nursing process does not explicitly recognize or accommodate the human being's freedom to question, search, struggle, and create. The structure of the nursing process compels the nurse to think in a certain way based on comparative judging (Mitchell, 1991). Even if persons would speak of their freely chosen way of living with the pain, it would be categorized and labeled. Chances are that if a traditional nurse heard of Mr. L's plans to pretend his wife was still alive, the nurse would judge that statement as abnormal and label Mr. L with denial or dysfunctional grieving.

This chapter has explored dimensions of human freedom that have meaning for nurses who intend to participate with others in their living of health. Whether nurses honor and integrate views of persons as free, as co-authors of their personal becoming, depends on their scientific-theoretical beliefs. Practice with Parse's theory of human becoming advances the tradition of human science that originated more than a century ago. For nurses who accept the challenge to honor human freedom in relationships with others, there is a call to bear witness and explicate the ways persons freely choose their human emergence in mutual process with the universe. The knowledge generated about human freedom will advance a nursing science that honors others just for being human.

REFERENCES

Allen, D. G. (1985). Nursing research and social control: Alternate models of science that emphasize understanding and emancipation. *Image: Journal of Nursing Scholarship, XVII*(2), 58–64.

Bauman, Z. (1988). *Freedom.* Minneapolis, MN: University of Minnesota Press.

Bernstein, R. J. (1983). *Beyond objectivism and relativism: Science, hermeneutics, and praxis.* Philadelphia: University of Pennsylvania Press.

Bronowski, J. (1956). *Science and human values.* New York: Julian Messner.

Carboni, J. T. (1991). A Rogerian theoretical tapestry. *Nursing Science Quarterly, 4,* 130–136.

de Beauvoir, S. (1991). *The ethics of ambiguity* (B. Frechtman, Trans.). New York: Citadel Press. (Original copyright, 1948, Philosophical Library)

Deegan, P. E. (1993). Recovering our sense of value after being labeled. *Journal of Psychosocial Nursing, 31*(4), 7–11.

Dilthey, W. (1988). *Introduction to the human sciences* (R. J. Betanzos, Trans.). Detroit: Wayne State University Press. (Original work published 1883)

Frankl, V. (1959). *Man's search for meaning: An introduction to logotherapy* (I. Lasch, Trans.). Boston: Beacon.

Gadow, S. (1979). Advocacy nursing and new meanings of aging. *Nursing Clinics of North America, 14*(1), 81–91.

Gortner, S. R., & Schultz, P. R. (1988). Approaches to nursing science methods. *Image: Journal of Nursing Scholarship, 20*(1), 22–24.

Gulino, C. K. (1982). Entering the mysterious dimension of other: An existential approach to nursing care. *Nursing Outlook, 30,* 352–357.

Hall, B. A., & Allan, J. D. (1986). Sharpening nursing's focus by focusing on health. *Journal of Nursing & Health Care, 7,* 315–320.

Heidegger, M. (1962). *Being and time.* (J. Macquarrie & E. Robinson, Trans.). New York: Harper & Row.

Lapierre, D. (1991). *The city of joy.* New York: Warner Books.

Maslow, A. H. (1970). *Motivation and personality* (2nd ed.). New York: Harper & Row.

May, R. (1981). *Freedom and destiny.* New York: Bantam Double-day Dell.

Mitchell, G. J. (1991). Nursing diagnosis: An ethical analysis. *Image: Journal of Nursing Scholarship, 23*(2), 99–103.

Mitchell, G. J., & Cody, W. K. (1992). Nursing knowledge and human science: Ontological and epistemological considerations. *Nursing Science Quarterly, 5,* 54–61.

Moccia, P. (1988). A critique of compromise: Beyond the methods debate. *Advances in Nursing Science, 10*(4), 1–9.

Norbeck, J. S. (1987). In defense of empiricism. *Image: Journal of Nursing Scholarship, 19*(1), 28–30.

Oldroyd, D. (1986). *The arch of knowledge.* New York: Methuen.

Parse, R. R.(1981). *Man-living-health: A theory of nursing.* New York: Wiley.

Parse, R. R. (1987). *Nursing science: Major paradigms, theories, and critiques.* Philadelphia: Saunders.

Parse, R. R. (1990). Health: A personal commitment. *Nursing Science Quarterly, 3,* 136–140.

Parse, R. R. (1992). Human becoming: Parse's theory of nursing. *Nursing Science Quarterly, 5,* 35–42.

Parse, R. R. (1994). *Human becoming: A theory of nursing.* Manuscript submitted for publication.

Polifroni, E. C., & Packard, S. (1993). Psychological determinism and the evolving nursing paradigm. *Nursing Science Quarterly, 6,* 63–68.

Rasmusson, D. L., Jonas, C. M., & Mitchell, G. J. (1991). The eye of the beholder: Parse's theory with homeless individuals. *Clinical Nurse Specialist, 5*(3), 139–143.

Riezler, E. (1940). In R. N. Anshen (Ed.), *Freedom—Its meaning* (pp. 538–554). New York: Harcourt, Brace.

Sartre, J-P. (1965). *Essays in existentialism* (W. Baskin, Ed.). New York: Carol Publishing Group.

Sartre, J-P. (1966). *Being and nothingness* (H. E. Barnes, Trans.). New York: Washington Square Press.

Skinner, B. F. (1971). *Beyond freedom and dignity.* New York: Alfred A. Knopf.

Tillich, P. (1952). *The courage to be.* New Haven, CT: Yale University Press.

Winstead-Fry, P. (1980). The scientific method and its impact on holistic health. *Advances in Nursing Science, 2*(4), 1–7.

Chapter 4

The View of Suffering Within the Human Becoming Theory

John Daly

Suffering is an ineluctable aspect of life. Suffering as a phenomenon is linked in the literature to many life events including bereavement, grief, poverty, and pain. This chapter provides a selective review of the literature related to the phenomenon of human suffering. The major focus is explication of the concept of suffering from the perspective of Parse's human becoming theory. Experiential aspects of suffering are elucidated and interpreted using theoretical principles and concepts drawn from Parse's theory. Overall, this chapter represents a focused hermeneutical analysis, guided by human becoming theory, which sheds light on the meaning of suffering. Prior to proceeding to an analysis and interpretation of the phenomenon of suffering from the perspective of Parse's (1992) human becoming theory, an overview will provide general notions, specific definitions, and other theoretical perspectives regarding human suffering.

THE STATUS OF HUMAN SUFFERING

Suffering is a phenomenon which forms part of the tapestry of life for all human beings, yet the essential nature of this ineluctable aspect of life has in some respects received little attention in the literature. While the literature is replete with use of the construct "suffering" per se, attempts to illuminate the experiential aspects including the personal meaning of the phenomenon have been limited (Cassell, 1982; Kahn & Steeves, 1986). Some authors suggest that the suffering phenomenon is avoided and ignored by researchers and practitioners involved in the helping professions as the phenomenon is linked to personal existence and vulnerability (Copp, 1974, 1990a, 1990b; Goldberg, 1986). It is suggested that recognition and exploration of another's suffering may threaten personal integrity (Kahn & Steeves, 1986). It seems that acknowledgment of another's suffering "cuts too close to the bone" for many. Suffering of course may escape notice or scrutiny; Cassell (1982) notes that the nature of suffering is essentially private and experiential. Similarly Goldberg (1986) points out that suffering is often "borne silently and alone" (p. 97). Moreover, Goldberg (1986) speaks of a "silent conspiracy about sharing of suffering, as if suffering should be kept a private matter" (p. 98). This silent conspiracy may result in the silencing of the voice of the sufferer. Such a conspiracy may deny persons the opportunity to move beyond the suffering through dialogue with health care professionals or even family and significant others. As long as such a situation prevails, the suffering person is left to live the experience ignominiously. Copp (1990b) discusses the way in which health professionals often ignore and eschew human suffering; she infers that the phenomenon of suffering is treated in this way because of professional inadequacy. Parker and Gardner (1991) provide another perspective which suggests that nurses, for example, do assist people to cope with experiences such as suffering, pain, and disfigurement by making such events seem ordinary. These authors posit a process or strategy labeled "making ordinary" which essentially involves treating the extraordinary as ordinary. Parker and Gardner contend that this process, which is said to assist people in finding meaning in their lives, is largely invisible, as it is not documented nor recognized by other health professionals or even nurses themselves.

It is acknowledged that the phenomenon of suffering has not been adequately described and consequently a number of authors speak to the need for research into the nature of the suffering experience (Cassell, 1982; Copp, 1990a, 1990b; Kahn & Steeves, 1986; Morse & Johnson, 1991). Specifically, phenomenological research approaches have been recommended to build knowledge and understanding of human suffering (Kahn & Steeves, 1986).

SELECTED DEFINITIONS AND THEORETICAL PERSPECTIVES

Suffering has been defined in a number of ways by various authors and theoreticians. *The Australian Concise Oxford Dictionary* (1987) defines suffering as "undergo martyrdom." The verb "suffer" is defined as "undergo, experience, be subjected to pain, loss, grief, defeat, change, punishment, wrong" (p. 1133). Suffering is therefore linked to experiences of ailments, bereavement, or harmful injunction, on some level, which is directed toward the person (the sufferer). Suffering has often been linked to the experience of pain and defined in parsimonious terms (Cassell, 1982; Travelbee, 1966), though as Cassell (1982) has acknowledged, pain and suffering "are phenomenologically distinct" (p. 641). Perspectives on human suffering have been provided by a number of theorists including, among others, Travelbee (1966), Cassell (1982), Charmaz (1983), Copp (1974, 1990a, 1990b), Goldberg (1986), Heller (1987), Kahn and Steeves (1986), Mitchell (1991), and Morse and Johnson (1991).

Some perspectives on human suffering clearly associate suffering with the experience of pain. The experience of suffering is often linked to the experience of pain as though the relationship between these phenomena may be linear (Copp, 1974; Davis, 1981; Travelbee, 1966). Copp (1974), for example, presented the following definition of suffering: "a state of anguish of one who bears pain, injury or loss" (p. 491). Travelbee (1966) also saw a connection between pain and suffering stating, "To suffer is to be immersed in a black ocean of pain" (p. 89). More recently it has been acknowledged that simply anticipating pain can lead to the experience of suffering (Cassell, 1982; Copp, 1990b). Also, recent writings acknowledge that there is not necessarily a linear relationship between pain and suffering per se. Perspectives which link the experience of suffering to pain or loss alone appear to trivialize a complex phenomenon which is not related just to medical contexts (Kozrelecki, 1978). Suffering exists outside of those contexts; further, the phenomenon has its own particular qualities and structure which surely differentiate it from concepts such as pain or loss.

Other perspectives of suffering suggest that suffering results when the "self" is threatened in some way or one experiences significant loss. Some theorists advance the view that suffering emerges as an existential experience when one perceives the "self" to be under threat for some reason (Cassell, 1982; Kahn & Steeves, 1986), when self-integration is compromised (Goldberg, 1986), or when one experiences "loss of self," which occurs in numerous contexts (Charmaz, 1983). Goldberg (1986) contends that the nature of suffering is an amalgam of the following phenomenological components: "dreaded lost sense of self, the feeling that self is crumbling away without a new valued self emerging which leads to living restricted lives, experiencing social isolation, regarding oneself as discredited and believing oneself to be a burden to others" (p. 102). The link between the notion of threat to self and suffering is reflected in Kahn and Steeves' (1986) theoretical definition of suffering: "an individual's experience of threat to self and . . . a meaning given to events such as pain or loss" (p. 623). These perspectives, however, do not describe what the elaborated meaning of these events may represent for the sufferer.

More specifically, existential views of suffering are provided in the literature also. Such perspectives look to personal meaning as a source of suffering. Heller (1987) provides a view of suffering which is centered on meaning for the person, that is, the sufferer. She asserts that "meanings without a 'meaning to life' is precisely what suffering is all about. Animals can be 'in pain.' But suffering is a human privilege. To attribute virtue to suffering is a tribute paid to the human condition" (p. 21). A number of scholars speak of the meaning one ascribes to life experiences or events, such as encounter with pain. Goldberg (1986) states that "organisms experience pain but pain does not become suffering until it is translated into a category of meaning" (p. 97). Kahn and Steeves (1986) concur with Goldberg; commenting on the relationship between pain and suffering, they state, "Suffering . . . is not grounded in the same cause or stimuli but derives from the individual's evaluation of the significance or meaning of the pain experienced" (p. 625). Mitchell (1991) views suffering "as a lived experience which is multidimensional and which can be understood only from the perspective of the individual living it" (p. 101).

Efforts to explicate more global perspectives of suffering are evident in recent literature; for example, Morse and Johnson (1991) report that suffering may be "conceived to be a comprehensive concept incorporating the experience of both acute and chronic pain, the strain of trying to endure, the alienation of forced exclusion from everyday life, the shock of institutionalization and the uncertainty of anticipating the ramification of the illness" (p. 338). The literature on suffering, however, reflects a dearth of experiential accounts of the phenomenon.

HUMAN SUFFERING: A VIEW FROM PARSE'S THEORY

From the perspective of Parse's theory of human becoming (1992), suffering may be regarded as a chosen way of being with a situation. To choose suffering as a way of being with a situation does not necessarily mean that persons reflectively choose to have pain, illness, loss, or anguish. It does, however, mean that persons make certain choices explicitly and tacitly that cocreate the suffering, and they choose the meaning given to these experiences. Further, it means that to suffer is a way of living moments by dwelling in the suffering, by pretending that it does not exist, by dramatically changing a situation, by moving away to another reality, or by some other way. Parse posits that the meaning assigned to personal experience reveals one's value priorities. Suffering is a value priority and is meaning itself, a way of being with a situation.

Further, from Parse's theoretical perspective the person who is suffering is living choices which are personal beliefs and values. For Parse, suffering cannot be predefined; it is a lived meaning assigned by individuals to life situations. The lived meaning arises with the human-universe connectedness and is peculiar to the person living the suffering. Therefore, the suffering experience can be described only by persons who believe they are suffering. Suffering is an imaged value languaged through the experience of anguish. The phenomenon of suffering unfolds in the process of human becoming. It reflects choice in terms of the meaning of one's situatedness, at the pre-reflective and reflective realms of being all-at-once. It is the contextual living of personal values. Suffering, then, may be construed as a chosen way of becoming, incarnated through the human-universe interrelationship.

Simply living one's values cocreates suffering in context, for example, if one lives values which are not shared by others, and others exact retribution through some means. If one seeks to be valued by others and is not, suffering is a possibility in the pattern of becoming. Choosing to suffer, to experience discomfort, pain, anguish, or fear may reflect an affirmation of self, an intention of moving on in a new and different way with self and others.

This author's synthetic definition of the concept of suffering is: *Suffering is an agonizing heaviness prompted through being with and apart from others, objects, and situations unfolding in an unburdening lightness.* This synthetic definition emerged through dwelling with data related to the meaning of suffering for persons who have lived this experience. An example of how one person conveyed the meaning of suffering follows.

A middle-aged woman, Betty, recently lost her husband; he left her, because he wished to live alone and away from her. She had devoted herself in the main to life as a loving partner to her husband. Betty responded to the loss of her husband by plummeting into what she described as a state of black depression and suffering. From her perspective, her life was empty and she felt engulfed in what she described as "the angst of existential aloneness." Betty wrote a poem about herself and her situation. In the poem she saw herself as a distressed, beached whale, no longer buoyant in the sea but trapped on the sand, a creature alone with no volunteers available to help refloat it. The whale struggled, a leaden weight on the sand. Its struggling against the sand and shingle, in efforts to shift back into the sea, caused painful tears in the flesh of the mammal. Still the whale struggled in desperation and exhaustion, trying to find its own way back into the sea to comfort, sustenance, and safety. Betty stated that she felt extremely sad and alone, though she knew that her friends and children cared about her. Eventually Betty was able to move on. She surrounded herself with new objects, including a houseboat located on a secluded river. For Betty this houseboat represented a haven which moved gently on the water providing a peaceful, private, and comforting environment.

A hermeneutical interpretation of Betty's description and others like it resulted in creation of the synthetic definition of the concept of suffering as provided in this chapter. The synthetic definition of suffering yielded the following three sub-concepts:

1. an agonizing heaviness
2. being with and apart from others, objects, and situations
3. unfolding in an unburdening lightness.

To illuminate further the nature of suffering from Parse's perspective it is possible to connect each of the three identified sub-concepts to a principle of the theory of human becoming.

Principle 1. *Structuring meaning multidimensionally is cocreating reality through the languaging of valuing and imaging* (Parse, 1981, p. 69). Parse's first theoretical principle "means that human beings construct a personal significance by choosing options from the various realms of the universe, as speaking and moving unveil the cherished beliefs lived explicitly and tacitly all-at-once. What is real for each individual is structured by that individual" (Parse, 1992, p. 37).

Suffering is the meaning given to the situation by the person who is living the experience of suffering. "Meaning" here relates to how one sees a situation and how one moves with that situation. The meaning ascribed to the lived experience of suffering by the sufferer incarnates the health of the person at the moment. Parse (1987) states, "Health is an expression of values at the moment, the meaning given to a situation" (p. 163). Choosing to value suffering and all that it may represent for the person is related to the human's struggle to create new ways of becoming. The meaning ascribed to the lived experience of suffering will vary, but as Mitchell (1991) has noted, the ascribed meaning "may involve feeling rotten, awful, alone or slapped in the face" (p. 101). In structuring meaning multidimensionally in the cocreation of reality, the human lives values at the prereflective and reflective realms of being all-at-once. Through languaging imaged values the person conveys the experience of suffering; this process involves imaging, which is symbolizing one's knowing "through a frame of reference which is the individual's own value priorities. New knowledge and new experience are sifted through the frame of reference" (Parse, 1992, p. 37).

Suffering may unfold if one's values (cherished beliefs, dreams, and worldview) are rejected or threatened by self or others. As Parse states, reality is cocreated; therefore, the meaning of the situation unfolds in interrelation with others and the universe. Change in the area of personal values unfolds in multiple possibles; such change may unfold in a personal struggle to move beyond the now moment with hopes and dreams. Parse (1981) states that valuing gives "meaning to multidimensional experience" (pp. 45–46).

Suffering may be construed as *an agonizing heaviness*. It represents a painful, weighty, agonizing anguish which unfolds in mutual interrelationship with others, objects, or situations. The decision to live suffering unfolds in choosing the experience from the multidimensional realms of being all-at-once. The reality of the phenomenon unfolds for the sufferer through the mutual human-universe process. It is a cocreated lived experience. Suffering may give rise to change in images of who one is, which relates to Parse's concept of imaging. In suffering, persons may experience a shift in the way they see themselves as being-in-the-world through living personal values. Seeing self as "in agony," "heavy," or "stuck" in context reflects the languaging of imaged values, as was the case with Betty in the narrative. Suffering may mean that one is struggling to move with shifting images of self in the light of what was, is, and will be valued. Living suffering may mean that one is struggling to move on in affirming cherished beliefs which were and are but may not be in the not-yet. This struggle may give rise to utter anguish and sequestered torment. Weighty anguish moves one to dwell with the pain and agony of confronting shattered beliefs and values. Suffering means dwelling with an agonizing weight. Experiencing weighty agony in context may unfold in communing with not-yet images in the struggle to move on. Hopes and dreams reflect a cherished image, an envisioning of the not-yet, and the meaning of one's situatedness changes when one can move to a valued place of comfort.

Betty's description of her suffering captures the idea of an agonizing heaviness. The described meaning of how Betty saw herself in context and how she moved with suffering was the languaging of imaged values for Betty as she expressed her experience of anguish at the moment. The meaning of the situation for Betty emerged in interrelationship with others; that is to say, the reality of the experience of suffering was cocreated. Suffering was the meaning which Betty ascribed to her being-in-the-world following the loss of her husband. Through the use of the metaphor of the beached whale she languaged how she was living-with-suffering. Betty had been living her values, including her cherished beliefs as the partner of her husband. The loss of her husband may have meant she could no longer live harmoniously all of the same cherished beliefs. For Betty, the meaning of *being* changed, unfolded in the phenomenon of suffering and the painful struggle toward new possibles, including the possibility of moving to a phase of comfort, sustenance, and safety.

Principle 2.   *Cocreating rhythmical patterns of relating is living the paradoxical unity of revealing-concealing and enabling-limiting while connecting-separating* (Parse 1981, p. 69).

Parse's second theoretical principle speaks to her perspective on human-to-human and human-universe process. Parse posits the process as rhythmically cocreated cadences. Patterns of relating, which are rhythmical, are paradoxical in that they encapsulate "apparent opposites" all-at-once (Parse, 1981, 1992). Parse (1992) states, "These rhythmical patterns are not opposites; they are two sides of the same rhythm that coexist all-at-once. Both sides of the rhythm are present simultaneously" (p. 38). Related to the process of human becoming, these rhythmical paradoxical unities represent the continuous coconstituting of actualities and potentials all-at-once. Situations which unfold in human-universe process are cocreated and inherently involve complementary aspects of rhythmical patterns of relating. Parse specifies these rhythmical patterns of relating with the concepts of revealing-concealing, enabling-limiting, and connecting-separating (Parse, 1981). Other paradoxical rhythms may surface in becoming through suffering; for example, from this author's view the experience involves the paradoxical unity of comfort-discomfort. Comfort and discomfort relate to the experience of release from weighty anguish and movement with feelings of harmony, buoyancy, and aliveness. Discomfort may relate to experience of pain or anguish which unfolds in suffering. Descriptions of the phenomenon of suffering, including Betty's, often include discussion of uncomfortable feelings such as anger, pain, sadness, and excruciating anguish. Most accounts of suffering encapsulate uncomfortable feelings.

The concepts used by Parse to specify her second principle invite speculation regarding the cocreated rhythmical patterns of relating which emerge in human suffering. It is speculated that in becoming through suffering one reveals and conceals aspects of self in interrelation with others and the universe; "one reveals-conceals all at once the who that one is now, which incarnates the who that one was and will be" (Parse, 1992, p. 38). Suffering is cocreated and lived as a private agony which is centered in one's world. The weighty burden of suffering may not be shared explicitly but is always languaged by the sufferer. The person living the personal agony of suffering conceals and reveals meaning through ways of being through suffering moments. As suffering reflects choice in terms of one's situatedness, it surfaces opportunities and limitations all-at-once. As Parse (1992) states, "In choosing, there are an infinite number of opportunities and an infinite number of limitations. Moving in one direction limits movement in another" (p. 38). The choice one makes incarnates options and limits all-at-once in enabling-limiting.

In choosing to suffer one is connected with others while separated from others all-at-once. This relates to Parse's concept of connecting-separating. Parse (1992) states, "In moving together with one phenomenon, the individual moves away from other phenomena. In moving together there is both the closeness of togetherness and the distance of moving apart with the same phenomenon" (p. 38). Moving with the phenomenon of suffering emerges in moving away from other phenomena. In moving with the phenomenon of suffering there is a complementary closeness with and distancing from the phenomenon itself. In suffering one withdraws and engages with harmonious, buoyant interrelating with others as well as sorrowful anguish.

The second sub-concept of the synthetic definition of suffering, *being with and apart from others, objects, and situations,* emerged from Betty's description of her experience of suffering. Betty experienced paradoxical feelings related in the main to how she was with others during her suffering. She experienced "the angst of existential aloneness," though she knew that she had friends and children who cared about her. This reflects the paradoxical nature of Betty's pattern of relating with others, especially as related to Parse's concept of connecting-separating. The sub-concept *being with and apart from others, objects, and situations* represents in a sense the concept of connecting-separating

at a lower level of discourse. In the poem she wrote, Betty saw herself as a beached whale trapped in painful struggle on the sand
trying desperately to find her own way back into the sea for comfort, sustenance, and safety. The agonizing heaviness reflected in
the metaphor of the beached whale may represent her all-at-once
connection and separation with suffering. Betty was moving with
the phenomenon of suffering in connection with others in her
world. In suffering, Betty felt with and apart from others. The
paradox evident in this rhythmical pattern of relating sheds light
on the all-at-once experience of being with and apart from others,
objects, and situations. Related to the meaning of *an agonizing
heaviness*, this rhythmical pattern appears to interrelate withdrawal with simultaneous awareness of communion with others.
This withdrawal-communion occurs all-at-once in suffering.
The sense of dread and weighty anguish that is suffering gives
rise to engaging resolutely with this phenomenon. This experience is languaged through use of terms such as "stuck" or
"trapped." Betty, for example, also spoke of being engulfed in
"existential aloneness." This way of being-in-the-world and interrelating with others involves choice and a decision; thus, it reflects
a valuing of closeness and distancing. There is evidence which
suggests that Betty lived the paradoxical unity of comfort-
discomfort in suffering. She saw herself as a whale writhing in
desperation and agony, and yet she was able to incorporate a view,
an imaged experience of comfort in the not-yet. Perhaps evidence
of this is Betty's envisioning of finding a place which could give
rise to comfort, sustenance, and safety. On the basis of this analysis it appears that connecting-separating may represent a significant element of the change in pattern of relating which may
accompany suffering.

Parse's (1981) third principle, *cotranscending with the possibles is powering unique ways of originating in the process of transforming* (p. 69) assists in further illuminating experiential
aspects of the suffering phenomenon. This principle suggests
that humans are oriented toward the not-yet, reaching beyond
with hopes and dreams. Cotranscending with the possibles involves reaching and propelling with the not-yet (Parse, 1981,

1992). The third sub-concept derived from the synthetic definition of suffering, *unfolding in an unburdening lightness,* may be linked to all of Parse's concepts in the third principle, powering, originating, and transforming. This sub-concept reflects transformation emerging, as creating new ways of viewing the familiar moves one to different horizons.

Suffering involves a struggle in moving with the tension of pushing-resisting; this may be further conceptualized as struggling to move with competing values or options. Parse's concept of powering has relevance here, as pushing-resisting relates to the struggle to affirm self in light of the possibility of non-being. The threat of non-being may relate to not truly living cherished beliefs in interrelationship with others, and this may unfold in suffering. Suffering in this context may reflect an affirmation of self, an intention of moving on in a new and different way with self and others. Parse's concept of originating has relevance in the context of human suffering, as it appears that the sufferer is faced with the challenge of finding new and unique ways of becoming. These new ways are imaged value priorities related to connecting-separating with others. The suffering experience unfolds cotranscendence through powering, originating a transforming. Transforming relates to change and moving on in the process of becoming, the changing pattern of one's life.

Moving again to the story of Betty, the struggle she lived to affirm self in suffering is clearly conveyed in her description of her situation. Through her suffering it appears that Betty, in cotranscending through transforming, shifted value priorities and imaged new ways of viewing the familiar in moving on to a place of comfort. Through the painful struggle that is suffering, Betty was eventually able to find ways of moving on which gave rise to feelings of comfort, buoyancy, and aliveness.

CONCLUSION

Parse's human becoming theory offers a rich, creative, and humanistic avenue for the exploration of universal health-related phenomena. This Parsean analysis of the concept of suffering has shed light on possible experiential patterns associated with the lived experience of suffering. This discussion highlights the need to explore the meaning of the context for the individual sufferer, provides some ideas regarding the patterns of rhythmical interrelating which might unfold in suffering, and demonstrates an appreciation of the all-at-once anguished struggle and joy of mobilizing transcendence in the process of becoming through suffering.

REFERENCES

The Australian concise Oxford dictionary. (1987). Melbourne: Oxford University Press.

Cassell, E. J. (1982). The nature of suffering and the goals of medicine. *The New England Journal of Medicine, 306,* 639–645.

Charmaz, K. (1983). Loss of self: A fundamental form of suffering in the chronically ill. *Sociology of Health & Illness, 5,* 168–195.

Copp, L. A. (1974). The spectrum of suffering. *American Journal of Nursing, 74,* 491–495.

Copp, L. A. (1990a). The nature and prevention of suffering. *Journal of Professional Nursing, 6,* 247–249.

Copp, L. A. (1990b). Treatment, torture, suffering and compassion. *Journal of Professional Nursing, 6,* 1–2.

Davis, A. J. (1981). Compassion, suffering, morality: Ethical dilemmas in caring. *Nursing Law and Ethics, 2*(5), 1–2, 6, 8.

Goldberg, C. (1986). Concerning human suffering. *The Psychiatric Journal of the University of Ottawa, 11,* 97–104.

Heller, A. (1987). The human condition. *Thesis Eleven, 16,* 4–21.

Kahn, D. L., & Steeves, R. H. (1986). The experience of suffering: Conceptual clarification and theoretical definition. *Journal of Advanced Nursing, 11,* 623–631.

Kozrelecki, J. (1978). Suffering and human values. *Dialectics and Humanism, 4,* 115–117.

Mitchell, G. J. (1991). Nursing diagnosis: An ethical analysis. *Image: Journal of Nursing Scholarship, 23,* 99–103.

Morse, J. M., & Johnson, J. L. (1991). *The illness experience: Dimensions of suffering.* Newbury Park, NJ: Sage.

Parker, J., & Gardner, G. (1991). The silence and the silencing of the nurse's voice: A reading of patient progress notes. *The Australian Journal of Advanced Nursing, 9*(2), 3–9.

Parse, R. R. (1981). *Man-living-health: A theory of nursing.* New York: Wiley.

Parse, R. R. (1987). *Nursing science: Major paradigms, theories, and critiques.* Philadelphia: Saunders.

Parse, R. R. (1992). Human becoming: Parse's theory of nursing. *Nursing Science Quarterly, 5,* 35–42.

Travelbee, J. (1966). *Interpersonal aspects of nursing.* Philadelphia: Davis.

Chapter 5

The House-Garden-Wilderness Metaphor: Caring Frameworks and the Human Becoming Theory

Lois S. Kelley

*I*n this chapter, a *house-garden-wilderness* metaphor conceptualized by the author is used to explore the ways in which Parse's (1981, 1992) theory of human becoming sheds light on nursing as a philosophy of caring (Boykin, 1990; Dunlop, 1986; Watson, 1985, 1990). Each of the two perspectives, caring and human becoming theory, has at its root a belief system related to the heritage of nursing. Within the context of the house-garden-wilderness metaphor, caring frameworks foster nurturing encounters with persons primarily in a *garden,* a protected place for learning and growing. Parse's theory of human becoming fosters journeying and sojourning with persons in the *house-garden-wilderness* of their personal worlds. Each approach suggests that the nurse seeks to engage with persons in the context of their human existence, to touch its depths, and to connect with the continuity of being at home in the world.

Metaphorically, all persons are in search of a *home*—that is, all persons seek grounding for their own being-becoming while also taking part in projects with others. Home represents the feeling of being in one's own place in the world (Mayeroff, 1971, p. 68), which flows from selecting what is right for oneself, while cocreating with others patterns of living that are paradoxical in nature. One may be both "at home" in a situation, yet seeking the feeling of home in other ways at the same time (Parse, 1981, 1987).

Nurses, with a societal obligation to care (Chinn, 1991), are in a unique position to assist persons or groups in seeking home (from the caring perspective), and to journey and sojourn with persons (from Parse's perspective). Parse's theory of human becoming invites nurses to move beyond the boundaries of the garden to engage with the unitary experience of the house-garden-wilderness.

Persons in search of home seek to know themselves and their worlds and to live in-the-world *as* they know themselves. This means living, growing, moving with house-garden-wilderness multidimensionally, with security and risks inherent in the chosen structure of the house, the relation of the garden to the house and wilderness, and the opportunities and dangers within. Creating a home experience calls on personal knowledge of the world that is both subjective and intersubjective all-at-once. Personal knowing is prereflective - reflective awareness of what is individually right, which stands apart from the shadows of societal expectations, meanings, and values.

Parse's human becoming theory reaches beyond the caring frameworks to embrace the paradoxical in lived experience and to explore unique personal truths that emerge in cocreated life situations. The human becoming theory specifies the domain of nursing science as the humanly lived experience of health. Humanly lived experiences are essentially *unitary* phenomena which are intelligible to others by virtue of a shared humanity. Human-to-human relating reveals the universality of the human condition and the uniqueness of the individual all-at-once (Dilthey, 1883/ 1988; Mitchell & Cody, 1992). Individuals and groups coparticipate in casting shadows and light at every moment, disclosing and hiding the possibilities for what one can become in coparticipation with the universe. Thus, there is certainty and uncertainty in journeying through the world, selecting where and how one will build one's house, what one will grow in one's garden, and how one will be with the house-garden-wilderness.

THE METAPHOR OF HOUSE-GARDEN-WILDERNESS

The house-garden-wilderness metaphor arose within the author through contemplation of the notions of home, being-in-the-world, caring, and becoming. The seeking of home involves the interplay of images, patterns of living, and forces that energize individuals and groups in creative living. Creativity emerges out of participating with others in infinitely complex universal rhythms while journeying and sojourning in the house, in the garden, and in the wilderness, as described here.

The House

The house can be seen as being built or structured from among the available visions and values related to "houses." Yet, the house represents the structure of meanings and values the individual chooses to live. The structure is a place of rootedness for the person, a place to dwell, rest, and recuperate. Familiar patterns of living, customs and rituals, help to run the house and to create the feeling of home. The house is a place for starting out on journeys and for coming home to, for the visible structure of the house is what the person considers actual and real.

The house also has niches, crannies, and rooms furnished long ago and not often visited. In secret corners of the house are riches and treasures not always recognizable if viewed solely from within the matrix of sociocultural values. The person knows or senses this richness as an awareness of something indefinable, yet magically inspiring, that leads the person onward. These special places and secret treasures represent the personal values and possibilities, kept "with" one always, some of which will become something more, some of which will be forgotten, but all of which are the person's own. Even the basement, which is usually thought of as a place of darkness, has within it souvenirs and "finds," personal treasures largely unrecognizable as such by others who may see only the shadows. Usually other persons come into one's house by invitation only, although sometimes there may be intruders; yet no one can know the house like its proprietor.

The Garden

The garden is a structure close and connected to the house; it is partially open to the untamed elements essential to its purposes, yet it is also bounded and controlled to some extent. The garden symbolizes a place of intentional relating with the world and with other persons, a protected place for walks and talks and feeling connected with the earth. A garden is a nurtured venture, a loving commitment, and a risk, yet one that draws on the known and must be carefully planned. In the garden one can learn from nature to wait or to be patient, to view the seed as resting, to abide with the flow of time as one cultivates and tends the garden. And, sometimes one must let go of that which is wilted, perhaps using the petals to make rose water.

The garden may be a place to plan or review encounters with the world or wilderness, but by its purpose it is constrained from surrendering to the wilderness itself; dispositions, attitudes, and potentials are cultivated here to forge pathways and bridges. It is also a place for honoring the dead and dying through its very commitment to life. The rituals of tending the garden allow one to witness the rhythms of the wilderness, to play and practice with them, yet to remain relatively distant and safe within the boundaries of the garden, to not be overwhelmed. Interchanges in the garden help the person grow in discipline and confidence and invite the person to recognize and welcome new possibilities, to nurture them into the probable, and finally into the real. The garden plot can be seen from beyond the garden walls; passers-by and visitors can observe the design, the full-grown plants, the fallow beds, and the wilting stems, but only by knowing the gardener can they know its history or its meaning for the person.

The Wilderness

The wilderness, boundless and largely unknown, lies both within and beyond the horizon. Populated with creatures great and small, it seems sometimes just beyond grasp, despite the expansiveness one glimpses from the window. What cannot be seen clearly in the moment, but is strongly felt, is the unrealized possibility, especially the possibility for which no pathway or bridge, either for the individual or the group, has yet been created.

Despite the artificial boundary of the garden wall, the wilderness is vital to becoming with the world and has a certain relation (for each person) to "home." Its rhythms may be recognized and honored along one's path in serendipitous happenings that seem beyond reflection and logic but which may energize personal choices.

Knowledge of the wilderness may emerge as a forceful perspective that can change customary personal and interpersonal rhythms. Changes in the rhythms of life evolve as the possibles of the person and wilderness meld to create a new cadence, which will change again. Thus the house-garden-wilderness provides an experience of seeking home amidst the interplay of safety and risk, known and unknown, custom and exception, and self with others.

NURSING PERSPECTIVES

Exploration of the metaphor of house-garden-wilderness may reveal in symbolic form nursing's evolution toward, and opportunities for articulating, its unique substantive domain. Both the caring and Parse perspective offer horizons for reflection. The word "horizon" suggests limits to what one can see or grasp. But to see what is beyond the horizon requires that one *move*, for example, by walking you, the reader, through the images of house-garden-wilderness.

Caring Perspective

What drives the person within the caring perspective is primarily a moral force (Watson, 1985, 1990) and rests on the belief that caring is the human mode of being (Roach, 1987). The images associated with the person here include focusing on the beauty and light within the person, responding to calls for caring, and taking action in the recasting of the personal light. The house is envisioned as a circle without hierarchy or levels (Boykin, 1990) with many people moving in and out (Watson, 1990).

This perspective focuses on the nurse offering care within the garden, rather than in the larger world or wilderness. Nurturing (Geissler, 1989), supporting (Gardner & Wheeler, 1981; Lane, 1987), using multiple ways of knowing (Carper, 1978), offering knowing, being with, doing for, enabling and maintaining belief (Swanson, 1991) occur within the walls of the garden which obligate the nurse: (a) to be in touch with her/his own person or private living, (b) to place the welfare of the person above the nurse's own in the moment of encounter, and (c) to offer authentic presence as substantive expertise. Within these protecting walls, the person is free to wander within a relationship of mutual exchange until the person hears a call from the wilderness for caring. The persons are then guided by the nurse to more fully express their caring capacities for self and others.

Within this perspective, the wilderness has been described as a moral landscape (Watson, 1990), as a community that calls (Roach, 1987), and as having culturally specific ways for expressing care (Leininger, 1980). The wilderness is generally seen as a complex place (Swanson, 1990) with distorted rhythms which are non-supportive (Greenleaf, 1991) and disconnected (Clayton, Murray, Horner, & Greene, 1991). The possibility of distorted rhythms is also reflected in questions such as "can you care too much?" (Gemma, 1989) or "does caring lead to conformity rather than creativity?" (Sherman, Cardea, Gaskill, & Tyan, 1989). The force for changing the rhythms arises from good intentions, intuition based on the senses, and the imperative to care for self and others.

Parse's Human Becoming Perspective

In Parse's theory (1981, 1987, 1992), the person is energized by the courage to be oneself, reflecting the belief that the person is always becoming, knows what is right, and chooses how to live from infinite possibilities cocreated with others. The images associated with the person are not predefined but are those of the person's own vision of becoming with the world, inclusive of beauty and ugliness, light and darkness, the push and pull of tensions in being like and unlike others. The person lives the interplay of house-garden-wilderness all-at-once and can be "located" only through attentive listening—for "*this* is where I am now," however it may be languaged. There is no spatial dimension per se to the house, garden, or wilderness, when it is interpreted through the perspective of human becoming.

The house has a visible structure in the moment but is always evolving with the person. It is built of personal history yet open to the possibility of emerging designs, replete with ups and downs, twists and turns, views from the front window, or explorations of secret passageways at will. The house has no absolute beginning or end but moves and breathes with its landscape.

Parse's human becoming theory and its congruent practice methodology (Parse, 1987) guide the nurse to live *true presence* with the person, journeying and sojourning in the person's house-garden-wilderness as it *is* for that person. True presence is intentional human-to-human relating, open to the emerging truths of the person in the moment. The nurse bears witness to the person's truths and moves with the person's struggle (Parse, 1987, p. 167) in creating home, wherever it may lead. "Gardening" may be one way of connecting with the person and for the person to try out new ideas in a relatively safe place.

Strolling or toiling in the garden may lead the person in planned cultivation or to the darkest corners of the house or to uncharted wilderness. The Parse nurse knows that house-garden-wilderness is a unitary, multidimensional experience where predecessors, contemporaries, successors, and individuals and collectives (peoples, cultures) intermingle all-at-once. The wilderness is always with the person, no matter how or when it may come to the fore; distant or unfamiliar rhythms bespeak possibilities. The outcomes of choices are unpredictable, and so the nurse is concerned not with any predefined schema for house-and-garden but with the meaning of home in the context of house-garden-wilderness for the person. The nurse's goal is the quality of the house-garden-wilderness experience from the perspective of the person.

The person, with the nurse, makes explicit what is appearing in her/his world in the moment (Parse, 1987, p. 168). The nurse moves with the person's struggle, with the rhythms set by the person. With the nurse, the person moves "beyond the meaning moment to what is not yet" (p. 169). The nurse guides the person not in what to do or how to be, but simply to focus on the meanings and values inherent in the lived experience. The force for changing the rhythms comes from the person's own way of knowing and connecting, which reflects the person's interrelationship with others and the universe. The nurse reveres and honors the person's own timing and pace for cocreating rhythms in tune with what is right for her/him.

Comparison of the Two Perspectives

The house-garden-wilderness metaphor can be used to shed light on transformational moments lived in nursing practice within two belief systems. The primary difference between the caring and the Parse perspective occurs in the way the person is viewed in seeking a home.

The caring perspective views the person as needing assistance in finding a place in the world, whether at home in the world or not. The nurse is believed to have expertise that can lead the person home. The tendency is to *explain* the person's seeking of home with reference to the *world*. The person waits for specific calls from others and then responds.

Transformation occurs between a nurse living a caring philosophy and a person who needs assistance in expressing caring, primarily in the "in-between" garden, where the transcendent "caring-healing moment" (Watson, 1988, p. 179) is fostered. It is the caring, with "informed moral passion" (Watson, 1990) expressed by the nurse in the garden, which allows the person to hear and respond to calls from the wilderness and from established institutions which invite care within a specific role (such as nurse).

The Parse perspective views the person as active and enterprising, always already with the world as experienced, and exploring in personal ways the possibilities reflected in houses, gardens, and wildernesses. The universe (house-garden-wilderness) is understood in relation to each person's own meaning of "home." The person, living house-garden-wilderness multidimensionally, dialogues with others in cocreating reality, using both the gifts and challenges of other persons and groups to live the universal interconnection uniquely.

Within the human becoming perspective, transforming unfolds in living out one's possibles prereflectively - reflectively all-at-once. There is no absolute division between articulate and prearticulate knowing; one *knows* the meaning of house-garden-wilderness for oneself. "Where" one's truths may lead shows one's values and is not to be judged as rational or irrational. The person cocreates in every moment through interrelating with house-garden-wilderness. The person does not "adapt" but follows a personal way, sometimes far from the usual path, to discover and name what it is that speaks to the person.

Comparing Unique Substantive Domains

Both the caring and human becoming perspective may foster, metaphorically, "being at home in the world." Both perspectives have moved beyond describing the substantive domain specific to nursing as merely the person, environment, health, and nursing (Fawcett, 1989). The caring perspective describes the essence of nursing's unique domain as caring (Leininger, 1984; Roach, 1987; Watson, 1985). Parse's human becoming perspective goes beyond the general consensus of four core elements and a singular essence of caring to posit the lived experience of health as the unique domain of nursing (Parse, 1981; Smith, 1990).

Within the caring perspective, substantive expertise is described as authentic caring presence between nurse and person utilizing the caring frameworks posited as unique in nursing. *But such caring practice is nowhere adequately described in a substantive way by current caring theories.* The extant caring theories embrace a deep philosophical commitment to care yet have not sought to break down the garden walls of traditional nursing practice to create a wholly new way of nursing in the world of the person. The challenge that remains is to articulate a theory of caring unique in nursing that embodies more clearly a perspective (house-garden-wilderness), to provide both a guide to practice and a congruent research method to build nursing science. In the absence of such a caring theory and research method, nursing within a caring perspective is guided by multiple theories from various disciplines and emerging mid-range theories (Swanson, 1991). In research, attention is given primarily to specific aspects of caring in various "garden" situations, and a variety of methods may be used (Watson, 1985). Leininger (1980) proposes that the collective values of a given cultural group should guide nursing practice and research while Watson (1985) and others propose an enrichment of traditional biopsychosocial nursing through a greater emphasis on a philosophy of caring.

Within the human becoming perspective, the unique domain of nursing is the lived experience of health, which, though cocreated with others, is experienced uniquely by each individual (Parse, 1981, p. 30). According to Parse (1987), universal human experiences surfacing in the human-universe process are appropriate for study with her research methodology. These are "health-related experiences reflecting: being-becoming, value priorities, negentropic unfolding, and quality of life" (Parse, 1987, p. 174). Examples include phenomena such as struggling through a difficult time (Smith, 1990), grieving a personal loss (Cody, 1991), taking life day-by-day (Mitchell, 1990), struggling with going along when you do not believe (Kelley, 1991), and the lived experience of hope (Parse, 1990). Such research contributes to nursing science through expanding the theory and generating knowledge rooted in a nursing perspective that is available to nurses in practice.

While each person's lived experience is unique, humans do coexist and coconstitute reality with others. Parse's theory-guided research seeks to understand the essences of universal lived experiences of health; these are "qualitative" experiences and can only be understood as such. They cannot be measured, "normed," or judged by an observer as good or bad. For example, to understand the essence of "creating a home" is to understand the phenomenon as it is lived, not to judge its degree or the person's success in living it. Although creating a home is a human universal, it is lived uniquely, and each person chooses how to live it within the context of interrelating with others.

Within practice, the substantive expertise of the nurse is in living true presence with persons in their worlds (house-garden-wilderness all-at-once). True presence evokes exploration (Parse, 1987), as the nurse moves in attentive presence with the person wherever their personal journey may lead. The cocreation of "what-is-right" emerges from the personal dialogue with the universe.

CONCLUDING REMARKS

Nursing as elucidated by the house-garden-wilderness metaphor leads beyond natural caring (Noddings, 1984), or professional caring (van Hooft, 1987), to nursing guided by theory of sufficient breadth and multidimensionality to foster coparticipation with persons in cocreating quality of life in a universe of open possibilities. A brief review of Parse's (1981) three principles helps to illuminate possibilities for enriched nursing practice.

1. *Structuring meaning multidimensionally is cocreating reality through the languaging of valuing and imaging* (Parse, 1981, p. 42). This principle articulates a reverence for the person's own way of knowing, loving, and expressing that goes beyond superimposing "caring" on traditional nursing practice, by positing these processes of structuring meaning as *cocreating reality*. One's house-garden-wilderness experience does not emerge from a vacuum but is rather a coparticipative unfolding experienced and interpreted uniquely by each individual. It cannot be known by observation and cannot be kept safe and protected by any degree of caring. The nurse bears witness to the reality of each person's house-garden-wilderness as lived by that person.

2. *Cocreating rhythmical patterns of relating is living the paradoxical unity of revealing-concealing, enabling-limiting, while connecting-separating* (p. 50). This principle articulates the essential paradoxes of human-universe interrelating. The rhythms of self-disclosure, opportunity, and communion in the house-garden-wilderness experience cannot exist without their apparent opposites, nondisclosure, limitation, and solitude. "There is always the known in the unknown and the unknown in the known" (Parse, 1987, p. 164). The road not taken holds meaning and consequences for the person in every moment of living. Even persons in the direst circumstances give meaning and value to every aspect of their experience. Both sides of each paradoxical rhythm reflect human-universe process, and neither side of the rhythm can ever be completely subverted. While the caring frameworks guide nurses who foster *caring* to shift rhythms away from the unpleasant, the human becoming theory guides nurses not to show the way but to stay with the person on the journeys of discovery and invention, knowing that the hidden side of the rhythm is not ablated by any endeavor. Parse's theory provides a framework for understanding paradoxical experiences of living that the caring frameworks do not address.

3. *Cotranscending with the possibles is powering unique ways of originating in the process of transforming* (p. 55). This principle articulates the human-universe coparticipation in the ever-changing house-garden-wilderness experience. The courage to be as oneself inspires choices from among the myriad possibilities of house-garden-wilderness which cocreate innovative patterns of living. In this way the person is "cotranscending" with all that is in the house-garden-wilderness (the human-universe interrelationship) all-at-once. The ongoing dynamic process of human becoming is nursing's unique domain, the lived experience of health.

In this chapter, the metaphor of house-garden-wilderness was used to illustrate possibilities for nursing's evolution through articulating its unique, substantive domain. Challenges for nurses using Parse's theory include building the body of nursing science so that essences of universal lived experiences of health might be better understood, giving voice to the understanding that emerges from theory-guided research and to the importance of both sides of paradoxical rhythms in living health, and articulating essential advanced education for nurses that will enable them to appreciate the value in attending to lived experiences of health.

REFERENCES

Boykin, A. (1990). Creating a caring environment: Moral obligation in the role of dean. In M. Leininger & J. Watson, (Eds.), *The caring imperative in education* (pp. 247–254). New York: National League for Nursing Press.

Carper, B. A. (1978). Fundamental patterns of knowing in nursing. *Advances in Nursing Science, 1,* 13–24.

Chinn, P. L. (Ed). (1991). *Anthology on caring.* New York: National League for Nursing Press.

Clayton, G. M., Murray, J. P., Horner, S. D., & Greene, P. E. (1991). Connecting: A catalyst for caring. In P. L. Chinn (Ed.), *Anthology on caring* (pp. 155–168). New York: National League for Nursing Press.

Cody, W. K. (1991). Grieving a personal loss. *Nursing Science Quarterly, 4,* 61–68.

Dilthey, W. (1988). *Introduction to the human sciences* (R. J. Betanzos, Trans. & Ed.). Detroit: Wayne State University Press. (Original work published 1883)

Dunlop, M. J. (1986). Is a science of caring possible? *Journal of Advanced Nursing, 11,* 661–670.

Fawcett, J. (1989). *Analysis and evaluation of conceptual models of nursing* (2nd ed.). Philadelphia: Davis.

Gardner, K. G., & Wheeler, E. (1981). The meaning of caring in the context of nursing. In M. Leininger (Ed.), *Caring: An essential human need.* Thorofare, NJ: Slack.

Geissler, E. M. (1989). An exploratory study of selected female registered nurses: Meaning and expression of nurturance. *Journal of Advanced Nursing, 15,* 525–530.

Gemma, P. B. (May, 1989). Can nurses care too much? *American Journal of Nursing,* 743–744.

Greenleaf, N. P. (1991). Caring and not caring: The question of context. In P. L. Chinn (Ed.), *Anthology on caring.* New York: National League for Nursing Press.

Kelley, L. S. (1991). Struggling with going along when you do not believe. *Nursing Science Quarterly, 4,* 123–129.

Lane, J. A. (1987). The care of the human spirit. *Journal of Professional Nursing,* 332–337.

Leininger, M. (1980). Caring: A central focus of nursing and health care services. *Nursing & Health Care, 1*(3), 135–143, 176.

Leininger, M. (Ed.). (1984). *Care: The essence of nursing and health.* Thorofare, NJ: Slack.

Mayeroff, M. (1971). *On caring.* New York: Harper & Row.

Mitchell, G. J. (1990). The lived experience of taking life day-by-day in later life: Research guided by Parse's emergent method. *Nursing Science Quarterly, 3,* 29–36.

Mitchell, G. J., & Cody, W. K. (1992). Nursing knowledge and human science: Ontological and epistemological considerations. *Nursing Science Quarterly, 5,* 54–61.

Noddings, N. (1984). *Caring.* Berkeley: University of California Press.

Parse, R. R. (1981). *Man-living-health: A theory of nursing.* New York: Wiley.

Parse, R. R. (1987). *Nursing science: Major paradigms, theories, and critiques.* Philadelphia: Saunders.

Parse, R. R. (1990). Parse's research methodology with an illustration of the lived experience of hope. *Nursing Science Quarterly, 3,* 9–17.

Parse, R. R. (1992). Human becoming: Parse's theory of nursing. *Nursing Science Quarterly, 5,* 35–42.

Roach, M. S. (1987). *The human act of caring.* Ottawa, Ontario: Canadian Hospital Association.

Sherman, J. B., Cardea, J. M., Gaskill, S. D., & Tyan, C. M. (1989). Caring: Commitment to excellence or condemnation of conformity? *Journal of Psychosocial Nursing, 27*(8), 25–29.

Smith, M. C. (1990). Struggling through a difficult time for unemployed persons. *Nursing Science Quarterly, 3,* 18–28.

Swanson, K. M. (1990). Providing care in the NICU: Sometimes an act of love. *Advances in Nursing Science, 13*(1), 60–73.

Swanson, K. M. (1991). Empirical development of a middle range theory of caring. *Nursing Research, 40*(3), 161–166.

van Hooft, S. (1987). Caring and professional commitment. *The Australian Journal of Advanced Nursing, 4*(4), 29–38.

Watson, J. (1985). *Human science and human care.* Norwalk, CT: Appleton-Century-Crofts.

Watson, J. (1990). Caring knowledge and informed moral passion. *Advances in Nursing Science, 13*(1), 15–24.

Watson, M. J. (1988). New dimensions of human caring theory. *Nursing Science Quarterly, 1*, 175–181.

Part II

The Human Becoming Theory in Practice

Rosemarie Rizzo Parse

*T*his section of the book contains six chapters related to nursing practice with the human becoming theory. Chapter 6 specifies the human becoming practice methodology. It is followed by chapters on metaphor in human becoming practice, true presence through music, true presence with homeless persons, true presence with families with HIV disease, and true presence with a child and family.

Metaphors arise in day-to-day living as humans picture the possibles and offer symbolic representations to describe their ways of becoming. Banonis in chapter 7 shares experiences from her practice that shed light on meanings people give to experiences. Jonas is a flute player who cocreates true presence with people through her music. In chapter 8 she describes the difference between performing professionally as a flute player and being in true presence in nursing practice with others through flute music. She describes her experiences with persons who are living their dying. Rasmusson, in chapter 9, creatively describes her experiences with persons who are homeless. She shares how she has come to know the perspectives of these persons and how she respects their perspectives in her practice. In chapter 10, Cody describes true presence with families living with HIV disease. He discusses his way of becoming with a family, sharing the joys and sufferings of the family living their dying as he bears witness to it. In chapter 11, Cody, Hudepohl, and Brinkman describe a situation of being in true presence with a child and family.

Descriptions of the nurse utilizing Parse's theory in practice provide examples of ways of living the human becoming theory. As shown within these chapters its practice is an alternative to traditional nursing. The examples also demonstrate in general how abstract nursing theory can be translated into practice.

Chapter 6

The Human Becoming Practice Methodology

Rosemarie Rizzo Parse

*T*he practice methodology evolving from the ontology of the human becoming theory was constructed along with the theory (Parse, 1981). It was formally published in Parse's 1987 book. (For details related to methodology, see Parse, 1987, 1992.) The goal of practice with this theory is quality of life from the person's perspective. Since what constitutes quality of life differs from one person to another, the nurse living Parse's theory "respects each individual's or family's own view of quality and does not attempt to change that view to be consistent with his or her own perspective" (Parse, 1992, p. 39). The practice methodology is significantly different from the commonly used nursing process (assessing, diagnosing, planning, implementing, evaluating). This process requires the nurse to label the person's behavior and determine interventions to change the behavior. It is traditional practice and follows the ontology of theories in the totality paradigm. It does not focus on the meaning of experiences from the person's perspective (Parse, 1987).

Parse's practice methodology arises in the human-universe process as nurse, person, and family live true presence. True presence is the artful living of the human becoming theory. It is a special way of being with the other that recognizes the other's value priorities as paramount. The nurse centers with the universe, prepares, and approaches the other, attending intensely to the meaning of the moment being lived by the person or family. True presence is an invitation for person or family to explore the depths of ideas, issues, or events as they choose. The nurse takes what the person or family says or does as the meaning of the situation and moves with the person or family without judging, labeling, or specifying a nurse-generated change. The nurse risks a subject-to-subject engagement in order to cocreate new possibilities with persons and families. The course is not charted; in the practice of the human becoming theory there are no canned care plans pre-established for a particular "patient problem" as there are in traditional nursing practice. The content of a nurse-person or nurse-family process emerges through true presence and may lead to planning for changing health patterns. The process focuses on the person's or family's own thoughts and feelings about people, ideas, objects or events in the moment of coming together with the nurse. As the nurse and person or nurse and family move on to other activities, a *lingering* presence of their coming together continues and is woven into the pattern of living at all realms of the universe for the nurse and the person or family. The messages that were given and taken by the participants of the true presence continue to illuminate meanings in the rhythmical process of changing. The dimensions and processes of the practice method are lived through the true presence.

The dimensions and processes of Parse's (1987) method are:

1. Illuminating meaning is shedding light through *explicating* the what was, is, and will be, as it is appearing now. Explicating is a process of making clear what is appearing now through languaging.

2. Synchronizing rhythms happens in *dwelling with* the pitch, yaw, and roll of the interhuman cadence. Dwelling with is giving self over to the flow of the struggle in connecting-separating.

3. Mobilizing transcendence happens in *moving beyond* the meaning moment to what is not-yet. Moving beyond is propelling with the possibles in transforming.

These dimensions are lived as the meaning of the moment, for person and family arise in the true presence of the nurse. As persons share thoughts and feelings, new meanings arise, casting a different light on the familiar in a situation that shifts the rhythms, mobilizing movement. The thoughts and feelings that arise in true presence show the *timelessness* of moments in that what is discussed often includes persons, ideas, objects, and events that *were* or *will be*, but present themselves as *now*. Now is the *context* of true presence cocreated in the human-universe process. The retrospective and prospective are always there in the moment of the now.

The nurse dwells with the flow of the rhythms of the person and family as they discuss what is important to them. "Dwelling with the rhythm is like treading water; while one appears to be in the same place, different waves arise to create subtle movement and often gigantic leaps" (Parse, 1992, p. 40). The *movement* in true presence, whether subtle or gigantic, is an ebb-and-flow rhythm that surfaces new meanings and propels participants in the human-universe process to different hopes and dreams. All movement in true presence cocreates a pattern, the cotton wool in the emerging fabric of the day-to-day struggles with the ups and downs of joy-sorrow that emerge with life's vicissitudes. The Parse practice methodology is a human-universe process, wherein the nurse as living unity in true presence joins persons and families in the journey of illuminating meaning, synchronizing rhythms, and mobilizing transcendence. For examples of the theory in practice see Butler, 1988; Butler and Snodgrass, 1991; Cody and Mitchell, 1992; Liehr, 1989; Mattice, 1991; Mattice and Mitchell, 1990; Mitchell, 1986, 1988, 1990, 1991a, 1991b, 1992; Mitchell and Copplestone, 1990; Mitchell and Pilkington, 1990; Mitchell and Santopinto, 1988a, 1988b; Quiquero, Knights, and Meo, 1991; Rasmusson, Jonas, and Mitchell, 1991.

REFERENCES

Butler, M. J. (1988). Family transformation: Parse's theory in practice. *Nursing Science Quarterly, 1,* 68–74.

Butler, M. J., & Snodgrass, F. G. (1991). Beyond abuse: Parse's theory in practice. *Nursing Science Quarterly, 4,* 76–82.

Cody, W. K., & Mitchell, G. J. (1992). Parse's theory as a model for practice: The cutting edge. *Advances in Nursing Science, 15*(2), 52–65.

Liehr, P. R. (1989). The core of true presence: A loving center. *Nursing Science Quarterly, 2,* 7–8.

Mattice, M. (1991). Parse's theory of nursing in practice: A manager's perspective. *Canadian Journal of Nursing Administration, 4*(1), 11–13.

Mattice, M., & Mitchell, G. J. (1990). Caring for confused elders. *The Canadian Nurse, 86*(11), 16–18.

Mitchell, G. J. (1986). Utilizing Parse's theory of man-living-health in Mrs. M's neighborhood. *Perspectives, 10*(4), 5–7.

Mitchell, G. J. (1988). Man-living-health: The theory in practice. *Nursing Science Quarterly, 1,* 120–127.

Mitchell, G. J. (1990). Struggling in change: From the traditional approach to Parse's theory-based practice. *Nursing Science Quarterly, 3,* 170–176.

Mitchell, G. J. (1991a). Diagnosis: Clarifying or obscuring the nature of nursing. *Nursing Science Quarterly, 4,* 52–53.

Mitchell, G. J. (1991b). Nursing diagnosis: An ethical analysis. *Image: Journal of Nursing Scholarship, 23*(2), 99–103.

Mitchell, G. J. (1992). Parse's theory and the multidisciplinary team: Clarifying scientific values. *Nursing Science Quarterly, 5,* 104–106.

Mitchell, G. J., & Copplestone, C. (1990). Applying Parse's theory to perioperative nursing: A nontraditional approach. *AORN Journal, 51*(3), 787–798.

Mitchell, G. J., & Pilkington, B. (1990). Theoretical approaches in nursing practice: A comparison of Roy and Parse. *Nursing Science Quarterly, 3,* 81–87.

Mitchell, G. J., & Santopinto, M. D. A. (1988a). An alternative to nursing diagnosis. *The Canadian Nurse, 84*(10), 25–28.

Mitchell, G. J., & Santopinto, M. D. A. (1988b). The expanded role nurse: A dissenting viewpoint. *Canadian Journal of Nursing Administration, 4*(1), 8–14.

Parse, R. R. (1981). *Man-living-health: A theory of nursing.* New York: Wiley.

Parse, R. R. (1987). *Nursing science: Major paradigms, theories, and critiques.* Philadelphia: Saunders.

Parse, R. R. (1992). Human becoming: Parse's theory of nursing. *Nursing Science Quarterly, 5,* 35–42.

Quiquero, A., Knights, D., & Meo, C. O. (1991). Theory as a guide to practice: Staff nurses choose Parse's theory. *Canadian Journal of Nursing Administration, 4*(1), 14–16.

Rasmusson, D. L., Jonas, C. M., & Mitchell, G. J. (1991). The eye of the beholder: Applying Parse's theory with homeless individuals. *Clinical Nurse Specialist Journal, 5*(3), 139–143.

Chapter 7

Metaphors in the Practice of the Human Becoming Theory

Barbara C. Banonis

One picture is worth a thousand words! This time-worn cliche reveals a truth which can be useful to the nurse practicing from Parse's (1992) theory of human becoming. Language is a symbolic representation of the human experience. Human language is replete with metaphors and symbols which offer creative gateways to understanding lived experiences of health. The person in true presence with the Parse-guided nurse can illuminate the meaning of the health experience through exploration of metaphors and symbols. The purpose of this chapter is to discuss the value of metaphors and symbols in languaging the human experience and to illustrate the use of exploring metaphors and symbols as a way of illuminating meaning in the Parse practice methodology.

PARSE'S THEORY OF HUMAN BECOMING

Parse's (1992) theory of human becoming expresses a belief in the openness of human beings in mutual process with the universe. The human engages in "freely choosing ways of becoming as meaning is given to situations" (p. 37). Parse's practice methodology flowing from the theory consists of three processes in which the nurse coparticipates in true presence with the person or family: illuminating meaning, synchronizing rhythms, and mobilizing transcendence. The focus of discussion here is to illustrate how metaphors and symbols are ways of expressing unique meaning as persons and families illuminate meaning, synchronize rhythms, and mobilize transcendence in the true presence of the Parse-inspired nurse.

Illuminating meaning is "shedding light through uncovering the what was, is, and will be, as it is appearing now. It happens in explicating what is. Explicating is a process of making clear what is appearing now through languaging" (Parse, 1992, p. 37). In true presence with the person/family, the nurse invites the person/family to share their health experiences. In the telling of the story, feelings and thoughts are shared which "shed light" on the meaning of the experience. As the person, family, and nurse listen to the story together and dwell with the rhythms of the moment in true presence, new awarenesses can emerge, and all participants move on.

The human experience is complex, creative, and uniquely personal in meaning. It is not easily described in simple, straightforward language. Metaphors and symbols are creative language patterns that reveal and conceal a deeper meaning of the experience. An attuned listener will notice that metaphors and symbols are frequently used when people describe experiences. A Parse-guided nurse, whose focus is illuminating meaning, synchronizing rhythms, and mobilizing transcendence in the lived experience being described, can "tune in" to the metaphors and symbols used by the person/family as a way of explicating the meaning in the situation.

VALUE OF METAPHORS AND SYMBOLS IN LANGUAGE

Metaphors and symbols can shed light on the meaning of complex human experiences. Kopp (1971) says metaphor is "a way of speaking in which one thing is expressed in terms of another; this bringing together throws new light on the character of what is described" (p. 17). Metaphors invite a person to view an experience from a new perspective (Burke, 1984) where insight into actions and attitudes can arise (Lakoff & Johnson, 1980). Making connections between images and lived experiences is a creative process which serves to express the wholeness of meaning in the situation as uniquely lived by the person.

METAPHORS IN THE NURSING LITERATURE

Human language is replete with metaphors and symbols. This is particularly evident when persons are describing a lived experience. Recent literature documenting personal accounts of research participants provides the following illustrations:

> In a study on hope, a participant describes listening to music while his *thoughts travel* (Parse, 1990).

> A person who is the focus of a multidisciplinary team meeting commented, "That's one thing about living 86 years, you know how to *make it through the storms*" [italics added], and "I'll *close this door* [italics added] and work it out when I'm ready" (Mitchell, 1992).

> In describing uncertainty and dissatisfaction with school, work, relationships and physical symptoms, the participant states, "I'm just *ground into the ground*" [italics added] (Barnfather, Swain, & Erickson, 1989).

> In discussing recovery from addiction, a subject recalls thinking about situations that are routine: "not a *flash or lightbulb going on in my head*" [italics added] (Banonis, 1989).

The authors of the research and practice articles also use colorful metaphors in the context of their writing about human experiences. For example, in her discussion of literature on hope, Parse (1990) cites authors who describe hope as a "weaving of an experience now going forward," and "a waiting for the not-yet born" (p. 16). Banonis (1989) describes the experience of recovering from addiction as a lived experience of choosing the struggle to "pull self out of a well of darkness into the comfort of light" (p. 42). Santopinto (1989) uses images of "skirmish," "veiling intentions," "seeking shelter," and "taking flight inward" in discussing the "relentless drive" to be ever thinner (p. 33).

The participants and authors cited here were not focusing on the uses of metaphors or symbols in their studies or articles and did not address their use. Metaphors and symbols emerge naturally when human beings attempt to articulate the human experience.

METAPHORS IN PRACTICE

Within the author's employee assistance practice, persons frequently describe their experiences through the illustrative language of metaphors and symbols. Some examples include images such as: "It's spring and I'm blossoming" (used to convey growth); "Wheels are spinning in my head" (to convey thought); "I'm a runaway train going downhill" (to convey movement); "My feet are stuck to the ground" (conveying immobility); "feeling waves of sadness crashing over me," or "giddy as a goose in heat" (conveying sorrow-joy); "I can see the light at the end of the tunnel" (conveying new perspectives); "It's the dawning of a new day, or more like a new era for me" (conveying hopefulness).

The exploration of a metaphor or symbol used by a person in telling his or her story can bring about powerful insights and transformation in the person's view of self and the situation. An example is offered here to illustrate.

Mr. M came to the employee assistance program office complaining of headaches and dizziness, the cause of which several doctors had been unable to determine. Mr. M began the discussion with a recitation of all of his accomplishments: "My sons are grown"; "My work is completed"; "I have achieved all my goals"; "I'm ready to retire" (Mr. M was 55 years old). He punctuated the list of his accomplishments by stating, "I'm at the end of the road." When he was asked to repeat what he had just said, he repeated the words "I'm at the end of the road" and sighed. Then, looking the nurse directly in the eyes he remarked, "Do you think I'm dying?"

The nurse asked Mr. M to reflect on what it meant to him to be "at the end of the road." He commented on having completed his goals and not having anywhere else to go in terms of accomplishments. "Oh, *it is* the end of the road," he said with a deep sigh. The nurse then asked him what he saw when he imagined the end of the road. He paused to think, then proceeded with a tone of wonder in his voice, "The paved road is ended," (pause) "but there is a footpath that goes on." "Tell me more about the footpath," the nurse inquired. "Well, I have always wanted to write a book, and I have always been awed by nature." He began to expound upon nature, discussing butterflies and metamorphosis and finally stated, "Nature has always been a mystery to me. It's fascinating!" Mr. M's voice was full of enthusiasm as his eyes welled with tears. "I'm not ready to die," he said firmly.

During the remainder of the nurse-person session, Mr. M explored ways that he could pursue his dream of writing a book through the discovery of nature. He thought about how this would affect his relationships with his wife and sons. Considerations about space, time, and finances were raised by Mr. M. As he spoke, increased energy showed in his voice, eyes, and posture. He left the office with a progressive plan and new sense of the possibilities.

The nurse called Mr. M after 2 weeks. Over the phone, he indicated that the headaches were not completely gone, but he felt "much better." There was a lively discussion about his retirement plans and the space he was clearing in his home for collecting his notes and writing his book. Mr. M had taken the first steps on the newly discovered *"footpath at the end of the paved road"* of his life.

As the nurse in true presence with Mr. M engaged in illuminating the meaning and dwelling with the rhythm of the metaphor he was living—*"being at the end of the road"*—new possibilities emerged and new choices were revealed. The picture offered by the metaphor created a profound opportunity for Mr. M to explore the meaning of his experience. As he entered the image, he was able to creatively transform his story to expose hopes and dreams long put aside in his quest to achieve life goals. The new view energized Mr. M, mobilizing him toward his possibles.

The use of metaphors in practice is popular in counseling and psychology to stimulate transformational thought processes (Barker, 1985; Haley, 1978). Metaphors have also been used in pain relief with burn patients (Dobkin de Rios & Achauer, 1991) and in various nursing settings (Billings, 1991; Larkin & Zahourek, 1988). In each of these instances, metaphors are designed and suggested to the person as a way of stimulating a change process.

The use of externally designed metaphors to stimulate change in the person's thinking or behavior is not consistent with the role of the nurse practicing from a Parse perspective. The Parse-inspired nurse "respects each individual's or family's own view of quality and does not attempt to change that view to be consistent with his or her own perspective" (Parse, 1992, p. 39). Even though the interpretation of a metaphor is unique to each individual (Rico, 1983), it is important that the nurse, utilizing human becoming theory, not impose metaphorical possibilities through direct suggestion.

The Parse-educated nurse can illuminate meaning through metaphor and symbol in two ways: (a) "pick up on" the naturally occurring metaphors and symbols in the person/family story or (b) encourage the person to image or picture the situation/experience. Additionally, providing creative opportunities in the environment for writing, drawing, dancing, crafts, movement, or musical expression of the story can encourage imagining new ways of languaging one's experience.

Explicating the person's own images can shed a profound new light on the situation and the creative possibilities inherent in the picturing. As the nurse "tunes in" to the images offered by the person/family in true presence, the unique meanings of these metaphors and symbols can be explored. As in the situation described previously, asking the person to repeat the phrase encourages the person to become aware of the imaginative language being used. This can spark a new thought, moving deeper into the meaning. For example, Mr. M's case, when repeating "I'm at the end of the road" sparked "Do you think I'm dying?" The metaphor can also be explored directly: "Tell me more about [the metaphor]"; or "What does [the metaphor] mean for you?"

In one situation, a 28-year-old woman was talking to the nurse about her difficulty becoming independent from her family. As she told the story, she described having twice bumped into a hanging spider plant. The nurse asked her about the importance the spider plant might have in the story. The young woman reflected and then answered, smiling, *"There's only one baby left on the plant—the others were repotted in their own pots when they fell off."* She paused and then said, "This baby is not falling off; it may have to be cut from the mother to grow on its own." In subsequent sessions, the woman continued to find the use of this image, as well as others, helpful in describing the pain and joy of her separation experience.

When the person is having difficulty capturing the experience in words, the nurse can encourage the visualization of an image to help tell the story of the experience. The use of drawing or other types of picturing can facilitate the process. In one session a woman approaching her 40th birthday was describing the frightening experience of feeling that she did not know where she was at this age. She was having great difficulty putting her lived moment into words. The nurse asked her to draw a picture which might express her dilemma. When she looked at the picture, she saw that the left half of the paper was in dark colors and the right half was in light shades. There was a square area in the center. The nurse asked the woman to explain the picture. The woman looked closely at the paper and then, starting to cry, said, "It's the door." From this moment she was able to describe the experience of *"moving through a threshold."* By the end of the nurse-person discussion, she felt she had more clarity and hope about the transition she was experiencing. Although the future was not clear, she now knew where she was—"at the threshold."

SUMMARY

The use of metaphors in the Parse practice methodology provides a powerful and creative way for illuminating meaning, synchronizing rhythms, and mobilizing transcendence. Metaphors and symbols are prevalent in the languaging of the lived human experience. Metaphors provide persons and families in true presence with the Parse-guided nurse with rich opportunities to explicate the wholeness of meaning in an experience.

Metaphors may arise spontaneously in the description of an experience or may arise following encouragement by the nurse to express the experience through drawing, movement, music, writing and other means. In either case, metaphors and symbols provide a way of transcending limitations by revealing the deeper meaning in an experience which emerges through the picturing of images.

REFERENCES

Banonis, B. (1989). The lived experience of recovering from addiction: A phenomenological study. *Nursing Science Quarterly, 2,* 37–43.

Barker, P. (1985). *Using metaphors in psychotherapy.* New York: Brunner/Mazel.

Barnfather, J., Swain, M. A. P., & Erickson, H. (1989). Evaluation of two assessment techniques for adaptation to stress. *Nursing Science Quarterly, 4,* 172–182.

Billings, C. (1991). Therapeutic use of metaphors. *Issues in Mental Health Nursing, 12,* 1–8.

Burke, K. (1984). *Permanence and change* (3rd ed.). Berkeley: University of California Press.

Dobkin de Rios, M., & Achauer, B. (1991, July). Pain relief for the Hispanic burn patient using cultural metaphors. *Plastic and Reconstructive Surgery*, 161–164.

Haley, J. (1978). *Problem solving therapy.* San Francisco: Jossey-Bass.

Kopp, S. (1971). *Guru: Metaphors from a psychotherapist.* Palo Alto: Science and Behavior Books.

Lakoff, G., & Johnson, M. (1980). *Metaphors we live by.* Chicago: University of Chicago Press.

Larkin, D., & Zahourek, R. (1988). Therapeutic storytelling and metaphors. *Holistic Nursing Practice, 2*(3), 45–53.

Mitchell, G. (1992). Parse's theory and the multidisciplinary team: Clarifying scientific values. *Nursing Science Quarterly, 3*, 104–106.

Parse, R. R. (1981). *Man-living-health: A theory of nursing.* New York: Wiley.

Parse, R. R. (1990). Parse's research methodology with an illustration of the lived experience of hope. *Nursing Science Quarterly, 3*, 9–17.

Parse, R. R. (1992). Human becoming: Parse's theory of nursing. *Nursing Science Quarterly, 1*, 35–42.

Rico, G. (1983). *Writing the natural way.* Los Angeles: Tarcher.

Santopinto, M. D. A. (1989). The relentless drive to be ever thinner: A study using the phenomenological method. *Nursing Science Quarterly, 2*, 29–36.

Chapter 8

True Presence Through Music for Persons Living Their Dying

Christine M. Jonas

I walked into one room of the palliative care unit in an acute care teaching hospital and seated in the corner was an older Polish woman listening to her son speak of family news. Behind curtains on the other side of the room a frail, thin, older Chinese woman was sitting silently with her young daughter. I offered to play the flute for the people in the room as a way of being present with them. Everyone accepted. As I began to play the music, the Polish son and the Chinese daughter came to my side to sing. The older Polish woman watched and smiled. Then the elderly Chinese woman came from behind the curtain and sat down where she could see and be a part of what was happening. I then began to play a familiar waltz. As I played, the son and daughter continued to sing, but then the Chinese mother called her daughter to her. I continued to play. As I looked up from my music, I saw the older Chinese mother and her daughter waltzing in the middle of the hospital room. The nurses came by to look in and were moved by what they saw. Later that day I walked by the room again and saw the Chinese daughter teaching the Polish son how to waltz while their mothers looked on. Dancing with living while dying was the message I received that day.

Nursing practice with older persons living their dying in an acute care setting calls forth many challenges. The purpose of this chapter is to describe practice with older persons living their dying when the nurse is guided by Parse's (1981, 1987, 1992) theory of human becoming. The goal of practice with Parse's theory is quality of life from the perspective of persons and their families. The possibility of enhancing quality of life during dying is a particular challenge in a highly technologic environment that focuses primarily on medicine and cure. Older persons living their dying in institutions are often bombarded with invasive measures while struggling for comfort and choice about their dying. Unfortunately, dying often becomes medicalized and treated like an illness rather than being honored as a life experience.

I initially practiced from a systems model where I focused on problems that I believed could be fixed. The systems model, however, was inadequate for guiding my practice with persons living their dying. I realized I could not fix persons, and more importantly perhaps, I learned that often persons who were dying did not want to be fixed and they did not think of themselves as broken or deficient. I wondered what it was that I had to offer as a professional nurse. I felt frustrated with my inability to manage others' problems, and I did not know what to offer to persons living their dying. And yet I believed that nurses' relationships with people made a difference to their quality of life.

I then discovered Parse's theory of nursing, which gave me a theoretical base for my practice, a base that was congruent with my own beliefs about human beings and health. Through Parse's theory of nursing, I have learned how to live true presence with persons as they approach their dying alone and with others. True presence forms the base of an autonomous practice focused on meanings, relationships, and transcendence.

There are several aspects of Parse's theory that were especially important in my work with persons living their dying. First, the goal of practice with Parse's theory of nursing is quality of life from the perspective of persons and their families, rather than from the perspective of health care providers. Second, nursing practice is lived in relationships with persons and their family members. For Parse, nursing is not linked to task completion or problem management according to norms. Rather, practice is the artful living of knowledge in ways that change quality of living and dying as guided by others living their own desires, hopes, and dreams. Third, it is in the true presence of the nurse that persons illuminate meaning, synchronize rhythms, and move beyond the now moment. These processes change ways that persons live health as they clarify what and who is important for living in the moment.

Liehr (1989) states that from Parse's human becoming theory "true presence is crucial for . . . enhancing the quality of life with individuals and with families" (p. 8). Music has been described as a unifying, comforting, and uplifting experience by clients in a chronic care setting (Mavely & Mitchell, 1994). Playing the flute is a special way to be present with persons living their dying. A nurse may choose to be present through silence, discussion, or other creative ways as long as the intention is to be truly present.

In the example described above, I was truly present with the Chinese and Polish families through the music of the flute. Living true presence is an intentional way of being. I centered on being with the people in the room in an open and loving way. As I played my flute I intentionally centered on the people in the room and asked myself what life was like for them. I continued to play and synchronize the rhythm of the music with the rhythms of the people in the room. The persons set the rhythm for the music and moved with one another. The moment when the mother and daughter began to dance propelled each of us beyond the actual situation of sitting in a hospital room to another place. The moment of moving with the dance of life while embracing death showed each of us the mystery of transcendence.

Parse (1994) describes true presence as a free-flowing attentiveness where the person's quality of life shines through the moment as the person tells and does not tell of what is important. True presence is a powerful human-with-human connection experienced at all realms of the universe. Living true presence means being with the rhythms of the sounds and the silences, the visions and the blindnesses of the unity in motion. To be present with others requires purposeful preparation and intention (Parse, 1994). In true presence all that is said and not said is quality of life as lived by the person. True presence is not limited to the moment; it lingers and stretches through time as persons move on to different situations with others (Parse, 1994).

Lingering presence was evident as I walked by the room and witnessed the Chinese daughter teaching the Polish son how to waltz while both mothers watched. Also, the Chinese daughter returned after her mother's death to talk with the nurses about how important and wonderful it was to have had that dance with her mother. She said it was a day she would never forget, and one for which she would always be thankful. Parse suggests that an experience of true presence is weaved into the fabric of one's life as lingering presence. How a nurse is with a person makes a difference at many realms. In being present there is a valuing for human dignity and the freedom to choose one's way. These values are fundamental to living the art of the human becoming theory (Parse, 1994).

Nurses guided by Parse's theory related their concern about Mrs. B, a woman 101 years of age admitted to the hospital with pneumonia. She was alone and dying. Guided by Parse's theory the nurses wanted to know more about Mrs. B and her life, but she could not speak to them in words at this time. When the nurses called the nursing home where Mrs. B had lived for 25 years and discovered that she loved music, they requested that I come to play my flute for Mrs. B. The nurses and I were truly present with her as I played the music. One of the nurses gently held Mrs. B's hand and sang quietly with the music of the flute. Mrs. B opened her eyes, and when asked if she liked the music, she smiled and nodded. There was a loving feeling in the closeness we lived with Mrs. B as she moved toward her death. We left the room that day knowing we had contributed to Mrs. B's quality of life while she lived the last day of her life.

Another day I was told about a family member who was very angry about his father's approaching death. I was asked to see this family. I offered to be present through flute playing. The son requested that I play a particular song his father liked. As I played the music, the father lay peacefully on his bed, with his eyes closed and his daughter's hand in his; the son walked over to the window and began to cry. Before I left the room the family thanked me and said they felt connected to their father in a new way. He had squeezed his daughter's hand when she asked him if he heard the music. Later that evening as I left the hospital I saw the son outside getting some fresh air. He stopped me and thanked me for spending time with him and his family. He then talked about what this time meant for him and how he could not stop the tears. He spoke about how this time had called forth many moments of recent and past deaths in his life. He thanked me for listening and for being with him in his pain.

On another occasion, an older woman was in great pain and discomfort as she struggled with living out her last days. Martha was a very independent woman all her life; she loved to be in the country and had loved to dance before she had to have her leg amputated. Martha also loved music. As I played the flute in true presence with her, she moved with the rhythm with her eyes closed and then she said she moved to a place of calm. Martha said that the music took her away from her troubles and pain for a few moments. She said it took her to the open fields of the prairies where she loved to walk freely with the breeze blowing through her hair.

When Martha planned her funeral, she requested my flute playing because it had meant so much to her when she was living. Standing on the hill beside Martha's grave were her daughter, a priest who had befriended her at the hospital, the nurse manager, and myself. I played Martha's favorite song. Martha's daughter was so moved and thankful to be with the music that her mother loved. She said she could feel her mother's presence. As we connected and separated with Martha that day, I recalled her words. She had said that on the day of her funeral when she would hear the music she knew that she would finally be able to dance again.

The moments of being with others in true presence through music are laden with meaning. Many people talk about how presencing with music means love, freedom, joy, and a soothing. Others find the music lifts them to other places and moves them beyond their present situation. A room changes when the music is played. A tremendous loving feeling lingers in the room during the playing of the music and after the piece is finished. Persons are touched through the moments of true presence. The meaning of being touched is often revealed to me in discussion after the music is played. One man said he felt as though his insides were being squeezed and wondered if I could see the rainbow that was flowing from him. A woman said she felt a presence in the room that came from me out of the flute and into the room. Another man spoke about how he missed my presence, not my music.

I am careful to clarify that I am not entertaining with the music. Rather, I am using flute playing in my nursing practice to convey in my whole way of being a presence with others that changes how health and quality are experienced. Parse's theory guides my practice in a way of being with others as they live their dying—practice that goes beyond the traditional provision of comfort measures. The mystery of human becoming continues to surface as the meanings, rhythms, and ways of moving beyond through the music are lived with persons in practice.

An 86-year-old woman, Miss D, and her sister, who is a nun (whom I will call Sister Mary), were together when I walked into their dimly lit room on a cold December afternoon. Through the window I could see snow silently falling. The nursing unit was being closed for Christmas, so the halls now echoed with emptiness. Miss D was the last patient to be transferred because she was dying and the nurses did not want to move her. As I entered the room I saw Miss D, yellowed with jaundice, lying on her bed and breathing deep breaths intermittently. Sister Mary, dressed in her black habit, sat by her side. I bent down close to the bedside where Sister Mary sat on a chair with her feet barely touching the floor. I asked her how things were going. She said that she was fine, but it was hard to see her sister die. She also said she was thankful that her sister would soon be relieved of her discomfort.

Sister Mary said that Miss D was her last sibling to go. She said that she had watched many sisters and brothers die, and now she would be left alone. Sister Mary began to talk about the memories she had of her and her sister traveling across the ocean in large ships playing cards on the deck. She smiled remembering the times they had shared. As we talked, we paused to look and listen for Miss D's next breath. I then remembered for an instant the interdisciplinary rounds where Miss D's decision to receive no further treatment was altered when a young intern stated he did not go to medical school to watch people die. He assessed her as incompetent and too depressed to make her own decisions. Miss D was treated, but, despite the treatment, she chose to continue to live out her dying.

The nurses guided by Parse's theory lived true presence with Miss D and her sister as they struggled through the living-dying process. One of the staff nurses knew Miss D loved a special perfume and after her bath sprayed the perfume in her room. The scent of this perfume still lingered in the air. Sister Mary and Miss D asked to hear the flute music. Sister Mary requested one of her sister's favorite songs, one that would also be played at her funeral. I centered myself to be with Miss D and Sister Mary. I began to play the piece and could feel the room changing as we connected with Miss D through the music. Other nurses entered from behind the curtain to share in the music and presence. After the piece ended, I bent down next to Miss D and Sister Mary. Sister Mary looked down at me and said, "You know there are two things I want to do when I go to heaven." I asked her what they might be. She said with a smile, "I want to learn how to sing and I want a cigarette." I will never forget those moments with Miss D and Sister Mary. Miss D died later that day. It was an honor and a privilege to have had the opportunity to be with Miss D and her sister during the last hours of her life.

Being with persons who move beyond the now moment in the true presence of music is a mysterious process not easily expressed with mere words. Living true presence through music is different from performing for the public or playing with an orchestra. The intention of true presence is different from the intention in performing. When I perform music, I am not truly present to others;

rather, my focus is on the music and not on being with the people. In nursing practice my intention when I am flute playing is solely to go with the rhythms and meanings of a person and their family members. I move with them as they experience and cocreate their unique ways of becoming.

Nurses, physicians, social workers, and chaplains consulted with me and sent referrals for me to be with persons. The other professionals saw and appreciated the difference that the music of true presence made with persons. The mystery of human becoming continues to unfold through the meanings, rhythms, and ways of moving beyond with presence through music.

I feel honored and privileged to be with persons at this very important time in their lives, and I continue to learn from their experiences. I no longer wonder how to be with persons living their dying. I now know true presence through illuminating meaning, synchronizing rhythms, and moving beyond as a unique way of being with others that enhances quality of life for persons and families.

REFERENCES

Liehr, P. R. (1989). The core of true presence: A loving center. *Nursing Science Quarterly, 2,* 7–8.

Mavely, R., & Mitchell, G. J. (1994). Consider karaoke. *The Canadian Nurse, 90*(1), 22–24.

Parse, R. R. (1981). *Man-living-health: A theory of nursing.* New York: Wiley.

Parse, R. R. (1987). *Nursing science: Major paradigms, theories, and critiques.* Philadelphia: Saunders.

Parse, R. R. (1992). Human becoming: Parse's theory of nursing. *Nursing Science Quarterly, 4,* 35–42.

Parse, R. R. (1994). Quality of life: Sciencing and living the art of human becoming. *Nursing Science Quarterly, 7,* 16–21.

Chapter 9

True Presence With Homeless Persons

Diane L. Rasmusson

Many people see those who live on the streets as either helpless or worthless and lazy. As a nurse practicing Parse's (1981, 1987, 1992) theory of human becoming in a drop-in center for homeless people, I have found otherwise. My belief that human beings are the co-authors of their lives, that they continuously cocreate their unfolding, has taken away the boundaries of class and discrimination and promoted discovery of the richness that we share as human beings. When encouraged to express meaning and to make choices based on what is important, these people blossom like flowers with petals slowly opening up to the sunshine.

In being truly present with people in the drop-in center, the meaning of their lived experience is expressed. Many speak of feeling isolated from the "dominant street gang," the rest of society. To be alone means for some to be comfortable and familiar, yet disturbing . . . not "a part of." Friends who are not really friends are around, they say, when and if they have money. The only good friends, some say, are those that have been made in childhood. "A friend would be someone to share good times and bad, someone who would not share your secrets with others."

When living on the street, one cannot really trust anyone completely. That means that if there is some sort of concern or problem, joy, or sorrow, it is kept to oneself. "Life is not possible on the streets, just survival; you have to watch out for yourself."

Into this situation appears a nurse guided by Parse's theory of nursing. Although the environment of the streets is very foreign to some, from this nurse's perspective, health is evident there—in persons' living of what they see as important and their becoming of who they are (as described by each person). In the true presence of living Parse's theory, the unique individual meanings of shared life experiences on the street are discovered.

Parse's first principle is "structuring meaning multidimensionally is cocreating reality through the languaging of valuing and imaging" (1981, p. 42). Thinking about this principle when practicing with persons in the drop-in center guides the nurse to attend to the meanings persons express in their valuing and imaging. Parse says that human expression is lived at many levels, and languaging is how persons reveal and conceal what their worlds are all about. People on the street disclose the meaning of their lives in descriptions of fear, aloneness, and friendship. In discussing what is important to the person living on the street, love relationships, self worth, peace of mind, and family are frequently mentioned. They tell others what is important when they get upset about the ways others treat them and when they decide to keep their sorrows a secret. Parse's theory opens the nurse to the worlds of these persons in order to be with them, to dwell with them where they are, and to learn about meaning and reality.

Dwelling with people brings to light paradoxical patterns. Through synchronizing rhythms, the unique meanings of personal struggles come to light. Persons speak about their need for love and closeness amidst a fear of intimacy; a need for self worth, yet a feeling of worthlessness; a need for peace of mind coupled with an inner torment. Parse's theory proposes that human beings relate with the universe in rhythmical, paradoxical patterns.

The second principle of Parse's (1981) theory states, "Co-creating rhythmical patterns of relating is living the paradoxical unity of revealing-concealing, enabling-limiting, while connecting-separating" (p. 50). Practice with persons who are homeless affirms the inherent paradoxes of lived experiences. In the true presence of the nurse these people reveal and conceal who they are. In the context of their own lives, their own unique realities, the homeless persons identify the opportunities and limitations they face every day. And, their patterns of connecting-separating are of great concern in their living of joy and sorrow amidst the communion-aloneness of living on the street.

In speaking of hopes and dreams and plans for the future, the person with the nurse thinks about the possibilities of going beyond the now moment. The moving beyond is witnessed in the dreams of what might be, in the struggles to go on one more day, in the choosing of how one wants to be with others or participate in activities and life on the street. Moving beyond the now moment is linked to Parse's (1981) third principle which states, "Cotranscending with the possibles is powering unique ways of originating in the process of transforming" (p. 55). Believing that people are free to choose and that they are cocreators of their existence, the nurse bears witness to health as a process of human becoming through the structuring of meaning while rhythmically relating and moving beyond.

Becoming the who that one is involves freedom, and I am honored to be a part of such a process of life. In hope of sharing some experiences of practicing three years with this special way of being truly present and accepting others, I wrote the following:

All God's Children

A man is sitting on the sidewalk asking passersby for
    change.
Another drunken Indian, you say to yourself. Most people
    pass by as if he doesn't even exist.

But I know him. I know about the agony he went through
     as a child. I know about his parents and grandparents
     who were forced to give up their native culture in
     order to make room for the white man.
Their intense grief and pain was passed on to him.
Now, the man who is descended from a proud nation is
     pitied or looked down upon by society.

A tall, thin man walks by. Must be a crack addict, you
     think. Look at him, eyes half open, unshaven.
But I know him. He's in kidney failure. He lives on the
     street but spends three days a week on dialysis.
He speaks with deep sadness over the loss of his wife and
     son. She's getting remarried soon and he's worried he
     may not be able to see his son as often.
He also speaks of his father who died from alcoholism
     when he was a teenager.
The cocaine allows him to forget . . . for awhile.

A man comes into Emergency for the millionth time this
     week. What a mess he is, drunk, with scraggly hair
     and filthy clothes. He's such a pain, you think.
But I know him. When his sister called and told him her
     husband was dying of cancer, he signed himself into a
     detoxification unit for a few days and then went to
     visit her.
"She's my baby sister," he said. "She needs me now."

"Look at this," another man said as he showed me his
     umbilical hernia. "My doctor says I need an operation.
     He keeps using all these big words, so I never know
     what he's saying."
An an interpreter, I accompany him to the surgeon who
     gives the man a list of instructions. Too bad he's
     illiterate. He says nothing, and neither do I. Back at
     the drop-in, I do the interpreting.

He has needle marks in his arms. Sometimes he sniffs
glue, or whatever he can get his hands on.
But I know him. As a child, he was passed from foster
home to foster house, never fitting in anywhere.
Then one day he comes into the drop-in with a wild
sparrow on his shoulder, hiding in his hair.
"I think there's something wrong with his wing," he says.
He feeds him and cares for him, and a few days later the
bird flies away.

Another man is sitting on the sidewalk. People pass by.
He's probably just drunk. Look at him; he's so thin and
smells really bad.
But I know him. My colleague and I walk over to him. He
reaches out to us. Something doesn't seem right. His
hands are icy.
Two minutes later, we return with a blanket. Now he's
lying on the sidewalk, lifeless.
My colleague calls the ambulance and I start CPR. The
ambulance comes and takes him away to the hospital
where they work on him for another hour. He's dead.

The sacred tree holds on it green leaves of people who are
alive. The colored leaves are friends and family who
have died. When they fall to the ground, they become
part of the earth and give new life to the tree.
There is a place of dignity for everyone on this tree.
Sorrow is allowed to be expressed and true feelings of
love and a better time are spoken.
Everyone is equal here. Not as on the street. No one is
looked down upon or ridiculed. They are met where
they are without judgment and we work together to
discover hopes and dreams.

The next poem was written as I considered the persons with
whom I had been in true presence.

Who Am I?

When I was young
They said I was
another mouth to feed,
I was in the way,
a spoiled brat.

But I was young and scared
and lonely
and didn't understand
my world.

When I was a teenager
They said I was no good,
I didn't have a brain,
and I was nothing but trouble.
They said my friends were slime
and showed me the door.

But I was young and scared
and lonely
I didn't know
where I fit in,
or who I was.
I didn't understand
my world
So I left
looking for a new life.

Now that I'm an adult
They say I'm a bum, and lazy
and useless.
A burden on society
A waste of space
and money

But I'm still scared
and lonely
. . . and addicted
just like they were.

Maybe they were
right all along.
Maybe I am
good for nothing.

But I still believe
in love
in life
and yes, even in God . . .
whoever he or she may be.

I am many things,
But most of all,
I am me.
Sometimes happy
Sometimes sad,
sometimes frightened,
sometimes very angry
at the world
I was born into,
that I still don't
understand.

I still don't know where I fit in
or who I really am.

They say they know me
But they don't
How can they?
I don't even know myself.

I live with this person every day
year to year
. . . and still
I am a mystery
to me.

Who am I?
You can't tell me,
No one can.
I have to find out for myself.
And then, I hope to
be free
Instead of being trapped
in a person that everyone else
thinks I am . . .
but am not.

So, open up your mind
and give me a chance.
Let me be who I am.

Do not judge me on what I look like,
or who you think I am.
Open your eyes and let
me be me,
whoever that is . . .
and then accept me
for who I am;
An individual
with many different
moods and feelings.

Still lonely and scared?
In this world,
who wouldn't be?

REFERENCES

Parse, R. R. (1981). *Man-living-health: A theory of nursing.* New York: Wiley.

Parse, R. R. (1987). *Nursing science: Major paradigms, theories, and critiques.* Philadelphia: Saunders.

Parse, R. R. (1992). Human becoming: Parse's theory of nursing. *Nursing Science Quarterly, 5,* 35–42.

Chapter 10

True Presence With Families Living With HIV Disease

William K. Cody

*T*his chapter explores the art of true presence, as described by Parse (1981, 1987, 1992), in nursing practice with persons and families living with HIV (human immunodeficiency virus) and AIDS (acquired immune deficiency syndrome). In accord with Parse's theory, nursing is viewed herein as a human science and a performing art. HIV disease, including AIDS, is viewed in this context as an evolving nexus of constructed meanings.

As medically defined, HIV disease is a retroviral infection transmitted through direct blood or body-fluid transfer among humans. The proliferation of the virus over a period of months or years undermines the immune system, diminishes the body's ability to overcome infectious agents, and leads to multiple opportunistic infections which progress to multi-system failure and death. HIV disease is currently globally pandemic (Ehrhardt, 1992). "AIDS" in the language of medicine is the late stage of HIV disease, indicating frank illness, and is strictly defined by a long list of specific indicators (Buehler, 1992). There are few treatments for HIV disease, and none that is deemed highly effective; those that are available are likely to be costly, experimental, or both. Medical treatment mainly targets the numerous opportunistic infections associated with AIDS.

AIDS, for most people in everyday life, is very different from this objective description. The meanings of AIDS that people live with are intertwined with images and values related to death, sex, blood, sin, guilt, and stigma, among myriad others. For some people, AIDS is something virtually unthinkable hovering menacingly on the horizon. For others, the word bespeaks tragedy for "innocent" children but punishment for "guilty" adults. Among gay people, the word AIDS brings to mind the many tens of thousands of young gay men who have died and those who have the virus now, while at the same time the word resonates with societal attitudes of loathing and fear. For the families of these men, the word AIDS may symbolize their realization that their loved one was not quite the person they thought, had hidden much of importance from them, and was going to die or was already dead. For some intravenous drug users, AIDS (now believed to have been in the needles ten years before anyone knew) was one more reason to stop using, without sufficient means to do so, even as the prospect of infection and death became clear. For many mothers living with AIDS, it is a robber who robbed them of the chance to see their kids grow up. Yet for some who live very closely with the epidemic, AIDS is also an opportunity to reach out, to clarify what really matters, to connect more closely with those they love, and to focus on living precious values in the now. A number of authors have commented on the multiple meanings of AIDS.

> The link with sexuality and blood makes AIDS particularly susceptible to metaphorical use (Altman, 1987, p. 194).

> AIDS is a particularly good example of the social construction of disease. In the process of defining both the disease and the persons infected, politics and social perceptions have been embedded in scientific and policy constructions of their reality and meaning (Fee & Fox, 1992, p. 9).

> Yes, AIDS kills, but therein does not lie its significance. The latter lies rather in the understanding we come to acquire about the

world and our place in it, frail human hope, quixotic and eternal beauty, desire necessary and unfulfilled and still longing until extinguished with our breath (Schecter, 1990, p. 142).

These comments suggest even further meanings of AIDS, but they do not capture the experience of *living with* HIV disease, which is lived by real people in complex life situations, interwoven with their personal beliefs and values, their interrelationships with loved ones and others, their cherished patterns of daily living, and their hopes and dreams. Nurses who choose to work with persons and families living with HIV disease and AIDS are usually sensitive to these various meanings. They may have experienced "a calling," rooted in a deep sense of compassion, to care for this group of people whose experiences are, in the main, troubling to dwell with and poorly understood by society.

Such a value, to be a loving presence with persons in practice regardless of societal norms or approbation, is lived by the nurse in the nurse-person-family interrelationship when practice is guided by Parse's theory. But, Parse's theory-guided practice is not merely grafted onto the conventional tasks of nursing. It is a whole approach which provides a method of practice that is fundamentally rooted in the value for each individual as the who he or she is.

PARSE'S THEORY-GUIDED PRACTICE

In the belief system of Parse's (1981, 1992) human becoming theory, the nurse is not viewed as the "expert" on the health of the persons with whom he or she practices. Health is viewed as the quality of life experienced and described by the person (Parse, 1992). There is no separation between "biological," "psychological," "social" or "spiritual" aspects of health—the meaning given to a phenomenon as experienced by a person *is* the phenomenon for that person. There is no attempt by the nurse to fix, adjust, or manipulate any aspect of the person's health. The focus of practice as described by Parse is what the person is experiencing—what the person believes and values, how the person relates with other people and all that is in his or her universe, and how the person chooses to live—in short, the lived experience of health. The practice method is not different when working with *families.* Persons living a family relationship both share and do not share beliefs and values, and they make choices in life that are similar and dissimilar. In families, personal beliefs and values bring to light (and submerge) struggles and relational tensions, both subtle and pronounced, and the interplay of shared and unshared intentions cocreates the possibilities for each person in the family in synergistic becoming.

Scope and Goal of Practice

Nursing practice guided by Parse's theory is not limited to particular venues, age groups, populations, or body systems. Rather, the practice is consistent in relation to any group with whom the nurse practices and any situation in which the nurse practices. The Parse nurse's theoretical perspective of the human-universe-health process is rooted in nursing science and peculiar to nursing science. Thus, the nurse does not refer to "psychological," "sociological," or "spiritual" aspects of the human-universe-health phenomena, but, when called upon to articulate the theoretical perspective which guides his or her practice, speaks the language of Parse's nursing theory, which is differentiated, properly, from the language of any other theory.

Parse's theory focuses uniquely on personal, living realities. The nurse does not present his or her view of the situation to persons with whom he or she practices but, rather, moves with each person's view of the situation. The *specifics* of the situation are no less important than in more conventional practice; the specifics are, however, *identified from the perspective of those who live with them.* As a simple example, a T-cell count may be deemed important from either perspective, but the nurse guided by Parse's theory attends to the meaning of the T-cell count for the person. Family relationships are also clearly important from either perspective, but the nurse guided by Parse's theory attends to the meaning of the relationships for each person and is not concerned with predefined family dynamics or norms. The goal of Parse's theory-guided practice is *quality of life* from each person's perspective, and the goal is the same whether the practice is centered on the individual or the family.

True Presence

The central mode of nursing practice guided by Parse's theory is living true presence with others. True presence is described by Parse as "a special way of 'being with' in which the nurse bears witness to the person's or family's own living of value priorities." She further states, "True presence is an interpersonal art grounded in a strong knowledge base" (1992, p. 40), which reflects "the belief that each person knows 'the way' somewhere within self" (Parse, 1990, p. 139). To be engaged in true presence with others is like being wholly caught up in an activity one *loves*. All else recedes into the background as the nurse moves with the rhythms of the person or persons to whom he or she is giving full attention. The nurse offers presence in the person's universe *unconditionally* and is open to the reality the person lives. Engaging with persons in true presence may be likened to Gadamer's (1989) description of the action of a drama, which "exists as something that rests absolutely within itself [in nursing practice, the person in a situation; that is, the human-universe-health process]. It no longer permits of any comparison with reality as the secret measure of all verisimilitude. It is raised above all such comparisons—and hence also above the question of whether it is all real—because a superior truth speaks from it" (p. 112). The nurse is present to the truth the person lives, reverent in the presence of the person's long-confirmed truths, and equally sensitive to the truths emerging in cotranscending with the possibles.

True presence is a way of bearing witness. Bearing witness, according to the dictionary, means attesting to the authenticity of something through one's personal presence. In practice guided by

Parse's theory, the nurse bears witness, in true presence, to the lived experience of the person—the coherent whole of the person's life experience as it is appearing and evolving in the moment. That to which the nurse bears witness may be immediately apparent and eloquently articulated by the person but may also be languaged in silence by the person connecting with the always-present, pre-articulate, tacit dimensions of personal experience. The nurse does not "dig" for the meaning, nor seek to express or explain in verbal language an attitude or feeling that the person leaves unspoken but, rather, abides in the moment truly with the person, bearing witness to that which is real for that person. The art of true presence, like other arts, requires a strong knowledge base, love of the art, practice, and discipline.

Dimensions and Processes of Parse's Practice Methodology

Parse's practice methodology encompasses the topics discussed in the preceding paragraphs—the goal of quality of life from each person's perspective and the art of true presence—as well as the three dimensions and processes of the method, which are lived simultaneously. These are described by Parse (1992) as follows.

1. Illuminating meaning is shedding light through uncovering the what was, is, and will be, as it is appearing now. It happens in explicating what is. Explicating is a process of making clear what is appearing now through languaging.
2. Synchronizing rhythms happens in dwelling with the pitch, yaw, and roll of the interhuman cadence. Dwelling with is giving self over to the flow of the struggle in connecting-separating.
3. Mobilizing transcendence happens in moving beyond the meaning moment to what is not yet. Moving beyond is propelling toward the possibles in transforming (pp. 39–40).

True presence is described explicitly in the second dimension (preceding) but it is also the basic art underlying the entire methodology and is thus inherent in all the dimensions and processes. The method is congruent with the principles of Parse's (1981, 1992) theory, described in detail elsewhere in this volume. The nurse who lives this art form does not have to think continually "illuminating meaning," "synchronizing rhythms," "mobilizing transcendence." Rather, the dimensions and processes of the method are actualized in practice in the living of who he or she is as a nurse, an artist. The essence of the method is embedded in the knowledge base of the theory such that practice is the living expression of the beliefs articulated in the theory.

FOCUSING ON THE LIVING EXPERIENCE: NOTES FROM PRACTICE

Living true presence, clearly, is quite different from conventional nursing practice. The focus is the living experience of the person and family, the quality of life as experienced and described by each person. Conventional nursing practice does not have this focus, and conventional nursing education does not prepare one to practice in this way. It is rare for the traditionally educated nurse to be capable of speaking non-judgmentally about life as it is humanly lived. Thus, when nurses discuss "empirics"—actual practice experiences—the perspectives of the traditionally prepared nurse and the Parse nurse may be so divergent that they are talking about different things while referring to the same "facts." In this section, some commonly lived experiences among families living with HIV disease are discussed. These illustrations, gleaned from the author's experiences of living true presence with families living with HIV/AIDS, are offered as insights into commonly lived experiences among these persons and families and as illustrations of the focus on living experience in Parse's theory-guided practice.

Confronting Death

Confronting death is a universally lived experience, one that each person lives in a unique way. Among persons living with HIV disease there are recognizable threads of meaning woven into this experience. For many people, facing death itself is such a powerful experience as to overwhelm all other health-related considerations, like weight loss, difficult treatment regimens, societal disdain, or even HIV infection itself, and the closeness of death may color nearly every decision in daily living. The nurse knows that she or he cannot tell the person how to be with death. Rather, the nurse is truly present with the person as the person *is* with death. It is not always comfortable, but the truth of the experience for the person shines through. The *person* also knows that the nurse cannot tell him or her how to be with death and, in the loving presence of one who does not offer advice or consolation for the inconsolable, has the opportunity to reflect on the dying as his or her *own*. For people living with HIV disease, confronting death is not an abstraction but a reality; it is actually picturing one's dying. The nurse may ask, "How do you see it?" and offer true presence with the person as he or she explores the dreadful and beautiful images. In discussion, a person living with HIV disease may preface certain remarks by saying, "I have a terminal disease" and then proceed to discuss the specific priorities in his or her life in that light. The nurse stays with the person as he or she tells about what is and what is hoped for. "Having a terminal disease" often emboldens people to go against medical advice or the "rational" choice when it differs from their personal values. Very often, people with HIV disease find they have heightened priorities, find greater reasons for living, intently strive to enhance or renew their relationships, or place a greater value on not suffering and not seeing their families suffer than on merely living longer.

For others in the family, the news of impending death is often experienced differently—from the person with HIV and from one another. Even the person living with extremely complicated, debilitating HIV is likely to say, "I worry more about my family than

I do myself." The nurse in true presence does not try to refocus the person's energies, nor to resolve the struggles within the family but, rather, to coparticipate lovingly in their struggles to create comfort. For very young people this is perhaps the first death of a loved one they have experienced; it may be their first realization that everyone (including oneself) dies. The nurse knows that the personal meaning of this realization is unique to that person (though it is something each person must face), and stays with the person as he or she moves with the ramifications of the sudden understanding of mortality. The mothers of gay men with HIV have demonstrated devoted family caregiving to an extent that is well-known and admired in the HIV service community. Not infrequently, these are mothers who were distanced from their gay sons prior to "finding out" but rally to "be there for them" and labor intently to create comfort with them. The nurse bears witness to the love and commitment these women express with their very lives but is unwaveringly present, too, to the subtle dissonance of remembered and resurgent disharmonies.

Suffering

Living with HIV disease is a uniquely lived reality, but certainly for most people it includes innumerable unwanted experiences, such as severe pain, prolonged discomfort, insurmountable fatigue, frequent inconveniences, relational conflicts, tremendous expenses, and limitations in activities the person loves. "Suffering" (the abstract term) represents a uniquely personal lived experience in which it is clear that the meaning of the experience is the meaning given to it by the person living it. For many living with HIV disease, anguish and suffering are inextricably intertwined with the knowledge of impending death. Perhaps the sharpest pangs are those experienced in the transformation moment when the person's life changes from living free of HIV to living with HIV. It is common for persons living with HIV disease to say "it changed everything."

For many, suffering escalates as the discomfort, fatigue, inconveniences, expenses, and loss of abilities mount. Along with the numerous pharmaceuticals usually prescribed come their "side effects" (which often seem to the person worse than the ailment), the inconveniences of taking large quantities of medications, the interactions among these, and such things as surgically implanted central venous lines. Suffering, however, is inseparable from the will to overcome it, and persons with HIV find many ways to do so. These include taking charge of their own treatment (or nontreatment), even though their decisions may go against medical advice, or finding new reasons to persist, such as living to see a child graduate from high school or marry. For some, suffering is closely related to relational conflicts arising from the different meanings that close others give to AIDS—and attitudes toward being gay, toward "taking care of yourself," and the relationship itself. It is not uncommon to hear, "A lot of my friends don't come around much anymore," or "My father stopped speaking to me." In discussion, these experiences are almost always linked with further changes in the person's life: confirming beliefs, making decisions, and moving toward greater comfort with oneself. This may mean choosing to die rather than go on with the suffering. Not uncommonly, for persons "in the late stage" of HIV disease, there is suffering so intense that the person welcomes death. The Parse nurse views this experience as the person's way of living quality of life and is truly present with the person living her or his dying in a chosen way. The nurse invites the person to share that vision of dying and explores with the person ways of making the experience what the person hopes for it to be.

Loss and Grieving

Persons with HIV disease experience many losses, including the loss of life, the loss of close others, the loss of energy, the loss of attractiveness or sexual activities, the loss of employment or financial security, the loss of "the way things were" or "the way things might have been," the loss of hopes and dreams, and even losses that weren't evident before, like the loss of unknown others who have died or are dying with AIDS, with whom the person may feel a great kinship. People living with AIDS also say things like, "I grieve for the loss of *my future*. I had hopes, I had plans. It's not knowing how much time is left that hurts the most." This reflects the rhythm of certainty-uncertainty that emerges in the lives of persons living with HIV disease. There is certainty in some ways—that one's life has changed, is and will be different, and that one's death is likely to come sooner rather than later; but, there is also uncertainty as to when death will come and how that will be.

Grieving involves all those who are close in living with the losses, and the way each one lives with the loss weaves into the patterns of interrelating with those who are close. For much of the gay community, grieving for lost loved ones has become an attribute of daily living, with seemingly endless rounds of funerals month after month, or even the loss of one's whole personal network of friends. Each further loss, while experienced uniquely, echoes the others so resoundingly that there is also grieving for a time when death was rare. There are many shared meanings in the gay community related to the tremendous loss and overwhelming grief that AIDS has brought. Ways of being with one another and connecting with lost loved ones have been actualized through political action projects, group events, and special group endeavors like The Names Project (known as "the AIDS quilt" to the public and simply as "the quilt" in the gay community).

Telling and Not Telling

Telling and not telling is more than a matter of saying, "I have the HIV virus" to family, friends, and associates. Often the "telling" in this regard is merely the tip of the iceberg, and not infrequently the person who is to be (or is not to be) "told" already "knows." Often, many persons in a family are involved in pretending it was something else until the very end. Embedded in the possibility of "telling" is the disclosure-nondisclosure of something reflective of the whole person. The whole message may include, "I'm gay and

I'm afraid you won't love me anymore," or "I know you'll have a hard time knowing I'm dying and I can't bear to see *you* suffer," or "I don't want to be coddled, treated like an invalid, or buried before I'm dead." Often these meanings surface in discussion with the nurse either individually or in family group situations. More subtle aspects of an individual's experience also prompt the dilemma of telling and not telling. For a highly sexual person, to give up his or her active sex life is a major loss for which he or she grieves, yet the person is rarely in a situation to openly express grief in that regard and may be embarrassed to do so. With whatever gets "told" there is also the *untold*, and this rhythm evolves as persons share thoughts and feelings, which in itself changes the meaning of the situation, creating further issues of telling and not telling. Humor in moment-to-moment living with the family is a way of telling - not telling, and many families say it gets them through what would otherwise be unbearable.

Telling and not telling is an issue not only for persons who are HIV-positive, but also for family members of persons living with HIV/AIDS as they struggle with conflicting feelings about the whole experience. Sometimes the attempt to appear nonchalant and accepting conceals the love and concern that engender the effort, so that the possibility of saying, "I love you and I hate the thought that you're dying," diminishes in the daily pattern of being together doing mundane things, never saying what lies just below the surface. This too may be languaged with the nurse in true presence as the nurse invites the persons in the family to tell what the experience is like for them. There is also the possibility that the person for whom "telling" is an issue may never tell.

Making Hard Choices: What Really Matters

Like other "terminal illnesses," AIDS heightens the pressure in making choices in moment-to-moment living. Among the numerous choices confronting many if not most persons living with HIV and/or AIDS are the following: to take or not to take AZT; to pursue or not to pursue various types of aggressive or homeopathic treatments; to tell or not to tell specific persons about the HIV; to struggle with relationships with those who turn away or to let them go; to continue to work or to go on disability; and to plan for life, hoping for "the best," or plan for death, preparing for "the worst," or both at the same time. Those who are close to a person living with AIDS also make hard choices: to spend time with the person or stay away; to push the person onward when he or she feels weak or to let the person rest; to plan for a future with the person or to plan for the person's death; to reveal one's struggle to others or keep it quiet; and many others. Those who are widowed by AIDS, whether HIV-positive themselves or not, face difficult choices in moving on in life. Often they are more comfortable with another person widowed by AIDS, yet they doubt whether they can live through another illness and death.

The nurse guided by Parse's theory knows that only the person can make these decisions ultimately, even if others try to make them for that person. The nurse may ask the person to tell about the options when the person is facing a choice. The coparticipation of the nurse in this process is in prompting the person and family to shed greater light on the possibilities. In the presence of the nurse, who moves with their rhythms, persons and families explore the options and choose what is right for them.

Bearing Witness

For persons living with AIDS (or living close to someone with AIDS), there is a strong sense that "no one knows exactly what I'm going through." Conversely, persons in the same family openly say, "I'm not sure what it's like for him [or her], but I know it must be hard." The deeply personal experience to which these statements refer has to do with the dying or losing of someone close, the suffering for self and loved ones, the multiple losses and tangible limitations, and the whole complex of experiences tied up in living with AIDS. Families living with AIDS are not insulated from those persons in society who believe that AIDS is God's punishment for nearly unthinkable sins, nor from those who are terrified of catching this incurable, fatal disease, however unlikely this may be. Rather, persons and families living with AIDS do so every hour and every day virtually rubbing shoulders with such persons and painfully aware of their image in others' eyes—and, they often say, how very different it is from what they are actually experiencing.

Those who are authentically close to the person living with AIDS *bear witness* to the reality that the person is living, in the context of the love that means one suffers and grieves *for another*. Bearing witness has been described here, in the context of Parse's practice method. But, persons spontaneously bear witness to their loved ones' experiences in daily life; it is a dimension of the unconditional love that flows among persons coconstituting a family. There are likely many things persons in the family can do to help create comfort with one another; one can always bear witness to the reality of the lived experience of another, even if there is nothing "more" one can do and even if one does not agree with the path taken. Bearing witness occurs in ways great and small, known and unknown, and before, during, and after the person's death. The well-known Names Project—"the quilt"—is a clear example of bearing witness.

CASE STUDY: MIKE AND JOHN, LIVING MIKE'S DYING

What follows is a brief description of a practice situation in which the author participated as the nurse. Events and discussions within the situation flowed from the history and the values of the persons involved and are described in some detail. The nurse coparticipated with the family in this situation through dwelling with their unique rhythms as the events unfolded, inviting them to shed light on the *was* and *will be* as it was appearing in the moment, and moving with them beyond the now to the not-yet.

John and his lover of many years, Mike, lived a quiet life in a comfortable suburban home. They viewed their relationship essentially as a marriage and were deeply devoted to each other. Mike had two daughters, 18 and 20, who lived in a nearby small town. About a year earlier, John had found out that Mike had been involved with someone else. John was hurt and angry, but they decided to stay together. At John's insistence, they proceeded to have the HIV antibody test. Mike's test was positive; John's was negative.

Mike had had various ailments and injuries over the years that left him with chronic pain and an abiding distrust of the health care system. He decided early on that he would not seek aggressive medical treatment of any kind should he become sick. Mike's family was from a rural area where attitudes like his toward health and dying were not uncommon. Mike said he didn't want anyone to know that he had tested positive for the HIV virus. He didn't want to deal with the stigma surrounding AIDS, since he felt it would change his relationships with his daughters and with his family of origin. When he began to lose weight and to stay tired all the time, he told family and friends that he had cancer. This was accepted by his family, who, Mike said, ignored the obvious relationship between John and him whenever possible anyway.

John told the nurse he wanted to help Mike maintain a gratifying quality of life as long as possible. The nurse asked John to tell him what he saw as the alternatives. Meanwhile Mike ignored most of the available health care options and continued to smoke and drink. He ate less and less and spent his days watching television and sleeping. John worked full-time to support them, while at home he struggled to keep Mike going.

In spending time with John and Mike and discussing their situation with them, the nurse learned that Mike saw himself in a "masculine" role in the relationship with John, as a devoted, strong father to his daughters, and a good provider. In his work as a store manager, he had carried a revolver, and saw himself as a strong, intimidating presence. He very much valued his cigarettes and vodka, and, after having had back trouble and other ailments over the years, he was disinclined to follow medical prescriptions closely if at all. Although he had five siblings, he didn't talk with them at all about being gay or about his relationship with John. He was talking less and less but had made it clear that he was feeling very low lately and was going on with his journey toward death.

John described himself basically as a homemaker, but one with an appreciation of style and elegance; he was skilled in tailoring, cooking, carpentry, and gardening. He had embraced Buddhism as his religion and described his approach to life as accepting and pragmatic. He was also interested in the arts and customs of the Far East, and one of his pastimes was to copy the embroidery of the elaborate antique robes of Chinese nobility. He had several family members who lived locally but was really only close with one sister. The nurse made clear in discussing the situation with John that he (the nurse) was not there to tell them how to be with Mike's death or what to do but to truly "be there" with them, to invite them to explore the meaning of the experience, and to bear witness to their human dignity in living their choices.

Eventually Mike had to be cared for around the clock and was rapidly getting weaker. He stared at the television or into space, rarely moving or uttering a sound. When he was wet or thirsty or had slipped into an uncomfortable position, he would moan and fidget, occasionally calling John's name. Once in a great while he would realize John was doing something for him, smile feebly, and say, "Hey, John," then drift off again. The nurse moved with the rhythms set by John and Mike and assisted John in caring for Mike. He asked John to say what it was like for him to be living through this and what he was hoping for as Mike moved closer to death. John said, "I just don't want him to suffer any more. I know he wouldn't want anything done to prolong his life; he made that clear. I want to honor his wishes as much as I can, and he always told me to just let him go. He said that this was his time."

John invited Mike's two daughters and his sister, Jean, to be there with Mike as his death approached. None of them was fully comfortable with John and Mike's relationship, but they came to be with Mike as he died. As word spread among the family that Mike was dying, more siblings and friends began appearing at the door. John continually strived to be a good host to them all. The nurse moved with the rhythms that were happening in the household, centering on the quality of life for John and Mike, now sitting nearby as visitors bent over Mike to give an unacknowledged greeting, now talking with the other family members, now listening to Mike's young daughters talk about their feelings about what was going on.

The younger daughter, Amy, said, "I just hope he knows that we love him no matter what, that we always have loved him and we always will," her eyes welling up with tears. "John's a nice guy," she said. "I don't know if I could do what he's done for Dad." As the hours wore on, she would occasionally wander to the head of Mike's bed, lean over, kiss his forehead, and say, "I love you Daddy." Mike's sister, Jean, told stories about their childhood in the countryside, laughing at what a rebel Mike had always been and how fitting it was that he would even choose his own way to die.

As Mike's breathing got more and more shallow, his gaze more and more distant, John asked the nurse if he would sit with Mike while he took a quick shower. The nurse sat with Mike as promised, happening to check his pulse and finding it very thready and rapid but irregular and slowing. John emerged from his shower wearing all white, an Indian dhoti, and fragrant oils. He looked very calm and serene, and the nurse knew that he had prepared himself in a way that was meaningful to him to be with Mike when he died.

John approached the head of Mike's bed and began talking to him. Mike's breaths were slowing down and becoming very shallow. Speaking softly into Mike's ear, John said, "Find your peace, Mike. Find your happiness. We'll be all right here; you don't have to stay. You can be free now. Find your peace. Find your happiness. Go toward the light." He continued this way for a long time. Amy tiptoed in and took a seat a few feet behind John and sat there silently watching her father and the man she knew now was his lover. Eventually Mike's breathing became too slow and shallow to sustain life. When Mike had not breathed at all for a minute or more, John stopped talking to him and laid his forehead down on Mike's. Amy arose and walked over to the head of Mike's bed, where she stood sobbing quietly. After a moment John raised up, looking peaceful and composed, a faint smile fleetingly on his lips as his eyes met those of the nurse. Amy bent over, kissed Mike's forehead, and said, "Good-bye Daddy." John leaned over and gave the nurse a big hug. The nurse reached out to Amy nearby, and the three of them stood there a long while hugging.

As previously suggested, the goal of practice guided by Parse's theory is enhanced quality of life from each person's perspective. The art of living true presence is a subtle art and focuses on the person's and family's own values and patterns of living. The author cannot know what the quality of this experience might have been for John and Mike's family if the nurse had not been there. What is evident is that each person in this situation did what he or she chose to do and participated directly and intentionally in cocreating the situation lived by the family. The nurse's coparticipation with the family enhanced exploration of the personal meanings of the experience for each person. In the presence of the nurse Mike's family chose to relate in ways that enhanced comfort for Mike and for one another as Mike was dying, and in ways that they could talk about as meaningful for them. Mike and each person in his family chose how to move beyond the now to the not-yet and, in so doing, coparticipated in creating the will be.

REFERENCES

Altman, D. (1987). *AIDS in the mind of America.* New York: Anchor.

Buehler, J. W. (1992). The surveillance definition for AIDS. *American Journal of Public Health, 82,* 1462–1464.

Ehrhardt, A. A. (1992). Trends in sexual behavior and the HIV pandemic. *American Journal of Public Health, 82,* 1459–1461.

Fee, E. & Fox, D. M. (Eds.). (1992). AIDS: The making of a chronic disease. Berkeley: University of California Press.

Gadamer, H-G. (1989). Truth and method (2nd rev. ed.). (Translation revised by J. Weinsheimer & D. G. Marshall.) New York: Crossroad. (Original work published 1960)

Parse, R. R. (1981). *Man-living-health: A theory of nursing.* New York: Wiley.

Parse, R. R. (1987). Man-living-health theory of nursing. In R. R. Parse, *Nursing science: Major paradigms, theories, and critiques* (pp. 159–180). Philadelphia: Saunders.

Parse, R. R. (1990). Health: A personal commitment. *Nursing Science Quarterly, 3,* 136–140.

Parse, R. R. (1992). Human becoming: Parse's theory of nursing. *Nursing Science Quarterly, 5,* 35–42.

Schecter, S. (1990). *The AIDS notebooks.* Albany, NY: State University of New York Press.

Chapter 11

True Presence With a Child and His Family

William K. Cody

Jacqueline Hatfield Hudepohl

Kathleen Stentz Brinkman

*T*his chapter addresses the use of Parse's (1981, 1992) theory of human becoming in nursing practice with a child and his family. A practice proposition derived from the beliefs of the theory is introduced, explicated, and illustrated in the way the nurse lived the theory in being with the child and his family. The personal health description of the child, the nurse-person-family discussions through which the family situation was illuminated, and the nurse-person-family activities which emerged in the situation are described.

TOMMY'S SITUATION

Tommy was 11 years old and in the sixth grade. His mother, Sue, was a nurse, and his father, Frank, worked for an insurance company. He had two sisters, Lori, a college student, and Beth, a high school sophomore. His Aunt Elizabeth (his father's sister) lived with the family and stayed with Tommy while his parents worked. Their home was in the suburbs of a major metropolitan area. Tommy's parents and his teachers had voiced concern about Tommy's difficulty "getting along with his peers" and his "disruptive behavior" in school. They said he was "not achieving up to his potential." The parents asked the nurse to work with Tommy and the family in this situation.

PARSE'S PRACTICE METHODOLOGY

The dimensions of Parse's (1987, 1992) nursing practice method are illuminating meaning, synchronizing rhythms, and mobilizing transcendence. The processes are empirical activities, "explicating what is," "dwelling with the . . . interhuman cadence," and "moving beyond the meaning moment to what is not-yet" (Parse, 1987, p. 167). All dimensions and processes of the practice method unfold all-at-once with persons and families in life situations of all kinds. The practice is non-prescriptive and nonlinear.

The nurse elicits a personal health description from each person in the situation (Parse, 1981); this is a way of *illuminating meaning* and is actualized through the person's *explicating* the now. Health is conceptualized in the theory as the way the person *is*. Eliciting a personal health description does not mean asking the person to "tell me about your health." The description is elicited through questions like, "What's going on in your life now?" or even, "How are you?" As persons talk about their concerns, depth may be sought with questions such as, "What was that like for you?"

The nurse moves with the rhythms of the person and family in dialogue as they focus on the meaning of the situation. This reflects *synchronizing rhythms* and is actualized through *dwelling with* the varied struggles and joys of moment-to-moment family relating. The nurse is *truly present* with the family, which means moving with the ups and downs of the family rhythms while attending in a centered way to the meaning of the situation for each person. Through such nurse-person-family discussions, emerging patterns of health are identified from the perspective of each person. These emerge in conversation as the nurse consistently invites the person and family to tell about their perspectives of the situation.

The movement in changing patterns of health is chosen by each person through dialogue with the others in the family and the nurse (Parse, 1987). Nurse-person-family activities are planned by the family in the presence of the nurse and are not prescribed or delimited by the theory or the practice method. The person and family with the nurse *mobilize transcendence* through *moving beyond the meaning moment*. The family is *always* "moving beyond." The nurse moves with them in true presence with the goal in practice of quality of life for each person as he or she describes it.

A Proposition on Family Cocreation of Health

A proposition derived from Parse's theory shed light on this family situation and guided the nurse in practice. The proposition is: *changing views emerge while disclosing important personal beliefs.* This practice proposition describes a crucial dimension of family-cocreated health as viewed in Parse's theory and corresponds with the theoretical structure: *transforming unfolds in the revealing-concealing of valuing,* which interrelates three central concepts from the theory. It means that the way the persons living as family view their situation evolves through their telling and not telling about what really matters. *Changing views,* the first concept in the proposition, is a manifestation of transforming, from the principle of cotranscending with the possibles (Parse, 1981). Parse (Parse, Coyne, & Smith, 1985) states that transforming is "the changing of change," which "unfolds in the shift of view experienced when new light is shed on a familiar situation" (p. 15). This "new light" is not new knowledge but a new way of knowing a familiar situation.

Disclosing, the second concept in the proposition, is one side of the rhythm of *revealing-concealing,* a recognizable paradox of human becoming, from the principle of *cocreating rhythmical patterns of relating.* Parse (1981) says that while each person chooses to portray self in a certain way to others, each is also "more than and different from that which is seen by others" (p. 52). No human-to-human presence is without revelation *and* mystery.

Important personal beliefs, the third concept, refers to cherished connections and ideals in one's life and is conceptually linked with *valuing.* Valuing is a process of *choosing* from alternatives, *prizing,* and affirming the choice by *acting* (Parse, 1981, p. 45). Parse maintains that values are *lived;* one shows one's values in living day-to-day. Telling and not telling about what is really important to oneself within a family situation spins the warp and woof of the family's patterns of relating. The family with each individual evolves through this process.

LIVING PARSE'S METHOD WITH
TOMMY AND HIS FAMILY

When Tommy's parents, Sue and Frank, asked the nurse what her way of working with the family would be, the nurse told them that she would discuss the situation with Tommy and the family over time, but she would not tell them what to do. Frank and Sue felt they did not know "what was really going on" with Tommy, and they asked Tommy if he would spend some time with the nurse. Tommy did agree to this, but the nurse told Sue and Frank that she would not tell them about her time spent with Tommy. Telling and not telling would be for those in the family to decide, not the nurse.

Tommy's View: Nurse-Person Discussions

The process of surfacing a personal health description may be approached in various ways. The person's view may emerge explicitly in one-to-one discussions with the nurse or in small or large group activities. The nurse may ask the person to write a story about him- or herself or to draw something that he or she is interested in. The nurse and Tommy were together on a number of occasions—on walks, drives, various outings, and in quiet talks. In their first discussion, Tommy told the nurse he was not doing as well in school as his parents and teachers expected, that he had been in some fights with "bullies," and had received the first B's of his life on his report card. He said he felt all alone in school and "different from the others." He told how he was not included in games at recess and was singled out for teasing on the playground, which often resulted in fights. When fights occurred, he said the others claimed it was he who started the fights and he ended up getting punished for it. Tommy said he knew he could get good grades, "all A's," if he wanted, but sometimes he didn't want to do it "because that's all Mom and Dad expect—good grades, and I have all this other stuff to worry about!"

During this and subsequent meetings, Tommy said that his parents and teachers were "a lot more worried" about his problems at school than he was. He said things had been "kinda' rough" at school, on and off, since the third grade. He had "been tested" and had been to see the school psychologist before. He said that in his present situation, "the main thing" he was feeling was not being sure what he was "supposed to do." He said sometimes he felt that his mom and dad "don't care about me" and "they change their minds every 15 minutes." He said he felt "left out" and "not important," that his opinions didn't matter, and the things he did do were not appreciated as much as his older sister's achievements. He felt that comparisons to Beth were unfair, and that his mom and dad's desire for him to be a straight-A student was "too much pressure." He was involved with Boy Scouts, choir, and soccer but didn't have friends over to his house very often or play with other kids, aside from these activities.

Tommy said he spent a lot of time with his Aunt Elizabeth since his parents were "always working," but he always described her as working around the house and rarely talked about any interactions with her. He said he liked it when his father and he had something planned on weekends like building things together, going to Scouts, or learning to play golf. He also said he enjoyed having his family all together when his sister Lori came home from college for a visit. He said Lori "seems to make everyone have more fun, like they used to." He talked a great deal about the busy, overlapping schedules of everyone in the family but said that he felt left out of the planning most of the time. He said he seldom went outside because there was nothing to do, and he didn't ride his bike since "there's no one to ride with." Sometimes on Saturdays he would go to his father's office, but he just felt in the way, "like I'm just tagging along," since there was nothing for him to do there.

When asked what he liked to do, Tommy said, "I like math and science because I'm pretty good at them. I like to build things, too. I built an ant farm and I made my own skate board." He mentioned his enjoyment of cooking and told the nurse about copying recipes from TV. He said he liked to play the guitar and to practice hitting golf balls. The nurse listened in true presence and came to know Tommy as he presented himself and his world to her. She was not seeking to give Tommy a particular perspective on his situation or to change it in any way, though she knew it would change. Rather, her intention was to bear witness to Tommy's changing reality with unqualified respect for Tommy as a person.

Over time, the nurse gained an appreciation of Tommy's view of the others in his family. His father, he said, was "always talking to people and trying to sell insurance." He said his dad was good at answering his questions and building things and that he liked to play golf and soccer with him. Tommy said his mom "ran the house" and kept them all organized, with Aunt Elizabeth's help, but she worked a lot of overtime as a nurse and wasn't around as much. Sometimes she helped him learn to cook something new. Aunt Elizabeth was good at sewing, ironing, cleaning, and watching TV. He said that Lori liked to act silly and to make him laugh and that he missed her since she'd been away at college. Beth talked on the phone a lot, "laid out of school," and got away with it. She was always spending time with "her boyfriends," but got all A's and played basketball on the school team. He said things seemed easy for her, she did what she wanted, and everybody praised her. He hated being compared to her.

Parse (1981) says, "Perspectives of self emerge in human encounters as individuals view themselves as well as view themselves being viewed by others. The nurse asked Tommy, "If your
family members were describing you, what do you think they
would say?" And Tommy answered as follows:

> Dad would say, "He's good at building things and playing the gui-
> tar. He's a smart kid, but he doesn't try hard enough." Mom would
> say, "He does a lot of things well, but he needs to learn to concen-
> trate on his school work and not get into fights." Lori would say,
> "He's fun to fool around with. He laughs at my jokes and beats me
> at Monopoly." Beth would say, "He's a pest." And Aunt Elizabeth
> would say, "He straightens up his room when I ask him to and
> folds his own clothes."

Tommy felt he could talk to his father about most things. He could
talk to Lori, too, but she wasn't around much anymore. He was
hesitant to seek out other family members because he wasn't sure
they would really listen. He did not mention any friend with
whom he could talk. Tommy said he was happy when his family
did fun things together, which wasn't often anymore because of
their busy schedules. He was also happy doing anything with his
father. He said he remembered when he was in the first grade and
his mother took him shopping; they would look for antiques out in
the country and always buy a chocolate milkshake with two
straws before they came home. He said he was sorry when Lori
left for college and sometimes he got angry when no one listened
to him.

A Personal Health Description for Tommy

Health, in Parse's theory, is the quality of life as experienced and
described by the person (Parse, 1992). The major themes related
to quality of life that emerged in Tommy's discussions with the
nurse were as follows.

1. Tommy feels he can't and won't do all that Mom, Dad, and
   teachers want him to do in his studies and other activities.

2. He feels alone at school and "picked on," as some of the other students single him out for teasing.
3. He feels alone at home, since he is left out of planning schedules, and he doesn't think the others feel he is very important in the family.
4. He knows what he likes and what he is good at but isn't sure how his family sees him or how they feel about how he really is.
5. He enjoys spending time with his father, mother, and sisters, remembers times when they did a lot more things together, and wonders if those happy times are gone forever.

Emerging Patterns of Health

Three emerging patterns of health for Tommy were identified from the themes listed above.

1. Tommy knows his own strengths, limitations, and struggles in being himself with his own view of things, while being called to live up to the expectations of others.
2. He enjoys being with important persons in his life doing things they like, yet he spends much of his time alone.
3. While he is not unhappy with his relationships with close others, he dreams of times when less busy schedules allowed greater family togetherness.

The nurse dwelled with these emerging patterns as she and Tommy continued their discussions. In true presence with Tommy and sometimes with his family, the nurse explored the meaning of the situation for each of them.

Nurse-Person-Family Activities

The nurse met with Tommy and his parents over time, and they discussed each person's perspective in light of their shared values of being a family and loving and supporting one another. During this time Tommy's parents suggested that the whole family go off together to spend Christmas week at a relative's cabin in a remote northern area. This "retreat," as they called it, was agreed to by all and came to be viewed as an escape from schedules, work, telephones, television, and the day-to-day grind. In the nurse-person-family discussions, Tommy, his parents, and the others had brought to light that they weren't communicating as well as they once did and as they would have liked. Sue said that while writing Christmas cards to tell others how much they meant to her, she wondered when was the last time she had told those closest to her the same thing. The nurse asked if the family members could write one another "Christmas cards" to be opened at the cabin, telling one another what each meant to the other. The family members agreed among themselves that this would be "fun" and "a good thing to do."

After coming back from the trip, the family described to the nurse how in discussion of their messages to one another they had come to some realizations. Although they all loved each other greatly and thought about one another often, they had become so caught up in other activities that they weren't spending much time together, and as each of them changed in their interests, contacts, and activities, they didn't really know one another as well anymore. Sue and Frank led the family in a plan to set aside two to three hours a week for the family to be together.

Having liked the Christmas cards they had exchanged, they decided to use writing again for another family activity. Their plan may have been inspired by the nurse's way of being with them and her persistent questions of "What is that like for you?" and "How do you see that?" Each person in the family was asked to write a description of him- or herself and every other family member from his or her own perspective. They shared these descriptions during their time together. Although the family members did not share with the nurse all that was said in their private family times, they said that the activity had been rewarding and that it had helped to create family closeness anew.

The parents spoke of hearing things said that "we already knew but had chosen not to think too much about, for some reason." They had all enjoyed hearing what the others thought about them, although there had been tears as well, upon hearing of the pain in some of the relationships that they had not been aware of fully. They said they had started to refocus and to think about things differently. Beth and Tommy even planned an excursion to a museum and to lunch in a popular cafe, a first since Beth had entered her teens. Despite the hectic schedules that resumed after the Christmas trip, Frank and Sue also suggested establishing a new family tradition of dinner in a local restaurant once a week.

In further discussion of his thoughts and feelings with the nurse, and in light of his enjoyment of making things and the recent talk in the family about "not knowing each other," Tommy decided to put together a scrapbook about himself. He designed it to reflect his history in the family from his birth to the present, using photos, drawings, stories, poems, and letters. He decided to "interview" his parents, siblings, and relatives, about his babyhood and said the book would "document" their memories "not only of me, but of the way we all were," so they wouldn't "forget again." After some weeks when it was apparent Tommy was spending less time alone, he told the nurse he had started a diary. He said, "It's funny, now I feel like I need more time to myself to listen to myself think. So I write it down, just for me." Hearing that Tommy regarded the diary as "just for me," the nurse did not question him further about it.

Tommy gradually spoke less about teasing, rough times, and unpleasant experiences at school, although the facts of the school situation were said not to have changed. He still reported occasional teasing and unpleasantness, but in the nurse-person-family discussions and activities, Tommy focused on other priorities. As time passed, Sue and Frank rarely mentioned his grades, which, though improved, still included the occasional B+. The family was spending more time together and their togetherness seemed to have increased priority for everyone in the family. The various activities in which they had engaged to enhance their communication had let one another know he/she was loved, appreciated, and cared for.

In discussing evolving personal perspectives and meta-perspectives ("one's view of the other's view of self") Parse (1981) writes, "As one experiences these perspectives in the gaze, dialogue, and touch of others, the realization of what one envisions he is not, for self and others, simultaneously emerges with what one envisions one is and can become" (p. 64). In this situation, while each individual continued to evolve as the person he or she was, based on personal values, the shared value of being a family and caring deeply for one another also shifted priorities to enhance family togetherness.

CONCLUSIONS

This description of the situational experience of Tommy with his family relates to nursing-theory-based practice and to family cocreation of health. The practice proposition: changing views emerge while disclosing important personal beliefs, makes explicit the beliefs that guided the nurse in living true presence with Tommy and his family, bearing witness to their shared and unshared values in being individuals and family all-at-once. This empirical proposition reflects the theoretical structure: transforming unfolds in the revealing-concealing of valuing, drawn directly from Parse's theory. The cocreation of family health changed and evolved through focusing on emerging patterns of health. Though the nurse was most directly involved with Tommy in this practice situation, the complete involvement of the family in creating quality of life with Tommy was evident even (and perhaps most obviously) in their absence. Tommy's story thus illustrates how prereflective-reflective living of personal values in relation to others who are doing the same cocreates the individual, the family, and their health all-at-once, as described in Parse's theory.

REFERENCES

Parse, R. R. (1981). Man-living-health: A theory of nursing. New York: Wiley.

Parse, R. R. (1987). Man-living-health theory of nursing. In R. R. Parse, *Nursing science: Major paradigms, theories, and critiques* (pp. 159–180). Philadelphia: Saunders.

Parse, R. R. (1992). Human becoming: Parse's theory of nursing. *Nursing Science Quarterly, 5,* 35–42.

Parse, R. R., Coyne, A. B., & Smith, M. J. (1985). *Nursing research: Qualitative methods.* Bowie, MD: Brady.

Part III

The Human Becoming
Theory in Research

Rosemarie Rizzo Parse

*T*his section of the book contains eight chapters on research related to the human becoming theory. Chapter 12 sets forth the Parse research method. Chapters 13, 14, and 15 are reports of studies using the Parse research methodology. Chapter 16 is a hermeneutic research study on Walt Whitman's (1855) *Leaves of Grass,* in dialogue with Parse's (1981, 1992) human becoming perspective. Chapters 17, 18, and 19 are reports of research studies evaluating the human becoming theory in practice.

Mitchell's study in chapter 13 is on the experience of restriction-freedom for persons in later life. This is the first Parse method study specifically focusing on a lived paradoxical experience. Restriction-freedom is a paradoxical rhythm experienced in the human-universe process. Cody's study on grieving in families living with AIDS reported in chapter 14 is the first Parse method study with families. Family was defined broadly as close others from the perspective of the person with AIDS. It is Cody's second study on grieving; the first was published as "Grieving a Personal Loss" (Cody, 1991). The third Parse method study, reported here in chapter 15, is by Daly on suffering. Findings from all of these studies enhance the knowledge base of nursing by expanding the human becoming theory. Through hermeneutic dialogue, Cody in chapter 16 weaves the human becoming theory with *Leaves of Grass,* creating new understandings of human experiences.

The three evaluation studies reported here were conducted in Canada. Santopinto and Smith reported in chapter 17 on an evaluation study with both children and adults in an acute care setting. Jonas conducted an evaluation study in a family practice area, as reported in chapter 18, and the study by Mitchell in chapter 19 was conducted with adults in an acute care setting.

Findings from all three of these studies showed that with the introduction of the human becoming theory as a basis for practice, patients experienced nurses as more concerned about their opinions and more willing to listen to their views. Nurses' views changed from considering patients as problems to considering them as persons living distinct value priorities. The nurses reported greater satisfaction with practice when being truly present to people rather than focusing on assessing problems and deciding diagnoses. Nurse supervisory personnel and physicians were pleased with the nursing care that patients received, and nurse supervisors noted that nurses' attitudes changed toward patients, which led to enhancing the dignity of patients and their families. These three studies enhanced understanding of the theory in practice. The practice experiences led to development of learning modules for use in other evaluative studies on the Parse theory in practice and for all persons desiring to learn the theory (Jonas, Pilkington, Lyon, & MacDonald, 1992).

REFERENCES

Cody, W. K. (1991). Grieving a personal loss. *Nursing Science Quarterly, 4,* 61–68.

Jonas, C. M., Pilkington, B., Lyon, P., & MacDonald, G. E. (1992). Parse's theory of human becoming: Learning modules. *Parse's theory of nursing: A learning guide.* Toronto: St. Michael's Hospital.

Parse, R. R. (1981). *Man-living-health: A theory of nursing.* New York: Wiley.

Parse, R. R. (1992). Human becoming: Parse's theory of nursing. *Nursing Science Quarterly 5,* 35–42.

Whitman, W. (1855). *Leaves of Grass.* New York: Author [facsimile of 1st ed.].

Chapter 12

Research With the Human Becoming Theory

Rosemarie Rizzo Parse

*T*here are two types of research studies related to the human becoming theory. One type is *basic* research which may be on lived experiences, the findings of which expand the knowledge base of the science, or may be through an interpretive hermeneutic process which sheds light on the meaning of texts from the perspective of the theory. The other type of research is *applied* research used for evaluating the theory in practice. The findings of this type of research do not expand the knowledge base of the theory per se, but, rather, they shed light on what happens when the theory guides practice in various settings.

THE PARSE RESEARCH METHODOLOGY

The Parse research methodology was constructed in congruence with the ontological base of the theory, and the details of the method and its construction with examples have been published elsewhere (Parse, 1981, 1987, 1990a, 1992). The principles of methodology construction are:

- *The methodology is constructed to be in harmony with and evolve from the ontological beliefs of the research tradition.*
- *The methodology is an overall design of precise processes that adhere to scientific rigor.*
- *The methodology specifies the order within the processes appropriate for inquiry within the research tradition.*
- *The methodology is an aesthetic composition with balance in form.*

(Parse 1987, p. 173)

The basic assumptions underlying the Parse method are:

1. *Humans are open beings in mutual process with the universe. The construct* human becoming *refers to the human-universe-health process.*
2. *Human becoming is uniquely lived by individuals. People make reflective and prereflective choices in connection with others and the universe which incarnate their health.*
3. *Descriptions of lived experiences enhance knowledge of human becoming. Individuals and families can describe their own experiences in ways that shed light on the meaning of health.*
4. *Researcher-participant dialogical engagement uncovers the meaning of phenomena as humanly lived. The researcher in true presence with the participant can elicit authentic information about lived experiences.*
5. *The researcher, through inventing, abiding with logic, and adhering to semantic consistency during the extraction-synthesis and heuristic interpretation processes, creates structures of lived experiences and weaves the structure with the theory in ways that enhance the knowledge base of nursing.*

(Parse 1992, p. 41)

Here the methodology will be described only briefly, providing an introduction to the reports of the three studies that follow this chapter. The Parse methodology is generically phenomenological in that the entities for study are experiences as described by people who have lived them. These entities in the Parse method are to be universal lived experiences of health such as, grieving, feeling restricted - feeling free, and suffering. Participants are persons who can describe through words, symbols, metaphors, poetry, or drawings the meaning of the experience under study. The processes of the method are described below:

1. *Dialogical engagement* is not an interview but rather a discussion between the researcher and participant, in true presence, which focuses on the phenomenon under study as it is described by the participant. These dialogues are audiotaped and when possible videotaped.

2. *Extraction-synthesis* is culling the essences from the dialogue in the language of the participant and conceptualizing these essences in the language of science to form a structure of the experience. This process occurs through dwelling with the transcribed audio- and videotaped dialogues in deep concentration to elicit the meaning of the experience as described by participants. The structure arising from this process is the answer to the research question.

3. *Heuristic interpretation* weaves the structure into the theory and beyond (Parse, 1987, 1992). Structural integration and conceptual interpretation are processes that move the discourse of the structure to the discourse of the theory. (For details regarding the method, see Parse, 1987, 1990b, 1992.) The findings from studies conducted using the Parse methodology produced new knowledge and understanding of human experiences adding to the knowledge base of nursing on phenomena such as going along when you do not believe, grieving, hope, taking life day-by-day, and struggling through a difficult time. (See Cody, 1991; Kelley, 1991; Mitchell, 1990; Parse, 1990b, 1994; Pilkington, 1993; Smith, 1990.) The expanded knowledge base

enhances the Parse nurse's repertoire for practice and offers the nurse researcher opportunities for further study.

HERMENEUTICS

Hermeneutics is an ancient, yet modern and postmodern mode of inquiry. Its traditional focus is meaning, and its central processes are *interpretation* and *understanding*. In the broadest sense, hermeneutics is simply synonymous with interpretation, the word *hermeneutics* having been derived from the Greek word *hermeneuein*, meaning "to interpret." Hermeneutic research is a dialogical process uncovering meaning interpreted through a particular perspective. The notion is not without controversy. There are different perspectives on how hermeneutics is to be understood. Dilthey (1988/1883) and others (Ermarth, 1978; Polkinghorne, 1983) believe that lived experiences should be studied through human projects. Heidegger (1962/1927), Gadamer (1975), and Polkinghorne (1983), focusing more on ontology, believe that hermeneutics is a way of understanding human existence through the interpreter-text dialogue. Interpretation is the ontological incarnation of meanings arising as the researcher beholds and dwells with the text (Gadamer, 1975, 1976; Heidegger, 1962/1927; Hirsch, 1967; Madison, 1990). A hermeneutic study where the human becoming theory is the perspective is rooted in the basic principles of the theory with the view that humans structure personal meaning in cocreating rhythmical patterns while cotranscending with possibles. Any aesthetic work interpreted in dialogue with the human becoming theory will reflect the principles of the theory (see Parse, 1981, 1992). For example, if a researcher chooses to interpret from the human becoming perspective a literary work written years ago, that interpretation will emerge in the language of the theory. This is exactly what Cody (chapter 16) demonstrates in his hermeneutic study, which he specifies as dialoguing with Whitman and Parse.

THE RESEARCH METHOD FOR
PARSE PRACTICE EVALUATION

An applied research method compatible with the tenets of the theory is used to evaluate the human becoming theory in practice. A pre-project–post-project descriptive qualitative method is appropriate for the purpose of evaluating the theory in practice. Data-gathering strategies are: direct observation of documents to identify what nurses record about patients; tape-recorded interviews with nurses regarding beliefs about nursing, health, human beings, and nursing practice; tape-recorded interviews with patients and families regarding their experiences of nursing care; and tape-recorded interviews with head nurses, supervisors, and physicians regarding their views of differences in health care delivery following the initiation of Parse's theory in practice. A record of responses from these data sources is made by an evaluator (who is not engaged in the day-to-day activity of the setting) before the regular teaching-learning sessions on the human becoming theory begin, several months into the study, and at the end of the research project. A nurse specialist in Parse's theory instructs the nurse-participants about the theory after the pre-project data are gathered. These sessions are given on a regular basis depending on the time frame established for each study. After process and end-project data are gathered, each set of data is compared, analyzed, and synthesized for themes arising from each source. These themes are the findings of the study. At the end of the project a definitive answer can be given to this research question: What happens to nurses' beliefs and practices and patients' experiences of health when the human becoming theory is initiated?

The findings from these studies are valuable and add knowledge and understanding about the human becoming theory in practice. This knowledge is useful to health care settings in the integration of the theory as a guide to practice. It does not add to the knowledge base of nursing science per se but, rather, to knowledge about the effectiveness of nursing theory-based practice.

REFERENCES

Cody, W. K. (1991). Grieving a personal loss. *Nursing Science Quarterly, 4,* 61–68.

Dilthey, W. (1988). *Introduction to the human sciences* (R. J. Bentanzos, Trans.). Detroit: Wayne State University Press. (Original work published 1883)

Ermarth, M. (1978). *Wilhelm Dilthey: The critique of historical reason.* Chicago: The University of Chicago Press.

Gadamer, H-G. (1975). *Truth and method* (G. Barden & J. Cumming, Trans. & Eds.). New York: Seabury.

Gadamer, H-G. (1976). *Philosophical hermeneutics* (D. E. Linge, Trans. & Ed.). Berkeley: University of California Press.

Heidegger, M. (1962). *Being and time* (J. Macquarrie & E. Robinson, Trans.). San Francisco: Harper & Row. (Original work published 1927)

Hirsch, E. D. (1967). *Validity in interpretation.* New Haven: Yale University Press.

Kelley, L. S. (1991). Struggling with going along when you do not believe. *Nursing Science Quarterly, 4,* 123–129.

Madison, G. B. (1990). *The hermeneutics of postmodernity: Figures and themes.* Bloomington: Indiana University Press.

Mitchell, G. J. (1990). The lived experience of taking life day-by-day in later life: Research guided by Parse's emergent method. *Nursing Science Quarterly, 3,* 29–36.

Parse, R. R. (1981). *Man-living-health: A theory of nursing.* New York: Wiley.

Parse, R. R. (1987). *Nursing science: Major paradigms, theories, and critiques.* Philadelphia: Saunders.

Parse, R. R. (1990a). Health: A personal commitment. *Nursing Science Quarterly, 3,* 136–140.

Parse, R. R. (1990b). Parse's research methodology with an illustration of the lived experience of hope. *Nursing Science Quarterly, 3,* 9–17.

Parse, R. R. (1992). Human becoming: Parse's theory of nursing. *Nursing Science Quarterly, 5,* 35–42.

Parse, R. R. (1994). Laughing and health: A study using Parse's research method. *Nursing Science Quarterly, 7,* 55–64.

Pilkington, F. B. (1993). The lived experience of grieving the loss of an important other. *Nursing Science Quarterly, 6,* 130–139.

Polkinghorne, D. (1983). *Methodology for the human sciences: Systems of inquiry.* Albany: State University of New York Press.

Smith, M. C. (1990). Struggling through a difficult time for unemployed persons. *Nursing Science Quarterly, 3,* 18–28.

Chapter 13

The Lived Experience of Restriction-Freedom in Later Life

Gail J. Mitchell

Since Kuhn's (1970) cogent analysis of the nature of scientific development through competing paradigms, many scholars endorse the belief that all research flows from a value-laden ontology or paradigmatic perspective (Hesse, 1980; Laudan, 1984; Morgan, 1983; Parse, 1981; Polkinghorne, 1983). In nursing, this paradigmatic perspective has been likened to a lens through which the researcher is afforded a certain view of human beings and health (M. J. Smith, 1988). Smith stated, "The lens can be focused on the person to look at particulars—a zoom lens; to look at interrelationships—a wide-angle lens, or to look at process—a motion lens" (p. 94). The research here was guided by a motion lens furnished by Parse's theory of human becoming. The motion lens focuses on process in the human-health interrelationship, a process uniquely circumscribed by Parse's theory in the principles of human becoming. The specific phenomenon of interest in this research was the paradoxical experience of restriction-freedom.

159

PHENOMENON OF INTEREST

The paradoxical experience of restriction-freedom emerged in two prior phenomenological investigations conducted by this author. The first study explored the meaning of taking life day-by-day (Mitchell, 1990) and the second, the meaning of being a senior (Mitchell, 1993; 1994). One participant, in describing the experience of taking life day-by-day, said she saw herself fading while simultaneously seeing more for herself in the future. This participant described limitations related to loss of vision, and yet she saw opportunities for starting new relationships. Another person felt restricted because she could not perform as well as she did in the past, but she also described feeling uplifted and free to learn new ways to get the job done. The core concept that captured the experience, in the researcher's language, was *glimpsing a diminishing now amidst expanding possibles.*

A common element in 600 narratives written by older persons on the meaning of being a senior also reflected the experience of restriction-freedom (Mitchell, 1993, 1994). One commonality evinced from this study was: engaging the now while rolling with the vicissitudes of life. Older individuals wrote of "conceding decline in strength while asserting self in other ways" and of "using obstacles in life for constructive purposes rather than encumbrances." One participant said she did not have "enough money since retiring but she had freedom to use her time as wanted." The paradoxical patterns reflected rhythms of restriction-freedom as they were lived.

The restriction-freedom paradox is similar to one reported by Jonas (1992), who explored the meaning of being a senior with 45 elders living in Nepal. One theme reported in the study was "familiar patterns diminish amidst expanding moments of respite while regard from others affirms self." Jonas reported how elders described the opportunities and limitations encountered in daily life.

EXISTENTIAL AND PHILOSOPHICAL VIEWS OF RESTRICTION-FREEDOM

The restriction-freedom paradox is a basic tenet of existential thought (Frankl, 1959; Heidegger, 1962; May, 1981; Sartre, 1965, 1966). Existential features of the restriction-freedom paradox relate to three basic truisms. First, human beings are born as finite beings, meaning nonbeing always coexists as a possibility with being. Second, human beings are born with certain givens that provide a defined yet open ground for one's becoming in life. And third, all persons are born at a particular time and place in the historical evolution of the world. All three truisms mean that human beings live with certain unchangeable givens that may both enable and limit their journey through life. Heidegger (1962) referred to Dasein's "throwness" in the world. In being "thrown" one coexists with others as a finite being, and yet, one is pure potentiality-for-being and becoming according to one's own possibilities.

All human beings experience restriction-freedom in unique yet shared ways (Buber, 1965; May, 1981; Parse, 1981; Tillich, 1957). Indeed, freedom cannot exist without restriction, for each opposing force "breathes vitality into the other" (May, 1981, p. 66). The rhythm of the restriction-freedom pattern may vary throughout the life process, and in different cultures, but all persons experience situations that are restricting yet freeing. According to May (1981), "If there were no destiny to confront—no death, no illness, no fatigue, no limitations of any sort and no talents to pose against these limitations—we would never develop any freedom" (p. 95). Despite the universality of the restriction-freedom paradox, as an inherent aspect of human experience, there is no indication in the literature that the phenomenon has been studied as a unitary rhythm. Traditional views of aging have not adequately integrated human experiences of restriction-freedom.

TRADITIONAL VIEWS OF AGING
AND RESTRICTION

The majority of persons in later life live with multiple restrictions and chronic limitations (Butler, 1991; Cantor, 1991; Nadelson, 1990). Research conducted with persons in later life has primarily focused on identifying the restrictions associated with aging, disease, and functional disability (see for example Duffy & MacDonald, 1990; Estes & Binney, 1989; Wetle, 1991). Two areas of concern identified in the literature related to the prevailing objective-particularistic, problem-based approach have relevance for this research.

First, it is increasingly evident that research limited to the study of restrictions and problems has not illuminated ways older people experience health and quality in their lives in spite of limitations, hardships, and problems (Keller, Leventhal, & Larson, 1989; Miller, 1991; Nadelson, 1990; Robertson, 1991). Researchers are now asking questions about patterns. For example, Keller et al. (1989) ask, What changes do older people live with and how do they cope over time? Ainlay and Redfoot (1982–1983) advocate for "studies that encompass the person's whole being-in-the-world as it is experienced" (p. 13). Anecdotal and serendipitous accounts of health and quality of life indicate that older persons relate health to freedom (Berg & Gadow, 1978; Nadelson, 1990; Parse, Coyne, & Smith, 1985), doing what is wanted, humor, helping others (Bearon, 1989; Jackson, 1991), peace of mind, love, and self-affirmation (Parse et al., 1985; Staats & Stassen, 1987). These dimensions of health have not been explored in any depth from the perspectives of persons in later life.

Another consequence of the narrow focus on problems has been to distort the way health care professionals view older persons themselves. This is the second point of concern linked to traditional research that has relevance in this current study. Research findings indicate that health care professionals rate the health of older persons much lower than elders do themselves (Rakowski, Hickey, & Dengiz, 1987; Ward-Griffin & Bramwell, 1990; Wilson &

Netting, 1987). The focus on restrictions and problems perpetuates the negative attitudes and ageism so prevalent among health care workers (Hennessy, 1989; Luken, 1987; Nadelson, 1990). Negative ratings by experts influence decisions about treatment policies, as well as the expectations made of older persons to comply and conform with medical interventions (Becker & Kaufman, 1988; Rakowski et al., 1987; Wilson & Netting, 1987). The research reported here offers a different view of later life by describing the freedoms that coexist with restrictions as they are experienced by persons themselves.

NURSING PERSPECTIVE

All research flows from some theoretical perspective (Cull-Wilby & Pepin, 1987; DeGroot, 1988; Guba & Lincoln, 1989; Moccia, 1988; Parse, 1987). Thus, the nursing perspective is explicated so that others may follow conceptual linkages and lines of reasoning.

The nursing perspective from which this research emerged is Parse's (1981, 1987, 1992) theory of human becoming. From Parse's perspective human beings cocreate health in relationship with the environment in the unfolding process of living value priorities. Parse's theory has three principles which are explicated in chapter 1 of this book. The theory posits that human beings are unitary, in mutual process with the universe, and inherently free to structure the meaning of lived experiences and to move in unique ways toward possibles that are cocreated and lived with others. The first principle of Parse's theory guides nurses to recognize that each person's reality is a uniquely created experience involving the individual's chosen meanings, values, and imaginings. The second principle guides nurses to view human beings in their coconstituted patterns of being with the universe. The main concepts are revealing-concealing, enabling-limiting, and connecting-separating. The third principle contains the main concepts of powering, originating, and transforming. It reflects the belief that persons continuously reach beyond, to coconstitute and cocreate possibles in the multidimensional realities of life.

PURPOSES AND SIGNIFICANCE OF STUDY

The purposes of this research were intimately related to the significance. The first purpose was to generate the meaning structure of the restriction-freedom experience as described by older persons. A specific structure of the experience of restriction-freedom sheds light on how older persons cocreate health in harmony with limitations. Such knowledge is essential for nurses who intend to participate with others in their living of health and quality of life.

The second purpose was to explicate how the rhythmical pattern of restriction-freedom relates to health and quality of life. Findings show health as a changing process of the human-universe interrelationship, which is a view consistent with current theoretical conceptualizations (Hall & Allan, 1986; Moch, 1989; Newman, 1990; Parse, 1981, 1990a; Sarter, 1987). Traditional views of health have been expanded, but definitions are so broad and all-encompassing that they hold limited utility for meaningful interpretation of human experiences of health. Nontraditional views of health have been invented that do not require operationalization of multiple variables, but, rather, the explication of meaning and human experience (Moch, 1989; Parse, 1981; Sarter, 1987). Parse (1981) conceptualized health as an open process of becoming and a personal commitment (1990a). Health is a coconstituted interrelationship that reflects one's patterns of living value priorities and transcending with the possibles. From Parse's perspective, health cannot be defined, given, or managed by another. To understand health, nurses are guided to explore the ways in which individuals choose meaning and cocreate patterns of relating value priorities while moving toward hopes and dreams.

The third purpose of the research was to expand Parse's theory of nursing for guiding practice and further inquiry related to lived experiences. This research advances nursing science by expanding Parse's (1981, 1992) theory of human becoming. The theory of human becoming circumscribes the researcher's biases *that* human beings structure meaning, rhythmically relate, and transcend with the possibles. Research findings expand Parse's theory by specifying *what* meanings, patterns of relating, and ways of transcending are linked to the universal experience of restriction-freedom for persons in later life. The research question was: What is the structure of the restriction-freedom experience in later life?

METHODOLOGY

Researchers require methodological approaches that conceptualize process in order to adequately represent the human-health interrelationship. Additionally, a perspective rooted in a nursing theory is mandatory for contributing to the knowledge base of the discipline. The phenomenological method derived from Parse's (1981, 1987, 1992) theory of human becoming meets the above criteria for conducting theory-guided investigations of lived experiences.

Description of Participants

Twelve persons spoke in dialogical engagement with the researcher about their experience of restriction-freedom. Participants ranged in age from 75 to 92. Ten of the twelve seniors were over the age of 80. Three of the participants were men and three were African Americans. Three of the participants were residing in a rehabilitation hospital and were planning to return to their homes within a one-month period. Four participants resided in a high-rise apartment building specifically for seniors, and five participants lived in a public housing complex not specifically for older people. The dialogical engagements occurred in places of the participants' choosing and were tape-recorded and transcribed verbatim. The study was approved by an ethical review board, and all standard procedures were taken to protect participants' human rights. Specific information related to protection of rights covered the following points: freedom to withdraw without penalty, measures to ensure confidentiality, risks and benefits, and parameters of participation.

PRESENTATION OF FINDINGS

The central finding of this study was: **the lived experience of restriction-freedom is anticipating limitations with unencumbered self-direction while yielding to change fortifies resolve for moving beyond.** The structure contains three core concepts or central ideas shared by all 12 participants: anticipating limitations, unencumbered self-direction, and yielding to change fortifies resolve for moving beyond. The core concepts symbolize universal meanings stated in the language of science. Tables 13.1 through 13.4 show the extraction-syntheses and propositions that were completed for four of the participants. A careful reading of the essences and propositions will reveal that all the participants described the three universal concepts in similar yet unique ways.

Once the concepts were identified they were linked to Parse's theory through heuristic interpretation (see Table 13.5). Heuristic interpretation represents the researcher's understanding of the structure given the frame of reference specified by Parse's theory. Theoretical interpretation advances understanding for scholars who share a certain view of the human-universe-health process.

DISCUSSION OF FINDINGS

The concepts that were described by all participants (anticipating limitations, unencumbered self-direction, and yielding to change fortifies resolve for moving beyond) coexist all-at-once as lived experience. The first two concepts can be viewed as different rhythms of the same paradoxical rhythm. Participants' descriptions linked anticipating limitations with restriction while simultaneously linking unencumbered self-direction with freedom. It must be emphasized that both sides of the paradoxical rhythm coexist simultaneously with the third concept, yielding to change fortifies resolve for moving beyond. The structure can be explored in more depth to further specify the meaning linked

Table 13.1   Extraction-Synthesis for Participant 1

Extracted Essences (Participant's Language)

1. Used to doing her own thing, the participant now suffers with pain and is not able to do what she wants while fighting to keep going with ambition and the Lord's help.
2. Learning to live day-by-day and to let things go undone, the participant says she cannot do anything, yet she sees herself as getting along well and being active.
3. Not wanting to be confined or pinned down like a prisoner, the participant does her own thing and gets around with friends without being depressed.
4. Needing money and clothes, the participant does what she can to get by while feelings of happiness come from living and doing what is wanted.

Synthesized Essences (Researcher's Language)

1. Self-sufficiency wanes with intense discomfort while fortitude and faith emerge for moving beyond.
2. Engaging the now while yielding to change surfaces opposing views.
3. Considered limitations spur independence and uplifting connections with others.
4. Despite insufficient essentials, unencumbered self-direction gives rise to pleasure.

Proposition

The lived experience of restriction-freedom in later life is yielding to change in the now as self-sufficiency wanes with intense discomfort as uplifting connections and pleasure surface despite insufficient essentials, and unencumbered self-direction amidst opposing views and considered limitations fortify resolve for moving beyond with faith.

Table 13.2   Extraction-Synthesis for Participant 2

Extracted Essences (Participant's Language)

1. Missing former opportunities to do things and get around, the participant adjusts to restrictive rules and cultural differences while choosing social and family connections that give happiness.
2. Freed from loved responsibilities and community ties and being able to say things without dispute, the participant calmly expects inevitable restrictions.
3. Laughing with concern about her forgetful memory, the participant keeps busy doing what she wants, even with less strength, and feels free when playing the organ and sharing smiles and a laugh with others.

Synthesized Essences (Researcher's Language)

1. Absent liberties prompt resolve for yielding to change amidst joyous unions.
2. Release from cherished connections coexists with unchallenged expressions surfacing peaceful anticipation of limitations.
3. Humor tempers apprehensions for moving beyond and fortifies familiar activities with unencumbered self-direction surfacing pleasure.

Proposition

The lived experience of restriction-freedom in later life is yielding to change through joyful unions that fortify resolve for moving beyond while absent liberties and peaceful anticipation of limitations, amidst humor and unchallenged expressions, temper apprehensions as unencumbered self-direction and release from cherished connections surface pleasure.

Table 13.3   Extraction-Synthesis for Participant 6

Extracted Essences (Participant's Language)

1. Having the freedom to come and go and not restricting himself to anything that matters, the participant thanks the Lord for good health and appreciates living, even when it is difficult.
2. Doing what is good for him gives rise to pride as the participant limits desires to do what he is able to do well.
3. Recollections of many restrictions placed on black people surface feelings that, although some things are better, racism is degrading and breaks the spirit.
4. Believing freedom is for all people and that you have to look at the positive in life and not dwell on unfairness, the participant trusts God and looks for fairness while treating others as he wants to be treated.
5. Seeing oppressors and dictators restrict freedom, the participant tries to make the best of life by adjusting his living and doing the best he can on a limited income.

Synthesized Essences (Researcher's Language)

1. Unencumbered self-direction coexists with gratitude and resolve for moving on.
2. Harmonizing actions with areas of expertise shifts views enhancing self-regard.
3. Memories of imposed hardships highlight advancement despite deprivation.
4. Cherished ideals surface optimistic views amidst faith and justice when relating with others.
5. Aversion to domination guides decisions about anticipated limitations while yielding to change.

Proposition

The lived experience of restriction-freedom in later life is shifting views of self through unencumbered self-direction while memories of imposed hardship highlight cherished ideals and advancement despite deprivation, as aversion for domination surfaces optimism, faith, and justice amidst the anticipation of limitations, while yielding to change harmonizes actions and fortifies resolve for moving on.

Table 13.4   Extraction-Synthesis for Participant 7

Extracted Essences (Participant's Language)

1. Having the freedom to eat, sleep, clean, and have fun with friends, the participant feels a pickup when laughing and singing with others but is lonesome for long-gone children, animals, and loved ones.
2. Seeing freedom in everything and feeling blessed, the participant says her freedom is not having troubles and being in good health.
3. Restricted by death of loved ones and worries on her mind, the participant sometimes does not feel like moving yet she walks every morning and praises the Lord just to be living.
4. Not being able to get to church and wishing there was some place closer, the participant enjoys watching the train from her window and thinking about others.

Synthesized Essences (Researcher's Language)

1. Unencumbered self-direction and buoyant connections mingle with the pain of lost others.
2. Omnipotent liberties and thankfulness surface harmony with what is.
3. Despite constraining losses and concerns, resolve for moving on fortifies faith.
4. Anticipation of limitations prompts pleasurable yielding to change.

Proposition

The lived experience of restriction-freedom in later life is moving beyond loss and concerns by yielding to change while unencumbered self-direction and buoyant connections mingle with a thankfulness and faith that fortifies resolve for moving on amidst anticipated limitations and omnipotent liberties that foster harmony and pleasure despite constraints.

Table 13.5 Heuristic Interpretation of the Structure of Restriction-Freedom

---

Structure of the Lived Experience

The lived experience of restriction-freedom in later life is anticipating limitations amidst unencumbered self-direction as yielding to change fortifies resolve for moving beyond.

Core Concepts

Anticipating Limitations	Unencumbered Self-Direction	Yielding to Change Fortifies Resolve for Moving Beyond
Envisioning the Will-Be	Unrestrained Movement	Relinquishment Vivifies Advancement
Imaging	Originating	Enabling-Limiting

Propositions

Structural Integration
Restriction-freedom is envisioning the will-be with unrestrained movement while relinquishment vivifies advancement.

Conceptual Interpretation
Restriction-freedom is imaging the originating of enabling-limiting.

---

to restriction-freedom as a unitary experience and to clarify theoretical relationships.

The first core concept, **anticipating limitations,** was described by participants as a process of reflecting on restrictions in the now, as well as on how restrictions might be experienced in time to come. Persons expected that painful arthritis, poor vision, and hearing loss would continue to present restrictions. Falls were anticipated as possible happenings, as was the eventual relinquishment of caring for self and living independently, unless death came first. Some participants spoke about anticipated limitations in a matter-of-fact way. One participant stated, "Old age steals so much but you have to pay a price for your long life. . . . If I have to go to a nursing home, I will lose my freedom." Other participants voiced concern and uncertainty about anticipated possibilities. One woman said, "I've got no clothes or money and I don't know what I'm going to do, but I am not going to give up."

Anticipating limitations relates clearly to Parse's (1981) concept imaging. Persons construct reality through their reflective and pre-reflective imaging. The participants' reflective ponderings about anticipated limitations shed light on their experiences of reality as a whole. Parse (1981) suggests that imaging is an aspect of questioning as persons search for answers. This searching was affirmed by older persons as they pictured themselves in their present situations while contemplating possibles for what might be. Imaging relates to knowing and understanding, to a "process of assimilating new ideas. . . . as one structures meanings compatible with one's world view" (Parse, 1981, pp. 43–44). The older persons in this study who described possible limitations were already engaging the limitations and giving them meaning. For example, one person stated the following about going to a nursing home: "I would have thought about it long enough that I would be convinced that that was the thing to do." This woman's imaging was a way of structuring meaning and cocreating reality as Parse's first principle relates, "Structuring meaning multidimensionally is cocreating reality through the languaging of valuing and imaging" (1981, p. 42). In describing anticipated limitations all participants simultaneously spoke of unencumbered self-direction, the second core concept.

Unencumbered self-direction related to the various meanings assigned to freedom and choice. The concept was described in relation to daily routines and patterns of living. For example, persons said: "I have all the freedom I want here. I can go for a walk. . . . clean my house or sit and talk with friends"; "I can go whenever I have the opportunity. . . . I'm free to play the organ and to partake in social activities if I want." Meaning aspects of unencumbered self-direction were further explicated. Seniors spoke of the importance of not being pinned down, confined, or dictated to. Persons who lived alone liked not having to consult others about decisions and activities. Several participants spoke of choosing how to be with restrictions. For example, "I'm free to choose to let it worry me to death or I can choose to accept each day as it comes." A man spoke about having the freedom to restrict his own actions in order to do what he thought was best.

Unencumbered self-direction was linked most distinctly to Parse's concept of originating. Originating is a concept in Parse's third principle, "Cotranscending with the possibles is powering unique ways of originating in the process of transforming" (Parse, 1981, p. 55). Originating is a process of "unfolding while emerging in mutual energy interchange with the environment" and of "choosing a particular way of self-emergence through inventing unique ways of living" (Parse, 1981, p. 60). The creation of unique ways of living was also evident in the third core concept.

The third core concept to make up the structure of the experience of restriction-freedom was **yielding to change fortifies resolve for moving beyond.** This concept related to a complex rhythm of yielding or going along with change which fortified participants' resolve and energies for moving beyond. Change is a continuous process of unfolding, and living day-by-day is a way of moving beyond. Usually persons think of pushing and struggling to propel on. Participants in this study disclosed that at times, yielding is also a way to propel on. For some participants the yielding to change related to letting things go undone, especially things like housework and laundry. For others, there was a yielding to others' help because of diminished self-sufficiency. Older persons yielded to the loss of favorite activities and routines, like driving a car and gardening. The changing restrictions that were described by participants were accepted, embraced, and endured. Seniors spoke of deciding to accept, adjust, and go along. They said: "You just have to live day-by-day, and what you can't do you just have to learn to live with it"; "it's a matter of adjusting to change"; "one good thing about blind-ness is you can't see the dirt."

In yielding to change there emerged a fortified resolve for mov-ing beyond. Participants decided to laugh, to learn new ways, to count blessings, and to have a different attitude in order to keep go-ing. For example one person stated: "I'm not going to worry about the many things I can't do. Many times I'll get upset but I'm not go-ing to let it throw me. I'll just sit down and wait till I'm able to cope with it. You can choose to sit down and cry over spilt milk and go crazy, but you have to fight, fight back instead." Another said, "I count my blessings and try to forget my adversities . . . having a positive attitude toward things and go on smiling and pushing my giants away the best I can." Most participants also described the importance of faith and trust in the Lord for moving beyond through yielding to change.

The concept yielding to change fortifies resolve for moving be-yond, when linked with Parse's theory, relates clearly to the theo-retical concept enabling-limiting. Enabling-limiting comes from Parse's second principle, "Cocreating rhythmical patterns of re-lating is living the paradoxical unity of revealing-concealing and enabling-limiting while connecting-separating" (1981, p. 50). Enabling-limiting relates to the way persons are both enabled and limited in life situations as they "choose to be certain ways. . . . and move in one direction which limits movement in another way" (Parse, 1981, p. 53).

Participants' descriptions shed light on factors which both en-able and limit them in later life. Yielding to change was spoken of as a deliberate way of being. Persons said they learned how to live with change by adjusting and going along. In choosing to yield to change persons were both enabled and limited. The limitations were described as "not being able to do all that is wanted," "having to wait," "losing strength," and doing without cherished activities like going to church and visiting the grave site of a loved husband. Participants were also enabled through the choice to yield to change. The enabling aspects were linked to learning new ways, finding humor, experiencing enhanced faith and trust, finding peace of mind, and saving energy for important things. Parse suggests that with every choice persons discover some doors opening while others close. These closings and openings are not all known when choices are made, so there is also uncertainty with enabling-limiting as persons continuously unfold while becoming.

The restriction-freedom experience has been specified as *anticipating limitations with unencumbered self-direction while yielding to change fortifies resolve for moving beyond.* When linked to Parse's theory, restriction-freedom is *imaging the originating of enabling-limiting.*

LITERATURE RELATED TO RESTRICTION-FREEDOM

Findings from this study are linked to both theoretic- and research-based works. In order to explore related phenomena, the discussion begins with a selection of ideas from extant theoretical views about restriction-freedom.

Related Theoretical Views

Data from participants in this research uncovered shared meaning linked to the restriction-freedom experience. The shared meaning related to how the participants pondered anticipated restrictions and how they pictured themselves being with them. Older persons described the freedom to do what was wanted, the freedom to choose how to look at situations, and the freedom to limit their own freedoms. Also shared among participants was a choosing to go along, to flow with the changes encountered in later life while pushing on.

The ideas contained in the structure generated here have been linked to restriction-freedom by other authors. Tillich (1952) linked the ideas of anticipation, future, and freedom.

> In every encounter with reality the human being is already be-
> yond this encounter. A person knows about it, compares it, is tem-
> pered by other possibilities, anticipates the future as he/she
> remembers the past. This is freedom, and in this freedom the
> power of life exists. It is the source of vitality. (Tillich, 1952, p. 82)

Evident in these ideas linking possibility, anticipation, and choice
is the basic existential belief that persons are continuously moving beyond, becoming their choices, and transcending as their
life project or existence is created and shaped (Heidegger, 1962;
Merleau-Ponty, 1974; Sartre, 1965). The restriction-freedom phenomenon described here sheds light on how persons rooted in multiple restrictions simultaneously live freedom while transcending
toward what might be. According to May (1981), "New possibilities
beckon us in our dreams, in our aspirations, in our hopes and actions, and the possibility pushes us to acknowledge, encounter,
confront, engage, or rebel against our destiny" (p. 67).

May (1981) also related problems to possibilities in a way that
has relevance to findings presented here. He suggested that problems or restrictions are the manifestations of unused possibilities. This is consistent with Ross's (1981) view that "possibles
represent alternatives relative to a given situation" (p. 35). Thinking about the relationship between restriction and undefined possibility sheds light on its meaning in relation to participants'
descriptions recorded in this study. Restrictions did set the stage
for what alternatives might be possible. For example, one participant described failing eyesight and the related restriction of not
being able to shop. The anticipated possibles described by this
participant were specified in relation to the loss of vision. The
person might have to give up shopping by herself, or have to shop
with friends who have better vision, or she may consider finding a
grocer who delivers personal orders. Findings reported here support the belief that anticipated restrictions and fears, as well as
desires and values, contribute to originating or creating one's
unique possibilities. Findings also support the fluid-like quality
of human freedom. Participants in this research revealed many

different meanings related to freedom as lived experience. For some participants freedom was having the liberty to do what they wanted, when they wanted, and without encumbrance. Freedom was also described as choosing an attitude or perspective from which to view one's situation. Other persons spoke of freedom as something that could be lost or taken away. Freedom was described in relation to being able to pursue cherished activities like playing the organ, reading, and laughing with friends. Some people defined freedom as a specific phenomenon, for example, freedom is having respect for others. Freedom included actions that paradoxically limited other freedoms and opportunities, like freely choosing not to drive anymore. Feelings explicitly linked to freedom by participants included pleasure, peace, and wonder.

May (1981) suggests that "freedom involves the whole human being, not a part" (p. 9), and that "freedom comes from engaging destiny" (p. 47). Participants' descriptions of restriction-freedom consistently represented a unitary, whole perspective. Persons did not break themselves into parts when talking about restriction-freedom. Rather, the phenomenon was discussed as a complex set of patterns related to lived experience. Further, the restriction-freedom experience included past memories and future expectations, supporting Parse's view that lived experience incorporates what was, is, and will be, all-at-once. For example, one participant in particular spoke about a haunting restriction from childhood that related to loneliness. All other persons clearly embraced the not-yet in imaging potential restrictions-freedoms. Findings also support the belief that freedom is an illusive process that recreates itself in the presence of restriction. The lived experience of restriction-freedom does not resemble a continuum or polarity of opposing forces. Both sides of the paradox exist wholly at the same time. Participant descriptions repeatedly affirm the mutual coexistence of restriction-freedom.

An important aspect of the restriction-freedom experience was linked to yielding to change. Findings indicated that participants freely chose to yield to changing restrictions and in yielding there surfaced strength for moving on. Yielding to change, and to obstacles in one's path, is an important notion in the ancient Chinese philosophy contained in Lao Tzu's (1992) *Tao Te Ching*. Tao, defined as the whole of reality itself, exists in part because of its yielding nature. According to this philosophy living things are soft and flexible, while hard and unyielding things are companions of death (Tzu, 1992). Yielding is also linked to power (Tzu, 1992). In this study yielding was connected to vitality and strength.

These ideas about vitality and yielding are also related to Tillich's (1952) work in *The Courage to Be*. For Tillich, the courage to be is the willingness to affirm one's essential being in light of danger and the power of nonbeing. Knowing what to risk, what to avoid, and what to embrace requires courage. The courage to be is fueled by a creative vitality that springs from human freedom, according to Tillich (1952). The lived experience of restriction-freedom reflects this courage to be. Participants described situations of daring, avoidance, and yielding in order to propel their moving beyond.

Related Research

The researcher indicated previously that the restriction-freedom phenomenon was identified in three other qualitative investigations about meaning in later life (Jonas, 1992; Mitchell, 1990, 1993, 1994). This current research project was intended to build on prior findings by specifying the structure of the lived experience of restriction-freedom. Other studies about lived experience and aging identified similarities and differences with findings from this study.

Parse et al. (1985) reported findings about the aging experience as described by participants living in various settings. The researchers described a surrendering to the system, undeniably a loss of freedom, that was identified by informants in nursing homes. Older persons did not mention freedom in describing their experiences. A review of excerpts from data linked to domains of researcher inquiry did reveal many actual and anticipated limitations that were sometimes similar to those expressed by participants in this study. Elderly individuals in both studies described fears of going blind, concern about not being able to care for themselves, and the dread of having to depend on others. Some participants in the Parse et al. (1985) study linked limitations to loneliness and isolation.

A conspicuous difference between findings from the Parse et al. (1985) study and findings reported here relates to the preponderance in the former work of descriptions by nursing home residents about meaningless time, waiting for death, and pretending to be elsewhere. These phenomena were not mentioned by older persons in the current study. Some participants did, however, expect to end up in a nursing home, where it was anticipated that freedom would be taken away or lost. The phenomenon of surrendering to the system noted by Parse et al. (1985) was quite different from the yielding to change described by participants in the current research. Most notable was that the surrender coexisted with rage, while yielding coexisted with resolve and strength for moving beyond. More study is needed to explore the experience of restriction-freedom for residents of nursing homes.

Other qualitative explorations about the meaning of aging offer support for findings presented here. Thompson (1992) studied the subjective experience of aging with older Britons and reported that later life was a time of active challenge that required exceptional abilities to imaginatively and creatively respond to change. This image of strength, creativity, and change is consistent with findings from this research. Thompson also reported that older persons spoke of freedom and enjoyment. Quotes offered by Thompson about freedom were almost identical to those of participants in this study. For example, "I like it that I can do as I please, go when I want to, and if I can afford it, buy what I want to and eat what I want" (p. 37). Differing with findings reported here was Thompson's claim that freedom was dependent on adequate income, a functioning mind, and the absence of pain. As pointed out in this current study, those phenomena may bear upon restriction, but freedom still coexists and gives definition to the limitations and restrictions.

Additional researchers have also identified freedom to be an important aspect of aging and later life in other cultures. Ikels et al. (1992) reported on a cross-cultural analysis of perceptions about the adult life course from participants representing seven sites and four countries—the United States, China, Ireland, and Botswana. Respondents from Botswana viewed aging as a negative experience. The Chinese indicated old age to be a time of release from responsibilities and worries—the old were thought of as finished or done with the struggle of life. The old in China were also considered to have poor intergenerational and societal relations, physical decline, and material insecurities. Participants in the United States and Ireland identified freedom as the best part of old age. One woman spoke of the soaring freedom in later life. This is consistent with research by Keller et al. (1989) who reported 50 percent of their sample of older persons (n = 32) identified having more freedom in old age.

The relevance of the restriction-freedom experience for nursing is its relationship with health and quality of life. The second purpose of this research was to explore the relationships among restriction-freedom, health, and quality of life. Findings are now discussed in relation to these phenomena.

RESTRICTION-FREEDOM, HEALTH, AND QUALITY OF LIFE

There is mounting interest in health promotion and the development of theoretical views that conceptualize health as a co-created process, as opposed to a well-functioning organism or an idealized state. In nursing, Parse (1981, 1987, 1990a, 1992) has pioneered the belief that health is a process of living value priorities. She regards the human being as a creative co-author and the source of health. Parse suggests that health is a personal commitment that is "lived in rhythmical patterns of relating that incarnate the meaning that the human being gives to situations"

(Parse, 1990a, p. 137). The quality of one's life is a personal appraisal centered in the whole unitary person who is in mutual interrelationship with others and the universe (Parse, 1990a).

The structure of restriction-freedom in this study represents a process generated from descriptions of lived experiences and the researcher's theoretical perspective. The structure was identified as *anticipating limitations with unencumbered self-direction while yielding to change fortifies resolve for moving beyond*. The researcher will revisit the qualitative research on the lived experience of health to uncover similarities with the structure of restriction-freedom.

The phenomenological investigation of health conducted by Parse (Parse et al., 1985) with 400 persons aged 7 to 93 uncovered three themes of health, harmony, energy, and plenitude. These themes surfaced for all participants, although the meaning and patterns of relating varied among different age groups. For the 100 participants over the age of 66 three common elements were identified: harmony - synchronous contemplation; energy - transcendent vitality; and, plenitude - generating completeness. A review of descriptive expressions from the Parse study revealed that transcendent vitality was related to being able to do what was wanted, and synchronous contemplation was linked to freedom from worries, freedom to make decisions, and freedom to make one's own way. These expressions of health were evident in findings here when participants spoke about freedom to be with friends, to come and go, to rise and to retire, to weep, and to celebrate.

Dittmann-Kohli (1990) and Thorne, Griffin, and Aldersberg (1986) in their qualitative studies of health reported that older persons gave detailed descriptions of ailments and limitations, and yet they simultaneously described health and quality in their lives. Thorne et al. (1986) indicated that health in later life was linked to meaningful relations, independence, growth, and attitudes from within. Dittmann-Kohli (1990) noted that older people do anticipate illness, threat, and loss of autonomy, and yet they still have positive feelings about their lives and themselves. He concluded that "adversity is rendered less oppressive by its integration into a different framework . . . that allows for subjective well-being in old age" (Dittmann-Kohli, 1990, p. 291). Both of these studies support the belief that the meaning of health and quality of life is a personal creation and value.

Wondolowski and Davis (1991) explored the lived experience of health for the oldest-old. Three common elements formed the definition of health which was "an abiding vitality emanating through movements of rhapsodic reverie in generating fulfillment" (p. 115). The common element of interest in relation to findings about restriction-freedom is "abiding vitality." Wondolowski and Davis reported participant descriptions indicating that the oldest-old experienced an "invigorating strength that was present as a force" (p. 115). These ideas about strength, vitality, and force are closely related to descriptions from this study about unencumbered self-direction and how yielding to change fortifies resolve for moving beyond.

Parse (1990a) suggests that health is a flowing process of human becoming. It is a synthesis of values and the way a person is, in interconnection with the world. If health is a synthesis of values, then findings presented here about restriction-freedom suggest that older persons anticipate connecting with and separating from cherished values while freely choosing to live familiar patterns amidst shifting priorities that propel change. In light of restriction-freedom, health is the flowing movement of shifting values.

Parse further defines health as "a personal commitment that is lived through abiding with the struggles and joys of everydayness in a way that incarnates one's quality of life" (1990a, p. 138). The way of being with a situation is through meaning. In other words, assigning meaning to lived experiences is a personal way of abiding with the situation. Meaning is chosen from reflective and pre-reflective realms, but when made explicit, according to Parse (1990a), it surfaces one's personal commitment. Once aware of a commitment, persons can go on living with that meaning or they can choose to change the meaning, which changes health. Parse

(1990a) offers three ways of moving toward changing health, which she uncovered with her research on health, hope, and laughter. The three ways are creative imagining, affirming self, and the spontaneous glimpsing of the paradoxical. These ways of changing a commitment can be discussed in relation to the lived experience of restriction-freedom.

Anticipating limitations was a core concept of the restriction-freedom experience. The concept included ways participants imaged themselves being with limitations. Parse (1990a) describes creative imagining as "the picturing of what a situation might be like if lived in a particular way" (p. 138). Parse says in this structuring scenario change is already made, since living possibles in the imagination projects the potential meaning, allowing the person to try it out. Findings from the current study indicated that participants moved with anticipatory projecting in relation to possible restrictions. The participants imaged themselves not being able to get around as wanted, they pondered what it was going to be like to give up apartment living, and they also pictured themselves fighting, laughing, and struggling to get through and move on. Parse proposes that through this process of creative imagining, persons learn about themselves and their worlds while choosing from and cotranscending with the possibles. Anticipatory projecting is symbolic of motion and change, in that persons ponder and choose what will happen prior to actually living it.

Affirming self is another way of changing health (Parse, 1990a). Participants in the current study spoke in affirming ways about how they were going to be with situations. For example participants said, "I can hold my own with this," "I am not going to give in," and "I'm more determined to keep up and going." These phrases reveal persons' valued preferences and patterns of persistence in the midst of struggle and restriction-freedom. Parse (1990a) proposes that affirming self is also related to beliefs and to the way one views situations. For example, participants in this current research spoke about choosing positive attitudes rather than negative ones. In choosing to "look at the bright side" or to "not cry over spilt milk" participants confirmed their patterns of preference for living health. These patterns affirmed the "who" persons chose to be.

Spontaneous glimpsing of the paradoxical is a third way to move and change the living of health (Parse, 1990a). This phenomenon surfaces when individuals suddenly see the incongruence in a personal situation which may lead to laughter, new insights, and different views. It was not possible to recognize this phenomenon in recorded dialogues of the present study. Glimpsing the paradoxical may have been related to one participant's account of laughing at the seriousness of memory loss, but it is not possible to know without further exploration with the person.

The lived experience of restriction-freedom when linked to the concepts of Parse's theory was *imaging the enabling-limiting of originating*. Findings presented here expand these concepts, enhancing understanding about lived experience and extending the knowledge base of a process-oriented science.

EXPANDING PARSE'S THEORY OF HUMAN BECOMING

Parse (1981, 1987, 1992) wrote her process-oriented concepts at a very high level of abstraction, which is appropriate for a theory about the human-universe-health process. The theoretical proposition that relates to the lived experience of restriction-freedom has been defined as *imaging the originating of enabling-limiting*. Each of these concepts is considered in light of extant research guided by Parse's theory in order to explore the depth of knowledge development.

Imaging is the process through which persons construct reality, search for answers, and come to understand the world through the integration of new ideas (Parse, 1981). Findings from the current study specify the meaning of reality for 12 older persons experiencing restriction-freedom. Findings shed light on what phenomena older persons search for in their imaging and on how anticipated restrictions-freedoms are integrated into worldviews.

Parse (1990b) and Santopinto (1989) have also extended knowledge about imaging in relation to other lived experiences. Imaging was a concept in the theoretical structure of the lived experience of hope (Parse, 1990b). Parse described how all participants spoke about their experience of hope in relation to possibles, such as living without the machine, picturing themselves in other ways. Santopinto (1989) identified imaging to be a central concept related to the relentless drive to be ever thinner. He explored this phenomenon with women who described the agonies and ecstasies of relentlessly striving for thinness. The way the participants imaged themselves changed their patterns of relating with others. Santopinto reported that the women "pursued cherished images at any cost" (1989, p. 34).

Originating was the second theoretical concept to be linked to the restriction-freedom experience. Originating represents the unencumbered self-direction of the restriction-freedom experience. Parse (1981) described originating as a unique unfolding and a particular way of self-emergence. Participants described their unique ways of originating in the restriction-freedom experience. Originating was linked to the freedom of self-direction. The meaning of this freedom included release, action, silence, laughter, respect, singing, playing, and choosing how to be with others and situations. Thinking about all the ways of originating revealed in this study pushes understanding of freedom to new realms. No other published research has identified originating as a central theoretical concept, although it has been discussed in all studies guided by Parse's theory.

The final theoretical concept linked to restriction-freedom identified in the current study was enabling-limiting. Enabling-limiting relates to the opportunities and limitations inherent in making choices (Parse, 1981). Findings from this study add to the knowledge base about enabling-limiting in relation to the restriction-freedom experience. For participants in this study, enabling-limiting connected yielding to change and the opportunities and limitations that surfaced as a consequence of that yielding. Participants created new opportunities for themselves in order to be free and to create harmony with restrictions.

Parse (1990b) and M. C. Smith (1990) discussed enabling-limiting in theoretical structures of lived experience. Parse's (1990b) study of hope uncovered descriptions about the inherent limitations of situations that surfaced choices to create harmony and to focus on opportunity. M. C. Smith (1990) explored the lived experience of struggling through a difficult time for unemployed persons. Participants in her study described "feelings of being expanded by assets and restricted by obstacles all at once" (M. C. Smith, 1990, p. 24). In dialogue with the researcher about the struggles of unemployment, participants said they appreciated so many things, such as material possessions, unexpected opportunities, and loving relationships. A feeling of good fortune coexisted with an awareness of restriction related to the engulfment of inadequate finances and prejudicial treatment (M. C. Smith, 1990).

RECOMMENDATIONS AND REFLECTIONS

Murphy and Longino (1992) suggest that qualitative research is critical to the advancement of knowledge about aging. Further, these authors recommend that "research on aging should become value-based and not value-free" (Murphy & Longino, 1992, p. 147). Recognizing science as value-based science means fully acknowledging the critical role of theory for all interpretation, including that of objective findings.

The appeal to make science explicitly value-based is consistent with the works of nurse theorists who for several decades have been promoting the development of nursing theory-based practice and research. The research reported here is an example of value-based research. The values of Parse's (1981) theory, embedded in the assumptions of her theory, underpin this research. Parse's process-oriented theory generated the motion picture perspective presented in this research project. The motion lens records the story of restriction-freedom as told by the older persons participating in this study. Parse's theory is one horizon of nursing knowledge, and additional definition, light, form, detail, and color emerge from each study guided by the principles of human becoming.

Recommendations

This qualitative research successfully generated a structure of the lived experience of restriction-freedom as described by 12 persons in later life. The study of the same phenomenon with different persons might lead to different concepts and relationships that further extend knowledge and enhance understanding. There is no attempt to generalize findings or to make inferences for how older people should experience restriction-freedom. What the research shows offers a motion picture depicting a slice of life. The restriction-freedom structure is woven back into Parse's theory so that new relationships about the process of human becoming, which is health, might be illuminated.

The restriction-freedom experience should be explored with other groups of persons, especially with elders who are living in different settings, like nursing homes or other long-term care settings. It was suggested in the discussion of findings that older persons in different cultures also experience restriction-freedom. More inquiry is needed in this area in order to uncover the range of differences and similarities for different groups of persons.

The phenomenon of restriction-freedom could also be investigated with persons who are restricted in their movements, such as persons who are confined to wheelchairs or beds. It would be illuminating to explore the phenomenon with prisoners or other persons whose freedoms are limited in some known ways. Older persons have reported a sense of newfound freedom after the release from responsibilities related to work and family. The phenomenon of being released could be further explored as a related lived experience.

The core concepts also spark ideas of interest for additional research. In order to identify a phenomenon of study from within Parse's framework, the lived experience must be universal, and it needs to be stated in such a way that all persons can speak about the phenomenon in relation to their own lives. The concept anticipating limitations might be studied as the lived experience of thinking about something threatening or frightening, or the lived experience of being concerned about the future. Anticipating limitations was linked to Parse's concept imaging, which could be used to launch a study seeking depth of meaning in unconventional ways. For instance, older persons could be invited to draw a picture about what the future holds and to discuss the meaning with the researcher.

Unencumbered self-direction could be further explored through inquiry into the lived experience of freedom, or of being able to do what is wanted. Unencumbered self-direction also relates to being able to follow through with personal plans or making plans to move toward something important. The third core concept of the restriction-freedom structure, yielding to change fortifies resolve for moving beyond, is more complex and poses many lived experiences to consider for further study. For instance, what is the lived experience of putting up with something unpleasant in order to accomplish something more important.

Reflections

Smith and Hudepohl (1988) suggest that nursing's evolution as a discipline depends on the development of its unique theories and their use in practice and research. This statement is based on the belief that a discipline needs a body of knowledge, and the building of this knowledge is the business of science. As stated by Kockelmans (1985), "Each science receives its ground and research domain by the projection of the ontological structure of the beings which it examines" (p. 130). Parse's theory has provided the ontological structure for this research, and findings advance the knowledge base of nursing science.

Parse's theory of human becoming is unique in nursing for two reasons. First, it is the only theory having well-developed practice and research methodologies that is underpinned by the human science tradition. Second, it is the only theory that provides process-oriented concepts and principles for guiding interpretation of lived experiences as uncovered during research and practice activities. Parse's focus on process is germane for viewing and interpreting human phenomena with a motion lens, and it is precisely the motion lens that will generate knowledge about health as process, a goal of the discipline that has yet to be realized.

Parse's process-oriented theory provides a framework for interpreting the "living" knowledge that so concerned Wilhelm Dilthey (1833–1911) a hundred years ago. Dilthey was concerned that the natural sciences would strip life of all meaning, and he called for a human science founded on living knowledge. The subject matter of the human sciences, according to Dilthey (1976), is the "interrelation of life, expression, and understanding" (p. 175). It is proposed that the motion lens framed by Parse's theory of human becoming launches a new science of life, expression, and understanding about the human-health interrelationship that could dramatically change the discipline of nursing.

Science-as-process, rather than product, is rooted in the belief that there are multiple realities and multiple truths about human experience and health. All bodies of knowledge are considered creative interpretations (Kockelmans, 1985). Nursing science contributes to the world of knowledge by enhancing understanding through meaningful interpretation of the human-health interrelationship. Nurses require a knowledge base that explicates the full range of human experience so that new ways of theory-guided practice can be invented and evaluated from the perspectives of those receiving services.

Nurses endorsing the traditional empirical paradigm and its related causal approaches argue that understanding does not translate into doable interventions. This is true. A scientific base that enhances understanding will only change horizons, broaden perspectives, and expand respect for human diversity. These changes do not relate to what nurses do to people but to how nurses think about human beings and their unfolding health. Understanding changes patterns of relating, and it is precisely patterns of relating in the nurse-person process that influence quality of life.

This researcher believes that the view of knowledge and truth as process is a mystery to be celebrated and passionately respected. Whether knowledge evolves through scientific revolutions (Kuhn, 1970) or piecemeal integrations (Laudan, 1984) is immaterial to the overwhelming recognition that there is no objective reality or ultimate truth from which to compare or judge a person's or family's experience of health. Theories circumscribe different truths that compel belief, or not, depending on the values of members of a discipline.

The quest for knowledge through the creative interpretation of universal experiences will continue to reveal the depth of meaning as well as the unlimited potential for human beings to create and reach beyond in the spirit of discovery. As suggested by DeGroot (1988), "Creative interpretation and theory contain truth and beauty and contribute to the quality of human existence" (p. 5). This statement is worthy of serious consideration in promoting efforts to advance all value-based science and the creative interpretation of the human-universe-health interrelationship.

REFERENCES

Ainlay, S. C., & Redfoot, D. L. (1982–1983). Aging and identity-in-the-world: A phenomenological analysis. *International Journal of Aging and Human Development, 15*(1), 1–16.

Bearon, L. B. (1989). No great expectations: The underpinnings of life satisfaction for older women. *The Gerontologist, 29*(6), 772–778.

Becker, G., & Kaufman, S. (1988). Old age, rehabilitation, and research: A review of the issues. *The Gerontologist, 28*(4), 459–468.

Berg, G., & Gadow, S. (1978). Toward more human meanings of aging: Ideals and images from philosophy and art. In S. F. Spicker,

K. M. Woodward, & D. D. Van Tassell (Eds.), *Aging and the elderly* (pp. 83–91). Atlantic Highlands, NJ: Humanities Press.

Buber, M. (1965). *The knowledge of man* (M. Friedman & R. G. Smith, Eds. & Trans.). London: George Allen & Unwin.

Butler, M. (1991). Geriatric rehabilitation nursing. *Rehabilitation Nursing, 16*(6), 318–321.

Cantor, M. H. (1991). Family and community: Changing roles in an aging society. *The Gerontologist, 31*(3), 337–346.

Cull-Wilby, B. L., & Pepin, J. L. (1987). Towards a coexistence of paradigms in nursing knowledge development. *Journal of Advanced Nursing, 12*, 515–521.

DeGroot, H. A. (1988). Scientific inquiry in nursing: A model for a new age. *Advances in Nursing Science, 10*(3), 1–21.

Dilthey, W. (1976). *Selected writings*. (H. P. Rickman, Ed. & Trans.). Cambridge: Cambridge University Press.

Dittmann-Kohli, F. (1990). The construction of meaning in old age: Possibilities and constraints. *Ageing & Society, 10*(3), 279–294.

Duffy, M. E., & MacDonald, E. (1990). Determinants of functional health of older persons. *The Gerontologist, 30*(4), 503–509.

Estes, C. L., & Binney, E. A. (1989). The biomedicalization of aging: Dangers and dilemmas. *The Gerontologist, 29*(5), 587–596.

Frankl, V. (1959). *Man's search for meaning: An introduction to logotherapy* (I. Lasch, Trans.). Boston: Beacon.

Guba, E., & Lincoln, Y. (1989). *Fourth generation research*. Newbury Park, CA: Sage.

Hall, B. A., & Allan, J. D. (1986). Sharpening nursing's focus by focusing on health. *Nursing & Health Care, 7*(6), 315–320.

Heidegger, M. (1962). *Being and time* (J. Macquarrie & E. Robinson, Trans.). New York: Harper & Row.

192   The Human Becoming Theory in Research

Hennessy, C. H. (1989). Autonomy and risk: The role of client wishes in community-based long-term care. *The Gerontologist, 29*(5), 633–639.

Hesse, M. (1980). *Revolutions and reconstructions in the philosophy of science.* Bloomington, IN: University Press.

Ikels, C., Keith, J., Dickerson-Putman, J., Draper, P., Fry, C., Glascock, A., & Harpending, H. (1992). Perceptions of the adult life course: A cross-cultural analysis. *Ageing and Society, 12*(1), 49–84.

Jackson, L. T. (1991). Leisure activities and quality of life. *Activities, Adaptation, and Aging, 15*(4), 31–36.

Jonas, C. M. (1992). The lived experience of being an elder in Nepal. *Nursing Science Quarterly, 5,* 171–176.

Keller, M. L., Leventhal, E. A., & Larson, B. (1989). Aging: The lived experience. *International Journal of Aging and Human Development, 29*(1), 67–82.

Kockelmans, J. J. (1985). *Heidegger and science.* Washington, DC: Center for Advanced Research in Phenomenology & University Press of America.

Kuhn, J. S. (1970). *The structure of scientific revolutions* (2nd ed.). Chicago: University of Chicago Press.

Laudan, L. (1984). *Science and values.* Berkeley: University of California Press.

Luken, P. C. (1987). Social identity in later life: A situational approach to understanding old age stigma. *International Journal of Aging and Human Development, 25*(3), 177–193.

May, R. (1981). *Freedom and destiny.* New York: Bantam Doubleday Dell.

Merleau-Ponty, M. (1974). *Phenomenology of perception* (C. Smith, Trans.). New York: Humanities Press.

Miller, M. P. (1991). Factors promoting wellness in the aged person: An ethnographic study. *Advances in Nursing Science, 13*(4), 38–51.

Mitchell, G. J. (1990). The lived experience of taking life day-by-day in later life: Research guided by Parse's emergent method. *Nursing Science Quarterly, 3,* 29–36.

Mitchell, G. J. (1993). Time and a waning moon: Seniors describe meaning to later life. *The Canadian Journal of Nursing Research, 25*(1), 51–66.

Mitchell, G. J. (1994). The meaning of being a senior: A phenomenological study. *Nursing Science Quarterly, 7,* 70–79.

Moccia, P. (1988). A critique of compromise: Beyond the methods debate. *Advances in Nursing Science, 10*(4), 1–9.

Moch, S. D. (1989). Health with illness: Conceptual evolution and practice possibilities. *Advances in Nursing Science, 11*(4), 23–31.

Morgan, G. (Ed.). (1983). *Beyond method: Strategies for social research.* Beverly Hills: Sage.

Murphy, J. W., & Longino Jr., C. F. (1992). What is the justification for a qualitative approach to ageing studies? *Ageing and Society, 12*(2), 143–156.

Nadelson, T. (1990). On purpose, successful aging, and the myth of innocence. *Journal of Geriatric Psychiatry, 23*(1), 3–22.

Newman, M. A. (1990). Newman's theory of health as praxis. *Nursing Science Quarterly, 3,* 37–41.

Parse, R. R. (1981). *Man-living-health: A theory of nursing.* New York: Wiley.

Parse, R. R. (1987). *Nursing science: Major paradigms, theories, and critiques.* Philadelphia: Saunders.

Parse, R. R. (1990a). Health: A personal commitment. *Nursing Science Quarterly, 3,* 136–140.

Parse, R. R. (1990b). Parse's research methodology with an illustration of the lived experience of hope. *Nursing Science Quarterly, 3,* 9–17.

Parse, R. R. (1992). Human becoming: Parse's theory of nursing. *Nursing Science Quarterly, 5,* 35–42.

Parse, R. R., Coyne, A. B., & Smith, M. J. (1985). *Nursing research: Qualitative methods.* Bowie, MD: Brady.

Polkinghorne, D. E. (1983). *Methodology for the human sciences.* Albany: State University of New York Press.

Rakowski, W., Hickey, T., & Dengiz, A. N. (1987). Congruence of health and treatment perceptions among older patients and providers of primary care. *International Journal of Aging and Human Development, 25*(1), 63–77.

Robertson, J. F. (1991). Promoting health among the institutionalized elderly. *Journal of Gerontological Nursing, 17*(6), 15–19.

Ross, S. D. (1981). *Philosophical mysteries.* Albany: State University of New York.

Santopinto, M. D. A. (1989). The relentless drive to be ever thinner: A study using the phenomenological method. *Nursing Science Quarterly, 2,* 29–36.

Sarter, B. (1987). Evolutionary idealism: A philosophical foundation for holistic nursing theory. *Advances in Nursing Science, 9*(2), 1–9.

Sartre, J-P. (1965). *Essays in existentialism* (W. Baskin, Ed.). New York: Carol Publishing Group.

Sartre, J-P. (1966). *Being and nothingness* (H. E. Barnes, Trans.). New York: Washington Square Press.

Smith, M. C. (1990). Struggling through a difficult time for unemployed persons. *Nursing Science Quarterly, 3,* 18–28.

Smith, M. C., & Hudepohl, J. H. (1988). Analysis and evaluation of Parse's theory of man-living-health. *The Canadian Journal of Nursing Research, 20*(4), 43–58.

Smith, M. J. (1988). Perspectives of wholeness: The lens makes a difference. *Nursing Science Quarterly, 1,* 94–95.

Staats, S. R., & Stassen, M. A. (1987). Age and present and future perceived quality of life. *International Journal of Aging and Human Development, 25*(3), 167–176.

Thompson, P. (1992). "I don't feel old": Subjective ageing and the search for meaning in later life. *Ageing and Society, 12*(1), 23–47.

Thorne, S., Griffin, C., & Aldersberg, M. (1986). How's your health? *Gerontion, 1*(5), 15–18.

Tillich, P. (1952). *The courage to be.* New Haven: Yale University Press.

Tillich, P. (1957). *Systematic theology* (Vol. 2). Chicago: University of Chicago Press.

Tzu, L. (1992). *Tao te ching* (T. H. Miles, Trans.). Garden City Park, NY: Avery.

Ward-Griffin, C., & Bramwell, L. (1990). The consequence of elderly client and nurse perceptions of clients' self-care agency. *Journal of Advanced Nursing, 15,* 1070–1077.

Wetle, T. (1991). Successful aging: New hope for optimizing mental and physical well-being. *Journal of Geriatric Psychiatry, 24*(1), 3–12.

Wilson, C. C., & Netting, F. E. (1987). Comparison of self and health professionals' ratings of the health of community-based elderly. *International Journal of Aging and Human Development, 25*(1), 11–25.

Wondolowski, C., & Davis, D. K. (1991). The lived experience of health in the oldest-old: A phenomenological study. *Nursing Science Quarterly, 4,* 113–118.

Chapter 14

The Lived Experience of Grieving, for Families Living With AIDS

William K. Cody

*T*he purpose of this study, guided by Parse's (1981, 1992) human becoming theory, was to investigate the meaning of grieving for families living with AIDS. Living with AIDS commonly entails many losses, including strength, mobility, financial security, social support, patterns of living, plans and hopes for the future (Dreuilhe, 1988; Monette, 1990; Nokes & Carver, 1991; Weitz, 1991) which link the experience with grieving. Although associated with bereavement and death, grieving is believed to occur with any event *experienced* as loss (Cowles & Rodgers, 1991; Marris, 1974). Yet it has been studied primarily as a psychobehavioral response to predefined object loss (commonly widowhood) with predefined norms (Parkes, 1987; Sanders, 1989). In this study, an understanding of grieving was sought through dialogue with families who were living it.

The family constellation for persons living with AIDS often comprises lovers and significant others not related by birth or marriage (Walker, 1991), while the mainstream view in family theory remains based on the model of the nuclear family (Burr, Hill, Reiss, & Nye, 1979; McCubbin & Figley, 1983). From Parse's perspective, the family is a flowing configuration of interrelationships cocreated through experiential processes of human-to-human relating. With regard to both the phenomenon of grieving and the study of families, this investigation, guided by Parse's theory, offers the opportunity for insights that the conventional views do not encompass.

The specific aims of this study were (a) to enhance understanding of grieving as it is lived in families living with AIDS, (b) to contribute to the expansion and specification of the human becoming theory, and (c) to extend the use of Parse's (1987a) research methodology with families. The research question for the study was: *What is the structure of grieving for families living with AIDS?*

PARSE'S THEORY IN RELATION TO FAMILIES AND GRIEVING

The first assumption of Parse's (1981, 1992) theory is *"The human is coexisting while coconstituting rhythmical patterns with the universe"* (1992, p. 38). Thus, a basic premise of this study is that all humans are involved with others in their universe in the cocreation of reality. Parse says the human "is not alone in any dimension of becoming" (1981, p. 20). Yet the human is also posited as freely choosing personal meaning, which affirms the uniqueness of the individual. The human coexists with others, coconstitutes reality through intersubjective relating with others, and differentiates self as a unique being through relating personal value priorities (Parse, 1981, 1992).

Parse (1981) has defined family as "the others with whom one is closely connected" (p. 81). The first principle, *structuring meaning multidimensionally,* means that family interrelationships cocreate values that are lived as persons coconstituting the family language their perspectives of life situations (Parse, 1981, p. 81). The second principle, *cocreating rhythmical patterns of relating,* means that family patterns of interrelating generate opportunities and limitations as persons coconstituting the family reveal and conceal aspects of self in rhythmic involvement-noninvolvement with family and others (pp. 81–82). The third principle, *cotranscending with the possibles,* means that family interrelating energizes transforming with each family life situation through choosing unique ways of living from among the many possibilities available in the ever-changing health process (p. 82). The perspective of the family within Parse's theory, then, may be described as "synergistic family becoming" (p. 129).

In the original publication of her theory, Parse wrote:

> [The human] is touched by birthings and dyings, which are the rhythmical happenings in day-to-day living. These happenings are created as [the human] chooses the meanings of a situation and, through this choosing, the possibilities that [one] can become. Choosing meaning points to the birthings and dyings inherent in each decision. This means that, in choosing one thing, [one] gives up another and in this way is both enabled and limited. . . . Possibilities . . . are relational in that [the human] and environment coparticipate in their emergence.
>
> (Parse, 1981, p. 27)

Persons participate in cocreating loss through their involvement with the cherished. For the person experiencing loss, that which is cherished and lost is paradoxically absent yet present. Parse's theory is unique in its capacity to describe these complex, multi-dimensional and paradoxical aspects of lived experiences such as grieving.

Two previous studies of grieving guided by Parse's theory have been published (Cody, 1991; Pilkington, 1993). Participants in both studies spoke of involvements with the absent presence and with close others, sharing the meaning of the grieving and feeling grateful for others who were there for them. These patterns of relating were described as helping participants to move beyond the pain of the loss and to gain a new perspective of their life situations. Grieving was seen as abiding with the cherished in new ways as life rhythmically unfolds patterns of being with and apart from the absent presence and others. The present study expands this perspective of grieving.

SIGNIFICANCE

The significance of this study lies in four areas: (a) The study expands and specifies Parse's theory of human becoming by generating a structure of grieving for families living with AIDS. (b) This study answers a need for research illuminating family life experiences from a nursing perspective, specifically the human becoming perspective. Although the discipline of nursing historically has strived to address family health, family-centered research guided by theory specific to nursing science has been minimal (Gilliss, 1989). (c) The researcher also sought to make a methodological contribution in this study. Discussions of grieving with families were recorded using video, and this report illuminates these variations in the processes of method. (d) The findings of this study may enhance nursing practice with persons and families who are grieving.

REVIEW OF RELEVANT LITERATURE

Literature relevant to this study is presented below in two sections—first, an overview of selected literature on the conventional and emerging views of grieving, including the interface with the literature on change and transition, followed by selections from the growing literature on living with AIDS.

Grieving

Major scientific theories related to grieving (Bowlby, 1969, 1973, 1980; Engel, 1961; Freud, 1917/1957; Kübler-Ross, 1969; Lindemann, 1944; Parkes, 1987) have been developed with reference primarily to bereavement, death, and dying. A well-known feature of these theories is the postulate of normative, roughly sequential "stages" or "phases" in the grieving process. In recent years it has been increasingly emphasized that these stages or phases may vary widely in intensity, duration, and sequence. The normative stance of the conventional theories remains steadfast, however, since the view of health itself is one in which parameters of normality are assumed. Passage through the stages of grieving is seen as the transit to healthy acceptance, resolution, or dying. This view is rooted in the assumptions of objectivism and linearity and the values of homeostasis, prediction, and control. Grieving is judged as either adaptive or maladaptive, with the latter construed either as pathology or as leading to pathology (Bowlby, 1980; Parkes, 1987; Sanders, 1989; Schneider, 1984; Schoenberg, Carr, Peretz, & Kutscher, 1970). In overviews of research related to grieving, Parkes (1987) and Sanders (1989) each examined hundreds of studies, yet the firm conclusions that they drew were extremely few. Both authors found there was no clear separation between "normal" and "abnormal" grief "reactions," although the attempt to delineate such a distinction has been a major thrust of the existing research. The *human experience of grieving* remains poorly understood.

The research on grieving in families has focused primarily on the death of a child, parent, or spouse within the nuclear family (Davies, Spinetta, Martinson, & Kulenkamp, 1986; Knapp, 1986; Kuhn, 1977; Pincus, 1974; Reilly, 1978; Weber & Fournier, 1985). Such studies are characterized by the combination of a normative, prescriptive model of grieving with a normative, prescriptive model of the family. The lack of attention to the family in research on grieving and the combination of highly normative grief and family theories are additional reasons the phenomenon remains poorly understood.

The majority of the nursing literature related to grieving focuses on bereavement following a death and closely mirrors the voluminous non-nursing scientific literature. Demi and Miles (1986) reviewed studies of bereavement published from 1970 to 1984. Most looked at variables affecting bereavement outcomes, such as age, gender, mode of death, and social support. Demi and Miles endorsed the use of "a multivariate conceptual model of bereavement" (p. 119), as did Shirley A. Murphy (1983) in a review of grief theories (all non-nursing). Nursing authors have applied grief theories in many situations, such as spinal cord injury (Werner-Beland, 1980), chronic illness (Miller, 1983), divorce (Lambert & Lambert, 1977), and others, including AIDS (Flaskerud, 1987). Most of these works summarily adapt one of the major grief theories to the situation specified.

Loss, grieving, change, and transition have been increasingly interconnected in the literature. Marris (1974) saw the "grief response" as an aspect of any major change, whether the change was wanted or unwanted, and as "characteristically ambivalent" (pp. 4–5). He held that the process of grieving turned on the reformulation of the meaning of the loss. Schneider (1984) noted the potential for loss and grieving in *all* life's changes, including growth and achievement. An overly rigid stage model would be inadequate, since "losses continue to occur throughout life and not usually at times when people have managed to resolve all the others" (p. 75). Bridges (1980) described transition as "the natural process of disorientation and reorientation that marks the turning points on the path of growth" (p. 5). The two "great transitions" of life, he said, are the development of a separate self and "movement . . . to a deeper sense of interrelatedness" (p. 32). Transition is the process of *ending, dwelling in-between,* and *beginning anew.* The in-between time is a time of self-renewal which leads to inner awareness, motivation, hopes and dreams. Watzlawick, Weakland, and Fisch (1974) developed a systemic theory of change. "First-order change" occurs within the existing system. "Second-order change" is change in the system itself, reframing the situation and thus the nature of first-order change within it. Second-order change "operates on the level of *meta* reality, where . . . change can take place even if the objective circumstances of a situation are quite beyond human control" (p. 97).

Change and transition have also been posited as central concerns of nursing (Shirley A. Murphy, 1990). Chick and Meleis (1986) describe transitions as to some extent self-limiting, characterized by beginnings, middles, and endings. They emphasize "preserving continuity of meaning, either by reestablishing disrupted connections or by substituting new ones" (p. 250). DeFeo (1990) proposes that change evolves along two dimensions, the "horizontal," associated with continuity and stability, and the "vertical," associated with potentiality and transformation (p. 89). He likens these two dimensions of change to the two paradigms in nursing, totality and simultaneity (Parse, 1987b). The totality paradigm is concerned with stability and equilibrium, the simultaneity paradigm with evolutionary process and becoming. This study contributes to the knowledge base within nursing's simultaneity paradigm on grieving as a way of becoming.

Several qualitative nursing studies relevant to the present study have been published. Smith (1990), in a study of "struggling through a difficult time for unemployed persons," uncovered the core concept of "grieving the loss of what was cherished" (p. 22). She noted, "As participants engaged in the struggle, new meaning was given to the [many, varied] losses . . . [which] contextualized the pain of grieving so that although present, it was experienced differently" (p. 25). Carter (1989) analyzed 30 narrative accounts of bereavement. Themes included *being stopped, hurting, missing, holding* and *seeking.* "Metathemes" were identified as *change, expectations* (which referred to a sense of "a right way to grieve," (Carter, 1989, p. 357), and *inexpressibility.* Sowell, Bramlett, Gueldner, Gritzmacher, and Martin (1991) studied "losing a lover to AIDS" and placed themes into the categories of *isolation/disconnectedness, emotional confusion,* and *acceptance/denial.* Carmack (1992) investigated the process of coping with "AIDS-related losses" through interviews with various associates of persons with AIDS. The basic process identified was *"balancing engagement and detachment"* within the context of a "redefinition of values" (p. 11).

Cowles and Rodgers (1991), in a concept-development paper on grief, found the concept "plagued by vagueness and ambiguity" (p. 119). Based on their analysis of 74 articles in medicine and nursing, they defined grief as "a dynamic, pervasive, highly individualized process with a strong normative component," the "human response" to generic loss, rather than death alone (p. 121). They reported a consensus that "there are limits to grief, beyond which it becomes inappropriate, unacceptable, or revealing of underlying or associated pathology," leading to the characterization of grieving as "normative." They concluded that "the recognition of grief . . . is best directed toward the determination of an antecedent loss and the individual's self-reports of 'grief' " (p. 124).

Living With AIDS

The issues surrounding the HIV pandemic and AIDS are enormously complicated. HIV disease itself is a terminal illness, but "AIDS" goes beyond that. Innumerable influences have gone into what Weitz (1991) calls the "social construction" of AIDS, a complex interweaving of sex, drug use, death, secrecy, and bigotry. Major issues for persons living with AIDS have been identified as facing their own death, fear, stigma, loss of strength, loss of financial security, loss of attractiveness, loss of interpersonal contacts, loneliness, and bureaucratic incompetence and misinformation (Altman, 1987; Schecter, 1990; Shilts, 1987; Weitz, 1991). But the most revelatory descriptions of living with AIDS are firsthand reports, such as Emmanuel Dreuilhe's (1988), in which he wrote:

> I mustn't panic and go to pieces, but instead believe profoundly in my own values, which are traditional to me even though they don't correspond to those of the majority. . . . Oliver's death and endless agony . . . loosened all the ties that still bound me to the world of healthy people. Most of them would never have been able to understand what we went through. Oliver, his mother, and I . . . companions in misfortune on this nightmarish journey. (pp. 37–40)

Paul Monette (1990) authored an account of his life with his lover, Roger, who had the virus. In a sense, they were both living with AIDS. Monette wrote: "Whatever happened to Roger happened to me, and my numb strength was a crutch for all his frailty. It didn't feel like strength to me, or it was strength without qualities, pure raw force. . . . In a way, I am only saying that I loved him . . ." (p. 65). Roger lived a year and a half after his diagnosis. Monette described the way of life they created, as one loss after another ensued: ". . . mornings in the garden while I read him the paper, evenings reading Plato, the smell of anise when we walked at night. These brief, immediate goals of the day-to-day we had come to cherish, no matter how constricted our movements" (p. 307). Life became very centered on priorities. Monette said, "Loss teaches you very fast what cannot go without saying" (p. 227).

Rudd and Taylor (1992) edited a collection of writings by women living with HIV. They noted that although great pain and loss are reflected in the writings, "the pieces in this anthology are overwhelmingly affirmative" (p. 17), as in the following:

> I am so alone and at the same time have the feeling that I am never really capable of being alone. . . . I cannot come to a standstill in my inner development. . . . Every single day is filled with so many experiences that bit by bit I am forced to live a richer and deeper life. (pp. 83–86)

Qualitative research related to living with AIDS reveals similar themes. Allan (1990) studied self-care practices of HIV-positive men and identified *"focusing on living, not dying"* as the central theme (p. 56). The practices included staying busy, living each day to the fullest, finding a reason to live, and establishing priorities for living. Hall (1990) studied "the struggle to maintain hope" for HIV-positive men. She reported that although the men experienced "periods of shock, anger, and giving up hope . . . [with one exception] they all regained a measure of hope" (p. 181); some initiated new projects or rekindled relationships. Hall (1990) wrote, "Even people in the late stages of HIV disease do not want to use up the rest of their lives . . . coping with illness and preparing for death. Like everyone else, they want to live for as long as possible and not be set aside from the living" (pp. 182–183). O'Brien (1992) summarized the qualitative data from a larger study on living with HIV, noting "the importance of relationships with significant others . . . needing them to know; being pressed for time . . . uncertainty of prognosis; modification of long-term goals or stopping to smell the roses; and turning to religious faith for solace and support" (p. 205).

Klein and Fletcher (1986) studied gay men in a grief recovery group, who, they reported, often spoke of the difficulties of being the only "real" family of the deceased yet not acknowledged as such by others, including health-care professionals. Brown and Powell-Cope (1991) investigated "the experience of AIDS family caregiving," generating the theme of "uncertainty." Uncertainty about loss and dying related to being told things like, "He might die tonight, he might die in six months" (Powell-Cope, 1991, p. 342). Uncertainty about relationships centered on whether or not to continue as caregiver with the tremendous day-to-day difficulties and awareness of impending death, although most did continue. Nokes and Carver (1991) investigated "the meaning of living with AIDS." Participants described "multiple losses including friendships, family, employment, and hope for a long life," and reconsidering drug use, sexual practices and personal relationships. They spoke about their children and significant others, "hope for reconciliation" from estranged family members, and wishing for spiritual strength (Nokes & Carver, 1991, pp. 177–178). These themes were interpreted in light of Parse's theory and will be addressed later in this chapter. Beauchamp (1990), also guided by Parse's theory, investigated "the lived experience of struggling with making a decision in a critical life situation" for persons with HIV, which he described as

> . . . affirming self through confronting uncertainty in moving toward the not-yet, while risking disclosing self with important others, as vacillating between options unfolds through envisioning what might be in light of what was and is. (p. 73)

Although the present study's focus is *grieving*, it also illuminates experiences of persons and families living with AIDS.

PARSE'S RESEARCH METHOD WITH FAMILIES

The method used in this study was Parse's (1987a, 1990) research method. It is the first such study conducted entirely with families as participants. The processes of the method are (a) participant selection, (b) dialogical engagement, (c) extraction-synthesis, and (d) heuristic interpretation (Parse, 1987a).

Participant Selection

Families living with AIDS were invited to participate in the study through service agencies and advertising in newspapers. The selection criteria for participants were self-identification as "living with AIDS" by one or more persons per family, the ability to speak English, and willingness to participate in a discussion of their grieving and to have the discussion videotaped. Informed consent of participants in this study was considered evidence of a familial relationship. It was made clear that the discussion was to focus on whatever *their own* actual experiences with grieving were. The setting for the discussion, chosen by participants, was either the participant's home, the researcher's home, or a private office in a service agency. When redundancy became evident in the descriptions, recruitment ceased. The ten participating families included: three gay male couples; a husband and wife; a woman and man living together and her daughter; two pairs of companions; two sisters (twins); a gay man and his mother; and a woman, her lover, and her brother.

Dialogical Engagement

Dialogical engagement is "an intersubjective 'being with' . . . in which the researcher is truly present to the participant in discussion as the remembered, the now, and the not-yet unfold all at once" (Parse, 1987a, p. 176). In this family-centered study, the dialogical engagements involved at least two persons other than the researcher. Each discussion began as the researcher asked participants simply to tell about their experiences of grieving. The researcher centered throughout the conversation on the descriptions offered. All questions flowed from the description and were open-ended. The discussions concluded when participants indicated they had described completely their experiences of grieving. The discussions were videotaped, as suggested by Parse (1990, 1994b).

Extraction-Synthesis

The researcher dwelled with each description while immersed in the dialogue, listening to and viewing the tapes and reading the transcripts. "Dwelling with" means centering on the meaning of the lived experience through contemplative "dialoguing" with the descriptions (Parse, 1987a, pp. 176–177). Through this process, the researcher extracted essences of the lived experience. Meaning is revealed not only through speech but also through facial expression, touch, movement, and silence. The use of video therefore enhanced the researcher's immersion in the dialogue. There were no essential differences between extraction-synthesis as described by Parse (1987a, 1990) and the procedures in this study. The multiplicity of perspectives expressed in each family dialogue, however, complicated the process. A *narrative* was extracted from each dialogue to precede the extracted essences in the research report. The narrative, written in the language of the participants, discloses the richness and vigor of the dialogue and enhances the readability of the extracted essences (written at the same level of discourse). The researcher moved the description to the language of nursing science through synthesizing essences and formulating a proposition for each family. From *all* of the propositions, core concepts of grieving were extracted and synthesized into a structure.

Heuristic Interpretation

The findings were connected explicitly to the theory of human becoming and expressed in the language of the theory. "*Structural integration* is connecting the proposition and the structure of the theory" (Parse, 1987a, p. 177). "*Conceptual interpretation*" is specifying the structure of the lived experience within the

human becoming theory, "leading to a specific theoretical structure from the principles" (p. 177).

Ethical Considerations

This study was approved for protection of human subjects through
the usual process. Participation was based on voluntary contacts
by persons self-identified as living with AIDS. All participants
were informed of their right to end participation at any time and
were assured of confidentiality; all signed a consent form detailing
the measures taken to protect their rights. All transcriptions utilized pseudonyms. Although participants had the researcher's
telephone number and an invitation to call at any time should they
have concerns about the study, no calls were received and there
were no withdrawals.

PRESENTATION OF FINDINGS

Extracted narratives (edited for length) for four families are
presented below. Each is followed by the extracted essences, the
synthesized essences, and the proposition for that family (Tables
14.1–14.4). The propositions for the remaining six families follow. (See Table 14.5 on page 219.)

Family 1: Rob and Jeff

Rob, age 23, was told his HIV test was positive three years ago.
His lover, Jeff, also age 23, has had negative HIV tests. They live
with Jeff's mother.

Extracted Narrative.   Rob and Jeff see living with HIV as the loss
of everything all-at-once, including their hopes and dreams.
Though there are things they still can do, it's hard "to be confined
to a certain way of life" at a young age. They lost many friends,
which hurts Rob especially. He is faced with giving up a way of
life and particular involvements, like smoking, that may shorten

his life. When Rob's dying became real for Jeff he "cried for hours and couldn't stop." The faith that he had worked for has been taken away, and life is hell-like, a "constant battle to get some faith" in something. Still they say they are lucky, since they are together, and Rob has yet to experience the worst of AIDS. What's most important is staying together, and they are looking forward to a ceremony of holy union. For Jeff how he feels about Rob is more important than what others think. They hope to "prove people wrong" about them and to have something affirming to show for being together. . . . Jeff wants Rob to "live in a bubble" to safeguard his health; it would be okay since he would be in there with him. For Rob the boredom and inactivity would be hell. Jeff relentlessly looks for new sources of support, but they find that few people understand their relationship or share their beliefs. . . . It's hard not knowing about tomorrow. For Rob, there is "so much to do, so little time," he isn't sure what he's going to do next . . . while Jeff feels they have to do everything now. They wanted to go to Europe, but they're not sure they can afford it now or how Rob would do with the touring, since he tires easily. He sees himself with Jeff many years from now "sitting on the back porch watching the grass grow," though he knows he may not live to experience it. When friends die with AIDS, it scares the hell out of him, and when they survive a bout with illness, it gives him hope. (See Table 14.1 on page 211.)

Family 2: Alice, Joe, and Hannah

Alice, age 43, received a diagnosis of AIDS after experiencing a yearlong complicated illness. Alice lives with Joe, about the same age, her daughter, Hannah, 13, and a son, 8, who did not participate in the discussion; she also has an adult son and a grandchild.

Extracted Narrative.   During her illness, Alice felt life leaving her; she had lost her self; she felt empty, unable to share, and hopeless. She was ready to die and "death was warm and fuzzy." Joe felt

Table 14.1   Rob and Jeff

Extracted Essences *(Participants' Language)*	**Synthesized Essences** *(Researcher's Language)*
1. Facing overwhelming loss and his possible death prompts for Rob a hurtful striving to hold on to small comforts and for Jeff a hell-like battle to regain faith, while they feel fortunate for what they still have.	1. Anguished struggling toward a constricting-expanding not-yet surfaces gratitude for what is and what is not.
2. Being together and living each day fully are important, and Rob and Jeff hope to reaffirm their relationship, contradicting others' disapproval. Jeff busily seeks safety and support, while Rob isn't sure he wants to give up enjoyment for a longer life.	2. Shared and unshared priorities fortify commitment and clarify personal perspectives while distancing-relating surfaces aloneness with togetherness.
3. With tomorrow unknown, deciding what to do is hard for Rob, while Jeff wants to do everything now. Rob's fatigue, possible death and other losses render their plans unsure, while awareness of what could happen sparks fear and hope.	3. Possibilities envisioned with ambiguity pulse with ease-unease.

Proposition

For Rob and Jeff grieving is
anguished struggling toward a constricting-expanding not-yet
with gratitude for what is and what is not,
while clarifying personal priorities fortifies commitment
and distancing-relating surfaces aloneness with togetherness,
as possibilities envisioned with ambiguity
pulse with ease-unease.

anger and helplessness that nothing could relieve her suffering. . . . Hannah didn't want to leave her for fear she would die.
Alice was angry when she got better; it was like "being played with
by God." Now she misses the way the family used to be, but with
hope renewed she is grateful for every moment she can share
with her family; it is not always pleasant, but comfortable and
good. Joe appreciates day-to-day things and special happenings
more but worries whether he'll be there to guide his kids. Hannah
is calmer now and thinks about her feelings more. . . . She's not
sure of anything, knowing that anybody could get sick and die, but
says, "I'm mostly afraid for my mom." . . . Alice felt like a burden
and not a mother to her children, but with no energy there was
nothing she could do. Joe would never have walked away; "in a situation like that you need help." . . . But this is something she has to
do all alone. The others are not in the same mode, don't feel as
strongly as she does. . . . [Events] bring her to sudden tears and
anger, and they just back off. Joe doesn't deal much with pain. Alice
says he feels nothing while she feels everything. . . . Hannah tries
to do everything right so her mom will be happy, but she for-
gets. . . . She only thinks about it a few minutes at a time unless
she has to. They tease and joke even in talk of conflicts and dying.
In the short time they have on earth, it's best to laugh; it doesn't
hurt as much if you do. . . . Alice was going to see her grandchild
by autumn no matter what; now she has to say, "If there's any way
possible." She doesn't put her dreams into then, but lives them now.
Joe says they "just take small bites of the future and nibble on
them." AIDS took away freedom of expression and action and they
are all cautious now, but that changes the focus from dying of AIDS
to living with HIV. Alice cries at times because she can't be what
she hopes to be. But with attention to what's most important there
is "more freedom and unburdening" than she's ever experienced.
Since Alice found out she had AIDS, she's thought a lot about her
[deceased] Mama. . . . She wants to know that Hannah has that
same feeling when she's gone, and strives to make memories that
will last a long time. (See Table 14.2 on page 213.)

Table 14.2   Alice, Joe, and Hannah

Extracted Essences *(Participants' Language)*		**Synthesized Essences** *(Researcher's Language)*
1.	Alice felt life leaving her empty and she welcomed death, while Joe felt helpless and got angry, and Hannah lived in fear. Alice misses the way things were but is grateful to share today with Joe, who worries about their future, and with Hannah as she explores her feelings.	1. Struggling together through harrowing personal agony confirms endearment.
2.	Alice feels everything deeply while Joe and Hannah sometimes back off and keep quiet. Joe is committed to stay, and Hannah tries to make Alice happy as they tease and laugh so it doesn't hurt as much.	2. Bearing witness uncovers aloneness with togetherness in pulses of divulging-hiding and ease-unease.
3.	Alice has to live her dreams now and plan on an if-possible basis. In living with HIV they lost some freedom but shifted the focus from dying of AIDS. Alice cries over unrealizable hopes, yet attention to what's important brings freedom and unburdening as she strives to make lasting memories with Hannah.	3. Opportunities and limitations emerging with ambiguity evolve new perspectives.

Proposition

For Alice, Joe, and Hannah, grieving is
struggling together through harrowing personal agony
confirming endearment,
as bearing witness uncovers aloneness with togetherness
in pulses of divulging-hiding and ease-unease,
while opportunities and limitations emerging with ambiguity
evolve new perspectives.

Family 3: Beryl and Cheryl

Beryl and Cheryl are twins who appear to be about age 30. Beryl found out three years ago that her HIV test was positive. Beryl lives in a multigenerational household with her grandmother and several children. Cheryl lives nearby with her husband and child.

Extracted Narrative.   Beryl has lost hope, her best friend, and respect for herself. She is afraid. She doesn't want to die and worries about leaving her children. She tries not to think about it, but it still comes back to her. Cheryl is losing her only sister; it hit her hard. . . . She doesn't know what she is going to do without Beryl, just that she will be lonely. Beryl wrote a living will and gave it to her family. It took her a month to get the nerve to do it. . . . Now her grandmother will care for her kids when she's gone. Making the will gave her a scary feeling it was time to die. But life is too precious to think about dying. She's going to keep enjoying herself and taking care of her family. When it's time for Beryl to die, Cheryl sees herself there, holding her hand and praying for her. . . . For Beryl, her family doesn't talk about her HIV or dying. . . . Cheryl says sometimes they tell one another how they feel and cry together. . . . She tearfully tells Beryl she loves her and hates that she may die soon. Beryl didn't know Cheryl felt that way . . . and she really appreciates it. Beryl's family used to ask her how she was doing, and now they don't. When she grieves she goes to her room, shuts the door, and cries to herself. It hurts that they don't cry with her, but she's sure someday they'll tell her how they feel. Beryl felt better when her mother shed just a few tears because it let her know her mother had feelings about her, but Cheryl worries how their mother will be when she really starts the grieving. Cheryl doesn't want her sister to leave her, but knows there's "nothing anybody can do." She is glad that Beryl is okay now and likes the times when she is happy. Cheryl wants Beryl to fight if she can and to enjoy life while she's here, because they don't know how much time they have. She sees how Beryl suffers. . . . Even though they're twins, she can't feel her pain;

Table 14.3   Beryl and Cheryl

Extracted Essences *(Participants' Language)*	Synthesized Essences *(Researcher's Language)*
1. Beryl lives with loss, fear, and worry but feels better knowing she won't suffer and her kids will be cared for; life and family are too precious to think about dying now. Cheryl, losing a beloved sister, sees herself comforting Beryl when she dies but sees only loneliness when she is gone.	1. Anticipating possibilities while abiding with imminent death fortifies intentions emerging with mutual concern.
2. Beryl says they don't talk about dying, while Cheryl says they share feelings and cry. Cheryl tells Beryl she loves her and doesn't want her to die. Beryl knows her family cares and will wait for them to show it more, while Cheryl worries about how that will be.	2. The comfort-discomfort of divulging-hiding surfaces aloneness with togetherness.
3. Cheryl, not knowing how much time is left, enjoys being together and is glad when Beryl is happy but also sees her suffer. She can't take on Beryl's pain, but she'll always be there for her.	3. Bearing witness confirms endearment in the face of unwelcome change.

Proposition

For Beryl and Cheryl, grieving is
anticipating the possibles,
while abiding with imminent death fortifies intentions
and the comfort-discomfort of divulging-hiding
surfaces aloneness with togetherness,
as bearing witness confirms endearment.

she wishes she could take some of the pain for her, but she can't. She will be right there for her when she gets sick. . . . (See Table 14.3 on page 215.)

Family 4: Carl and Eric

Carl and Eric, who are now lovers, have each experienced the AIDS-related death of a prior lover and both have tested positive for HIV. They appear to be in their late 20s and are active in the HIV/AIDS support community.

Extracted Narrative.   For Carl, not being able to control the disease and not knowing what would happen were extremely disruptive. He had wanted his previous lover, Wayne, to die, "prayed for it," for Wayne's sake, but also to get on with his life. When Wayne died, Carl had dinner as if nothing had happened. Much later, the grief was suddenly passionate. Seeking help, he got therapy and told his parents everything for the first time. When Eric's previous lover, Brian, was diagnosed, he didn't know who to tell or what to do. They fumbled their way through. His worst fear was for Brian, not fear of death, but whether he could stay strong and what others' reactions would be. The fear turned into numbness; having emotions would have been admitting it was all true. After Brian died, he tried to keep busy, sought medical services and started finding out what he needed to do for himself. . . . While Wayne was dying, Carl isolated himself from any reminder, felt empty, and wondered if he was capable of living alone. Wayne was dead for Carl long before he actually died. . . . Eric thought Brian was coming home until the end; then he wondered whether he could make it alone. . . . Recently, Carl and Eric cared for a dying friend. Eric says they supported each other through it, while Carl says grieving is a private thing "you do in your head" and nothing from outside makes it easier. Carl withdraws, and Eric gives him his space, while Eric needs other people and is good at being there. . . . After Wayne died, Carl had picked up where he left off, almost reliving it. He's sorry it had to be horrible

Table 14.4 Carl and Eric

Extracted Essences *(Participants' Language)*	**Synthesized Essences** *(Researcher's Language)*
1. Carl prayed for Wayne's death and refused to grieve, while Eric didn't want to admit Brian was dying and stayed numb. Both were afraid of the unknown and limited their thoughts till it was over, when they sought what they needed.	1. Struggling with divulging-hiding in the midst of ambiguity surfaces personal priorities.
2. Carl isolated himself from Wayne's dying, believing he was already dead, while Eric thought Brian was coming home until the end, and each wondered if he could make it on his own. When they grieve Carl needs his space and says it's private, while Eric needs people and says they support each other.	2. Bearing witness to suffering prompts aloneness with togetherness.
3. Carl is sorry that dying was horrible for Wayne but feels he did his best in an impossible situation and became more compassionate, while Eric remembers good times with friends when Brian was dying and now feels deaths are easier to accept. They both became stronger by living through it.	3. The ease-unease of opportunities and limitations engenders self-affirmation.

Proposition
For Carl and Eric, grieving is
bearing witness to suffering,
which prompts aloneness with togetherness
as struggling with divulging-hiding in the midst of ambiguity
surfaces personal priorities,
while the ease-unease of opportunities and limitations
engenders self-affirmation.

for Wayne. . . . [but] now he sees it as doing his best in an impossible situation. He's glad it happened as it did because he's more compassionate and stronger. For Eric, Brian's dying seems quick now, but at the time seemed like forever. . . . It was a good time in his life in ways, with people coming by to visit. His grieving made him stronger and made others' deaths easier to accept. Carl says having support makes his own potential loss of self easier to bear. If he should lose Eric, having been through it before, he knows not to stuff or run or deny himself anything. (See Table 14.4 on page 217.)

Extracted Concepts and Structure

Four core concepts were extracted from all of the propositions. These concepts are as follows:

1. Easing-intensifying with the flux of change
2. Bearing witness to aloneness with togetherness
3. Possibilities emerging with ambiguity
4. Confirming realms of endearment

For the ten participant families in this study, the structure of grieving is:

easing-intensifying with the flux of change
through bearing witness to aloneness with togetherness
as possibilities emerge with ambiguity
confirming realms of endearment.

Heuristic Interpretation

Easing-intensifying with the flux of change is *pushing-resisting with diverse rhythms,* which is interpreted as *powering,* from Parse's (1981) third principle. Bearing witness to aloneness with togetherness is living the paradox of *communion-solitude,* which

Table 14.5   Propositions for Six Other Families

For Bonita, Faye, and Eddie

grieving is
evolving cherished involvements
through anticipating an absent
    presence
differently
as bearing witness to suffering
surfaces aloneness with
    togetherness
while limitations and opportunities
clarify priorities and fortify
    intentions
easing-intensifying mutual
    concerns.

For Max and Terry

grieving is
bearing witness to anguish through
dwelling with and apart from
    absent presences
confirming endearment
while mutual burdening-
    unburdening
intensifies and eases change
as personal visions of the not-yet
evolve with variant tempos
surfacing aloneness with
    togetherness.

For Leo and Phil

grieving is
confronting mortality
with fortified intentions
as bearing witness to loss
while anticipating personal
    possibilities
surfaces new perspectives
and comfort-discomfort
mobilizes distancing-relating
in light of what is cherished.

For Frankie and Jane

grieving is
surfacing new views
through expressing anguished
    struggling and
dwelling with and apart from
    absent presences
in pulses of ease-unease
as anticipating possibilities
in the midst of ambiguity
and bearing witness to suffering
confirm cherished involvements.

For Michael and Betty

grieving is
being with and apart from others
while abiding in faith
easing-intensifying
anguished struggling with
    mortality
as bearing witness surfaces new
    perspectives
and anticipating the not-yet with
    ambiguity
gives rise to cherishing the now
confirming mutual concern.

For George and Richard

grieving is
mobilizing intentions
through the harmony-discord
of personal anguish
while dwelling with and apart from
absent presences
surfaces aloneness with
    togetherness
as abiding with imminent death
clarifies priorities in light of what
    is cherished.

is interpreted as *connecting-separating,* from the second principle. Possibilities emerging with ambiguity manifest human-universe *evolving with certainty-uncertainty,* which is interpreted as *originating,* from the third principle. Confirming realms of endearment is *honoring the treasured,* which is interpreted as *valuing,* from the first principle. Thus, the structure of grieving when integrated with the theory is *pushing-resisting with diverse rhythms of communion-solitude evolving with certainty-uncertainty through honoring the treasured.* The theoretical structure is *powering the connecting-separating in originating valuing.* This progression is shown in Table 14.6.

Table 14.6   Heuristic Interpretation

For the ten participant families living with AIDS, the structure of grieving is:

(Structure)	(Structural Integration)	(Conceptual Interpretation)
easing-intensifying with the flux of change	pushing-resisting with diverse rhythms	powering
through bearing witness to aloneness with togetherness	of communion-solitude	the connecting-separating
as possibilities emerge with ambiguity	evolving with certainty-uncertainty	in originating
confirming realms of endearment.	through honoring the treasured.	valuing.

DISCUSSION OF STRUCTURE

The structure as written above answers the research question and is thus the major finding of the study. The structure interrelates four concepts.

Easing-Intensifying With the Flux of Change

The first concept, *easing-intensifying with the flux of change,* is the rhythmic interplay of struggle, conflict, suffering and anger, with harmony and comfort. This concept encompasses fortifying intentions in the face of opposition and imminent death, personal and shared struggles to be with loss in new ways, and moving toward comfort through self-affirmation. For example, in Family 7, Bonita, a young mother, said, "It gets me down every now and then, but I go on. . . . Today I'm willing to live." In Family 9, Michael, a young gay man, said he struggled with self-blame, tensions at work and within the family, until he learned to "start loving Michael" and things started to turn around. He said, "When you're going through it, you don't realize where it's coming from, this strength. And then you make it through, and you go, well, if I can make it through that, I can make it through anything."

Easing-intensifying with the flux of change is a rhythmical, multidimensional process unbounded by calendar time and geographic space through which families engage with the push and pull of unwelcome change. Grieving has often been described as a confusing panoply of emotions. Many attempts have been made at explaining these emotions as little more than physiological responses to unpleasant stimuli that are "normally" resolved through homeostatic processes (Parkes, 1987; Sanders, 1989). Approaching grieving as lived experience offers enhanced understanding of the meaning of the human struggles, changing intentions, feelings, and patterns of relating experienced in grieving, without reducing the complexity of the phenomenon to a sequence of responses.

Positing *easing-intensifying with the flux of change* as a core concept in grieving is also consistent with the broadening of the concept of grieving and its integration with the study of change and transition (Marris, 1974; Parkes, 1971). Participants explicitly stated they were grieving many losses, such as the anticipated loss of self, anticipated or actual loss of someone close, loss of career, money, friends, energy, freedom, hopes and dreams. The concept of *easing-intensifying with the flux of change* describes this rhythmic process of struggling with multiple losses in many realms all-at-once.

Bearing Witness to Aloneness With Togetherness

The second extracted core concept, *bearing witness to aloneness with togetherness*, is living true presence *multidimensionally*, attesting to the lived reality of simultaneous individuality-communality. This concept encompasses dwelling with and apart from the absent presence and others all-at-once, bearing witness to suffering, and "being there" for loved ones. Multiple close, significant relationships were discussed by every family, not only among those who actually lived together but also with loved ones from childhood, some who were estranged, and some who had been dead for years. The importance of being together was evident in every family, but the participants also described a strong, pervasive sense of *solitude* in grieving. Deeply personal meanings brought the aloneness of grieving to the fore, yet it coexisted with the family members' mutual commitment. For example, in Family 2, Alice stated plainly, "This is something I have to do all alone," while much of the family's discussion was devoted to their mutual concerns and their focus on sharing in the now. In Family 7, Faye (Bonita's lover) and Eddie (her brother) spoke about "being there" for Bonita, while she said, "I just stay in a little shell all the time . . . because nobody knows what I'm going through."

The concept of *bearing witness to aloneness with togetherness* sheds light on lived experiences of family interrelating in grieving. Persons who are closely connected in grieving find unique ways of being with loss, choose from options, and incarnate choices in daily living *with and apart from* others. It is this human-to-human relating that cocreates the family, as personal choices commit individuals to a relationship and thus to being truly present with one another during times of strife and struggle. Bridges (1980, p. 32) says that the two "great transitions" of life are the development of a separate self and movement beyond separateness to "a deeper sense of interrelatedness." From Parse's perspective, however, this profound interrelatedness is inherent in being human.

Parse asserts that the human "is not alone in any dimension of becoming" (1981, p. 20) as the human coexists with predecessors, contemporaries, and successors all-at-once (p. 26). Aloneness is relative and perspectival; presence is not merely bodily location in space but is intentional; the two are not mutually exclusive. Yalom and Greaves (1977) differentiated between interpersonal loneliness, which can be allayed through interpersonal contact, and *existential loneliness,* "which cannot be allayed or taken away" (p. 398). Parse's (1981, 1992) theory suggests that persons coparticipate in existential loneliness in that they *bear witness* to the other's becoming through personal presence. Similarly, Moustakas (1972) said that in loneliness help comes "not through words . . . but by the honest, full presence of real persons and by their respect for solitude and privacy" (p. 10). In solitude a *different kind of presence* is experienced. Following her mother's death, Cole (1992) wrote of experiencing "a tangible absence," even dialoguing with her. She said, "Although I could not converse with her in person, these dialogues brought us closer in ways I could not have imagined" (p. 185). *Bearing witness to aloneness with togetherness* offers a way of understanding such paradoxical lived experiences through acknowledging and exploring (rather than explaining away) their very reality.

Possibilities Emerging With Ambiguity

The third extracted core concept, *possibilities emerging with ambiguity,* is the arising of potentialities for choosing how to be in life situations while never knowing all that is yet to be. As new views surfaced in dwelling with loss, participants saw themselves as like and unlike others, and personal choices in light of close relationships moved them onward in life. The choosing of meaning and action engendered through envisioning multiple possibilities was sometimes similar but always subtly different for each person in the family. For example, for Family 6, Leo and Phil (both HIV-positive), knowing that their time might be limited sparked a mutual exploration of their personal possibilities that led to selling their business and setting out on a cross-country adventure. Leo said, "Life's too short. We want to enjoy the time we have, whether it's a year, whether it's thirty years." In Family 9, Michael described how the "ugliness" of AIDS sparked his efforts to "enhance mind, body, and spirit" and to address the question "If I get sick and go downhill . . . have I done everything I wanted to do?"

The concept of *possibilities emerging with ambiguity* is linked with the paradox of *certainty-uncertainty* within the concept of *originating*, which Parse describes as "choosing a particular way of self-emergence through inventing unique ways of living" (1981, p. 60). Faced with options in a life situation, one strives to envision what each choice would mean, while the *quality* of certainty-uncertainty bears on the decision along with the comfort-discomfort of the individual in being like-unlike others. The concept of *possibilities emerging with ambiguity* relates to a view of grieving fundamentally different from the conventional theories which emphasize prediction and management of grief. From the perspective of the human becoming theory, the lived experience of ambiguity, in grieving, is the continuous unfolding of opportunities and limitations within a context of unwelcome and welcome change and challenges to personal values. What constitutes opportunity or limitation is relative to the person experiencing it. For example, *living with AIDS* was described as both a severe limitation and an opportunity for self-realization by many of the participants. The emerging possibilities included potentially horrific outcomes—suffering, poverty, death—but as the families saw their situations in a new light, new possibilities—to tell or not tell, to stay or go, to plan for death or plan for life—were cocreated through living personal and shared values.

The ambiguity was linked to the simultaneous *absent presences* and *present presences* of the cherished in every family.

The uncertainty inherent in change has been a persistent theme in the literature on change and transition. Commonly these works suggest that successful transition includes the resolution of uncertainty and a return to stability (Bridges, 1980; Marris, 1974). The second-order change theory proposed by Watzlawick et al. (1974) differs in that one is seen as *participating* in change and *creating* reality rather than adapting to it. Mishel (1990) referred to uncertainty as "the natural rhythm of life," stating, "Belief in a conditional world opens up the consideration of multiple possibilities since certainty is not absolute" (p. 260). DeFeo (1990) described the view of change in nursing's simultaneity paradigm as an evolutionary process involving *choosing direction and risking*. The concept of *possibilities emerging with ambiguity* in grieving is consistent with the emerging view of change as a coparticipative evolutionary process.

Confirming Realms of Endearment

The fourth extracted core concept, *confirming realms of endearment*, is the prizing of cherished involvements (present and absent) and the clarifying and shifting of personal and shared priorities. This concept encompasses what participants were most concerned about in the grieving, what *mattered*, whom they loved, and what prompted gratitude and appreciation. These concerns were highly individual but often centered on *being with close others* and *living for today*. The concept of confirming realms of endearment relates also to the meanings of comfort-discomfort, suffering and joy, and the meaning of *loss* itself. The concept is linked to Parse's concept of *valuing*, the rhythm of which is appropriating-disappropriating, taking unto oneself and letting go. In Family 7, Bonita said, "I lost a whole lot by finding out I [had] HIV." Yet, she said she was glad that she could "be responsible . . . get out of the streets . . . and be a mother to my kids." In Family 10, George (a gay man, HIV-positive) described what it meant to lose many cherished friends to the epidemic, while Richard (his companion) described the imminent loss of "virtually *all* of my close friends." In the midst of their great loss, they celebrated their partnership with smiles and laughter.

For this study, participants were asked to discuss grieving in relation to any loss or losses they had experienced. Among those persons who focused on death and dying, their concerns still reflected *personal* values; different participants focused on the pain, the lost years, their loved ones' suffering, or their preparations for death. Many participants spoke about a variety of other losses, such as a career as a cook, an affluent lifestyle, and "a healthy immune system." They described many ways in which they continued to honor their treasured-but-lost involvements while reprioritizing connections in the now by focusing on *what really mattered*. This study provides empirical substantiation of the centrality of personal meanings in loss and grieving and of the belief that loss must be defined by those experiencing it.

The concept of *confirming realms of endearment* reflects the importance of family relationships in grieving. For those anticipating personal death, being with close others brought comfort and assumed a new importance in their lives. For those anticipating the loss of someone close, making the most of the time they had and prizing special moments became priorities. Those describing erstwhile loss and grieving said the experience brought them closer to others and brought the value of the commitment to the fore. The concept of *confirming realms of endearment* elucidates the cruciality of personal values in family interrelating while living with loss and grieving.

DISCUSSION OF FINDINGS RELATED TO THEORY AND RESEARCH

Grieving as a Process of Becoming

This study expands a theoretical perspective of grieving that is specific to the discipline of nursing, *grieving as a process of becoming*. From Parse's perspective, change is a continuous, unitary process of the human-universe interrelationship, manifested in rhythmical patterns. Within this process persons coparticipate in change, loss, and grieving through choosing meaning, relating with others, and reaching beyond what is, to what is not yet. This conceptualization of grieving is not restricted by parameters of normality and is open to the entire range of human experience.

Parse's (1981) first principle states, "Structuring meaning multidimensionally is cocreating reality through the languaging of valuing and imaging" (p. 42). The meaning of grieving for the families in this study was structured through the mutual reflection of cherished images of what was, had been, and was yet to be. This process cocreated the reality lived uniquely by each person in the family. What was, had been, and was yet to be continuously changed as cherished images evolved through living with the losses. The concept *confirming realms of endearment* was integrated with the theory by specifying this process as *honoring the treasured*, which relates to the concept of *valuing*.

The second principle of the theory states, "Cocreating rhythmical patterns of relating is living the paradoxical unity of revealing-concealing, enabling-limiting while connecting-separating" (Parse, 1981, p. 50). Grieving, for the families living with AIDS, involved living with opportunities and limitations, presence and absence, divulging and hiding all-at-once; but what surfaced foremost was the experience of the *true presence of close others while dwelling with personal loss (the absent presence)*. The concept *bearing witness to aloneness with togetherness* was integrated with the theory by specifying this process as *communion-solitude*, which relates to the paradox of *connecting-separating*.

The third principle states, "Cotranscending with the possibles is powering unique ways of originating in the process of transforming" (Parse, 1981, p. 55). Grieving, for the families in this study, involved agonizing struggles fluxing with joys while confronting the enigma of what was yet to be, which engendered innovative changes in patterns of living. The concepts *easing-intensifying with the flux of change* and *possibilities emerging with ambiguity* were integrated with the theory by specifying the processes *pushing-resisting with diverse rhythms* and *unfolding with certainty-uncertainty.* Pushing-resisting is the rhythm of *powering,* the self-affirming force in grieving. Certainty-uncertainty is a paradox of *originating,* the generative process in cotranscending with the possibles.

The structure of grieving for families living with AIDS was found to be consistent with and complementary to descriptions of grieving in the two previous Parse studies. The structure of "grieving a personal loss" (Cody, 1991) was "intense struggling in the flux of change while a shifting view fosters moving beyond the now as different possibilities surface in dwelling with and apart from the absent presence and others in light of what is cherished" (p. 64), and the theoretical structure was *"powering transforming through the connecting-separating of valuing"* (p. 66). Pilkington's (1993) structure of "grieving the loss of an important other" for mothers who lost their babies at birth was "anguished suffering in devastating void amidst consoling movements away from and together with the lost one and others while confidently moving beyond personal doubts," and the theoretical structure was *"valuing the connecting-separating in transforming"* (p. 132).

Commonalities among the three studies of grieving are evident in the linkage with the concept of *valuing,* from the first principle of the theory, and with the concept of *connecting-separating,* from the second. This study supports *valuing* as a central concept in grieving. The families described their grieving in terms of love, commitment, and personal desires challenged and threatened by HIV and other forces of opposition, intensifying the appropriating-disappropriating rhythm of valuing. For those who were HIV-positive, the very value of being alive changed in a way that few of them believed others could understand; at the same time, *shared* values and priorities were strengthened, which perhaps was to be expected since the participants were already living the shared value of being a family.

This study supports *connecting-separating* as a central concept in grieving. Both Pilkington (1993) and Cody (1991) found that grieving unfolds through being with and apart from the absent presence and others all-at-once. The findings here focused on a slightly different aspect of the grieving, bearing witness to aloneness with togetherness. This all-at-once experience of cherished presence with close others and suffering in solitude was a central theme in grieving for the families in this study.

With regard to the principle of cotranscending with the possibles in grieving, Cody (1991) specified the concepts of *powering transforming,* and Pilkington (1993) specified the concept of *transforming.* This is not an either-or question, as all of the processes in the human becoming theory are continuous and all-at-once (Parse, 1992). Powering is "the force of human existence and underpins the courage to be" (Parse, 1981, p. 57). Its relevance to grieving is in moving onward in life as the who one is while opposing forces coconstitute (with the person and family) the welcome-unwelcome changes. Thus, *powering* inherently interrelates with *transforming,* "the changing of change, coconstituting anew in a deliberate way" (Parse, 1981, p. 62). Transforming, in grieving, is coparticipating in this "changing of change." It does not have a beginning or an end as such. Rather, one's coparticipation in change encompasses the cherishing that makes "loss" possible in an ever-changing universe *and* the choosing of how to live one's separateness-connectedness throughout life.

The present study specifies *powering originating* from the principle of cotranscending with the possibles. Both of the previous studies mention the emerging possibilities and the certainty-uncertainty which were more focal in this study. Cody (1991) wrote of "different possibilities surfacing in light of what is cherished" (p. 65), while Pilkington (1993) wrote of "confidently moving beyond personal doubts" (p. 132). The emergence of *originating* as a central concept in grieving here is related to the family-centered approach of this study and the plurality of views in each family. Personal priorities evolved through living certainty-uncertainty and conformity-nonconformity as each person chose unique ways of living with loss and thus cocreated innovations in family patterns of living.

Lived experiences are never finalized and always open to possibility. Three studies have illuminated grieving as a lived experience of becoming. They bear witness to the love and courage through which persons and families struggle in their chosen ways with welcome-unwelcome changes of every magnitude and reach beyond, alone-and-together, to the known-and-unknown possibilities of the not-yet.

Findings in Relation to Family Theory and Research

This study sheds new light on patterns of family relating. The prevalent tendency in the family-centered nursing literature is to borrow theory from other disciplines (Whall & Fawcett, 1991). This study contributes to the expansion and specification of nursing's theory base in relation to families and shows that research guided by Parse's theory of nursing reveals a view of family phenomena not encompassed by any other theory. It supports the idea of family-cocreated health as specified by Parse (1981), through elucidating family coparticipation in grieving.

Participants named the others *they* considered family with no imposition of parameters from the researcher. Many of the relationships among persons in this study would not be considered "family" according to conventional family theory or would be typologized as various forms of "nontraditional" families (Macklin, 1980). Those who bore witness to suffering and lived committed relationships in their grieving were present by choice; some were related by birth or marriage, and some were not. It was each participant's view of the family relationship that was important.

A prominent feature of the nursing literature on family research is the insistence on "the family" as the unit of analysis (Feetham, 1984; Gilliss, 1983; Susan Murphy, 1986; Whall & Fawcett, 1991), which is associated with the hypostatized structure of the nuclear family (or "the family system") and with the problematics of measuring family processes. Moriarty (1990) and others have noted the difficulties in attempting to recruit "entire" families into research. In this study, participants "brought their families with them" in a different way, as cherished others, living and dead, near and far, coparticipated in the study. The meaning of "family," like other meanings, is personal, contextual, and changeable. The notion of an "entire family" is arbitrary and ill-fitted to research focusing on the meaning of lived experience. This study supports Parse's (1981) view of the boundless human-universe-health process, living multi-dimensionally with predecessors, contemporaries, and successors all-at-once.

Findings in Relation to Living With AIDS

The way in which this study reflects living with AIDS is consistent with published first-person accounts (Dreuilhe, 1988; Monette, 1990; Rudd & Taylor, 1992). While participants were asked to speak with the researcher only about their experiences of grieving, all participants did of course speak at times about HIV or AIDS. One area of overlap is the *loss* of friends and family members attributed to the diagnosis. AIDS-related "stigma" is frequently addressed in the literature. In this study, *losses* of friends and associates linked with the so-called "stigma" were among the losses grieved in many of the families. The focus of this study, however, was the meaning of the grieving experience, and stigma as such was not discussed. Several participants voiced the opinion that those who left or avoided them after their diagnosis were not really deserving of their commitment after all. Often, hating the virus and the forces of opposition went hand-in-hand with finding new ways of loving self and others.

Nokes and Carver (1991, p. 177), as mentioned earlier, identi-fied three major themes of living with AIDS in a study guided by Parse's theory: (a) *"Prevailing thoughts about mortality surface and subside,"* (b) *"relationships fluctuate as priorities change,"* and (c) *"shifting expectations lead to thoughts about spirituality"* (wherein "spirituality" refers to a higher power, purpose in life, and hope). The similarity of themes in the present study reveals that *families* coparticipate with and share in the experiential processes of living with a potentially fatal illness. Nokes and

Carver formulated a proposition on living with AIDS within the context of Parse's theory: "Living with AIDS is an abrupt shift in patterns of becoming, sparked by unpredictable changing relationships with others as different hopes and dreams unfold amidst suffering" (p. 177). The findings of the present study are consistent with this proposition.

In Beauchamp's (1990) study of *the struggle to make a decision in a critical life situation* for persons with HIV, he wrote that "individuals [with HIV] living the experience of struggling to make a decision in a critical life situation are affirming self through confronting the pushing-resisting of uncertainty in moving toward the not-yet" (p. 85). Although the two phenomena specifically investigated were different, the findings of this study are consistent with Beauchamp's description in relation to living with AIDS. In O'Brien's (1992) study of living with HIV, she noted the following comments:

> I learned to love myself and work on my self-esteem. I can be happy right now and be happy just being me.
>
> I started giving more value to people and to life; it made me more responsible and mature.
>
> In some ways it is a kind of blessing that I have had to change my attitude; now when I make choices I decide what is really important. (p. 161)

Participants in this study made many similar statements, such as Bonita's assertion, "I'm *glad* that I am HIV positive, because I can slow down and stay settled." As mentioned earlier in this chapter, self-affirmation is a common feature in many accounts of living with HIV/AIDS, as it was in the grieving described in this study. Self-affirmation does not always manifest in ways that norm-based theories would recognize.

A similar issue was raised by Hall (1990), who strongly refuted the notion that hope in the face of terminal illness is "denial" or wishful thinking. In her study, persons with HIV maintained hope by refusing to go to support groups where people talked of dying, avoiding talking and thinking about AIDS and "believing that they are never going to die of AIDS" (pp. 181–182). In the present study, many of the participants spoke of hopes and dreams that could be deemed unrealistic, like 23-year-old Rob picturing himself with Jeff as old men in rocking chairs. Hall proposed that the essentials of hope for persons diagnosed as terminally ill are "having a future life in spite of the diagnosis. . . . having a renewed zest for life. . . . [and] finding a reason for living, usually one that was not evident before" (p. 183). The findings of this study are consistent with her conclusions.

METHODOLOGICAL CONSIDERATIONS

This study confirms that using Parse's (1987a) research method with families illuminates the complexity of lived experiences in a unique way and enhances understanding of the notion that health is cocreated with the universe including close others. The choice of families as participants influenced the entire project. The conceptualization of "family" in the theory was carefully considered and made explicit. Participants were sought by addressing invitations "to Families Living with AIDS" while clarifying that "family members may include lovers and/or friends." Participants were asked to invite as many of their close others to attend the research session as was comfortable and feasible for them.

Dialogical engagements. These were carried out with the families in essentially the same manner as dialogues with individuals, with one difference, which was that persons in the families spoke with one another. Some participants described experiences in which another person present was involved, without comment from the other; some simply said more than others or frequently interrupted. There was no attempt to seek a standardized way of guiding the conversation. The researcher was engaged with the participants in true presence, and *silence* on the part of participants was understood as a way of languaging something, yet there was no effort by the researcher to imbue the silences with linguistic meaning—they were *there* in the rhythm of the dialogue. As with individuals in dialogue, the family participants often referred to close others who were not present. Most of the descriptions were lengthy and detailed, and *all* addressed issues of great significance to the families *from two or more perspectives.* An advantage of using video with families was that the videos clarified *who* was speaking and *to whom* that person was speaking. In addition, the video recorded smiles, silent laughter, tears, and significant gestures, none of which could have been captured using only audio.

Extraction-Synthesis.   Concentrating the descriptions in extracted essences proved to be very challenging. Efforts to preserve the uniqueness of the individual perspectives led to the inclusion of the pseudonyms and the use of phrases like "for Rob . . ." in the extracted essences. Both the guiding theory and the descriptions indicated that an appreciation of *individual* perspectives was crucial to understanding the experience of the *family.* Presentation of the descriptions in the form of a *narrative* offered the opportunity to share the richness of the dialogues and enhanced clarity in the extracted essences. There were many instances in which persons nodded, shook their heads, smiled, cried, or laughed in response to one another, and the video images helped to clarify these subtle patterns of harmony and conflict in the family. The researcher did not critically analyze the gestures of participants and avoided anchoring understanding of any participant's view solely on visible expressions. The researcher dwelled with *the sense of the whole experience.* Each synthesized essence and proposition reflects multiple views, sometimes in harmony, sometimes in conflict, leading to a family-centered structure of grieving that takes into account the unique personal perspectives of the individuals in the family.

Logistics.   Several practical issues arose in the use of video, which added complexity and expense to the project and required the involvement of more persons. There were added difficulties in finding willing participants and arranging research sessions. The use of a camera operator meant involving another person in recording the dialogues. When no camera operator was available, the researcher used a stationary camera set on auto-focus, which resulted in videorecordings of poor quality, as did, in some instances, the use of amateur camera operators.

CONCLUSIONS AND RECOMMENDATIONS

Through this study, the meaning given to the lived experience of grieving in families living with AIDS was uncovered and interpreted in light of Parse's (1981, 1992) human becoming theory of nursing. The view of grieving presented in two previous Parse studies of grieving (Cody, 1991; Pilkington, 1993) was expanded in this one, which represents an advance for nursing science in the substantive area of grieving. The human becoming theory base may be further enhanced by investigation of lived experiences related to the concepts in grieving that surfaced here, such as being with and apart from loved ones through a difficult time, doing the best you can in an "impossible" situation, and bearing witness to suffering.

This study contributes to the honing of Parse's (1987, 1990, 1994a, 1994b) method for use with families and confirms it as a viable mode of inquiry for family-centered research. It is recommended that researchers conducting family-centered studies guided by Parse's theory closely attend to the meaning of Parse's definition of family. For family-centered research focused on lived experiences and quality of life, it is most important to attend to the way the persons in the family view themselves and their own experiences. Researchers using Parse's method with families and groups are encouraged to be at ease with uneven rhythms and silences in the dialogues. What is revealed in true presence uncovers aspects of lived experience that would remain opaque to more intrusive questioning. Including an *extracted narrative* prior to the extracted essences preserved the richness and vigor of the original descriptions and enhanced the clarity and readability of the extracted essences. The use of extracted narratives is strongly recommended for future family-centered studies. The use of video enhanced the immersion in the descriptions and facilitated the extraction-synthesis process. It is recommended that video be used to record dialogical engagements, especially with families as research participants.

A practice proposition reflects the essential meaning of the structure of the lived experience under study at a level of abstraction appropriate to the immediacy of practice. The researcher's practice proposition on grieving states that *struggling with the ambiguity of change through bearing witness to the absent presence sheds light on what really matters as creating new possibilities shifts priorities.* This proposition is consistent with the findings of all three Parse studies of grieving and with Parse's (1987a) practice methodology. The nurse practicing from the human becoming perspective has the opportunity to be with persons and their families with this knowledge of grieving and may better understand the meaning of grieving as illuminated through this research.

REFERENCES

Allan, J. D. (1990). Focusing on living, not dying: A naturalistic study of self-care among seropositive gay men. *Holistic Nursing Practice, 4*(2), 56–63.

Altman, D. (1987). *AIDS in the mind of America.* New York: Anchor.

Beauchamp, C. J. (1990). *The structure of the lived experience of struggling with making a decision in a critical life situation, for a group of individuals with HIV.* Unpublished doctoral dissertation, University of Miami.

Bowlby, J. (1969). *Attachment and loss, Vol. I, Attachment.* New York: Basic Books.

Bowlby, J. (1973). *Attachment and loss, Vol. II, Separation: Anxiety and anger.* New York: Basic Books.

Bowlby, J. (1980). *Attachment and loss, Vol. III, Loss: Sadness and depression.* New York: Basic Books.

Bridges, W. (1980). *Transitions: Making sense of life's changes.* Menlo Park, CA: Addison-Wesley.

Brown, M. A., & Powell-Cope, G. M. (1991). AIDS family caregivers: Transitions through uncertainty. *Nursing Research, 40,* 338–345.

Burr, W. R., Hill, R., Reiss, I. L., & Nye, F. I. (1979). *Contemporary theories about the family* (2 vols.). New York: Free Press.

Carmack, B. J. (1992). Balancing engagement/detachment in AIDS-related multiple losses. *Image: Journal of Nursing Scholarship, 24,* 9–14.

Carter, S. L. (1989). Themes of grief. *Nursing Research, 38,* 354–358.

Chick, N., & Meleis, A. I. (1986). Transitions: A nursing concern. In P. L. Chinn (Ed.), *Nursing research methodology: Issues and implementation* (pp. 237–257). Rockville, MD: Aspen.

Cody, W. K. (1991). Grieving a personal loss. *Nursing Science Quarterly, 4,* 61–68.

Cole, D. (1992). *After great pain: A new life emerges.* New York: Summit Books.

Cowles, K. V., & Rodgers, B. L. (1991). The concept of grief: A foundation for nursing research and practice. *Research in Nursing and Health, 14,* 119–127.

Davies, B., Spinetta, J., Martinson, I., & Kulenkamp, E. (1986). Manifestations of levels of functioning in grieving families. *Journal of Family Issues, 7,* 297–313.

DeFeo, D. (1990). Change: A central concern of nursing. *Nursing Science Quarterly, 3,* 88–94.

Demi, A. S., & Miles, M. S. (1986). Bereavement. *Annual Review of Nursing Research, 4,* 105–123.

Dreuilhe, A. E. (1988). *Mortal embrace: Living with AIDS* (L. Coverdale, Trans.). New York: Hill and Wang.

Engel, G. L. (1961). Is grief a disease? *Psychosomatic Medicine, 23,* 18–22.

Feetham, S. L. (1984). Family research: Issues and directions for nursing. *Annual Review of Nursing Research, 3,* 3–25.

Flaskerud, J. H. (1987). AIDS: Psychosocial aspects. *Journal of Psychosocial Nursing, 25*(12), 9–16.

Freud, S. (1957). Mourning and melancholia. In J. Starchey (Trans. & Ed.), *The standard edition of the complete psychological works of Sigmund Freud, Vol. 14* (pp. 237–258). London: Hogarth. (Original work published 1917)

Gilliss, C. L. (1983). The family as the unit of analysis: Strategies for the nurse researcher. *Advances in Nursing Science, 5*(3), 50–59.

Gilliss, C. L. (1989). Family research in nursing. In C. L. Gilliss, B. L. Highley, B. M. Roberts, & I. M. Martinson (Eds.), *Toward a science of family nursing* (pp. 37–63). Menlo Park, CA: Addison-Wesley.

Hall, B. A. (1990). The struggle of the diagnosed terminally ill person to maintain hope. *Nursing Science Quarterly, 3,* 177–184.

Klein, S. J., & Fletcher, W. (1986). Gay grief: An examination of its uniqueness brought to light by the AIDS crisis. *Journal of Psychosocial Oncology, 4*(3), 15–25.

Knapp, R. J. (1986). *Beyond endurance: When a child dies.* New York: Schocken.

Kübler-Ross, E. (1969). *On death and dying.* New York: Macmillan.

Kuhn, J. W. (1977). Realignment of emotional forces following loss. *Family, 5,* 19–24.

Lambert, C., & Lambert, V. (1977). Divorce: A psychodynamic development involving grief. *Journal of Psychiatric Nursing and Mental Health Services, 15*(1), 37–42.

Lindemann, E. (1944). Symptomology and management of acute grief. *American Journal of Psychiatry, 101,* 141–149.

Macklin, E. D. (1980). Nontraditional family forms: A decade of research. *Journal of Marriage and the Family, 42,* 905–922.

Marris, P. (1974). *Loss and change.* New York: Pantheon.

McCubbin, H. I., & Figley, C. R. (Eds.). (1983). *Stress and the family* (2 vols.). New York: Brunner/Mazel.

Miller, J. F. (1983). *Chronic illness: Overcoming powerlessness.* Philadelphia: Davis.

Mishel, M. H. (1990). Reconceptualization of the uncertainty in illness theory. *Image: Journal of Nursing Scholarship, 22,* 256–262.

Monette, P. (1990). *Borrowed time: An AIDS memoir.* New York: Avon.

Moriarty, H. J. (1990). Key issues in the family research process: Strategies for nurse researchers. *Advances in Nursing Science, 12*(3), 1–14.

Moustakas, C. (1972). *Loneliness and love.* Englewood Cliffs, NJ: Prentice-Hall.

Murphy, Shirley A. (1983). Theoretical perspectives on bereavement. In P. L. Chinn (Ed.), *Advances in nursing theory development* (pp. 191–206). Rockville, MD: Aspen.

Murphy, Shirley A. (Ed.). (1990). *Holistic Nursing Practice* [topical issue on "Nursing care of clients in transition"], *4*(3).

Murphy, Susan. (1986). Family study and nursing research. *Image: Journal of Nursing Scholarship, 18,* 170–174.

Nokes, K., & Carver, K. (1991). The meaning of living with AIDS: A study using Parse's theory of man-living-health. *Nursing Science Quarterly, 4,* 175–179.

O'Brien, M. E. (1992). *Living with HIV: Experiment in courage.* New York: Auburn House.

Parkes, C. M. (1971). Psychosocial transitions: A field for study. *Social Sciences and Medicine, 5,* 101–115.

Parkes, C. M. (1987). *Bereavement: Studies of grief in adult life* (2nd American ed.). New York: International Universities Press. (Original work published 1972)

Parse, R. R. (1981). *Man-living-health: A theory of nursing.* New York: Wiley.

Parse, R. R. (1987a). Man-living-health theory of nursing. In R. R. Parse, *Nursing science: Major paradigms, theories, and critiques* (pp. 159–180). Philadelphia: Saunders.

Parse, R. R. (1987b). *Nursing science: Major paradigms, theories, and critiques.* Philadelphia: Saunders.

Parse, R. R. (1990). Parse's research methodology with an illustration of the lived experience of hope. *Nursing Science Quarterly, 3,* 9–17.

Parse, R. R. (1992). Human becoming: Parse's theory of nursing. *Nursing Science Quarterly, 5,* 35–42.

Parse, R. R. (1994a). *Human becoming: A theory of nursing.* Manuscript submitted for publication.

Parse, R. R. (1994b). Laughing and health: A study using Parse's research method. *Nursing Science Quarterly, 7,* 55–64.

Pilkington, B. (1993). The lived experience of grieving the loss of an important other. *Nursing Science Quarterly, 6,* 130–139.

Pincus, L. (1974). *Death and the family: The importance of mourning.* New York: Pantheon.

Reilly, D. M. (1978). Death propensity, dying, and bereavement: A family systems perspective. *Family Therapy, 5,* 35–55.

Rudd, A., & Taylor, D. (1992). *Positive women: Voices of women living with AIDS.* Toronto, Ontario: Second Story Press.

Sanders, C. M. (1989). *Grief: The mourning after.* New York: Wiley.

Schecter, S. (1990). *The AIDS notebooks.* Albany: State University of New York Press.

Schneider, J. (1984). *Stress, loss and grief.* Baltimore: University Park Press.

Schoenberg, B., Carr, A. C., Peretz, D., & Kutscher, A. H. (Eds.). (1970). *Loss and grief: Psychological management in medical practice.* New York: Columbia University Press.

Shilts, R. (1987). *And the band played on: Politics, people, and the AIDS epidemic.* New York: St. Martin's Press.

Smith, M. C. (1990). Struggling through a difficult time for unemployed persons. *Nursing Science Quarterly, 3,* 18–28.

Sowell, R. L. Bramlett, M. H., Gueldner, S. H., Gritzmacher, D., & Martin, G. (1991). The lived experience of survival and bereavement following the death of a lover from AIDS. *Image: Journal of Nursing Scholarship, 23,* 89–94.

Walker, G. (1991). *In the midst of winter: Systemic therapy with families, couples, and individuals with AIDS infection.* New York: Norton.

Watzlawick, D., Weakland, J., & Fisch, R. (1974). *Change: Principles of problem formation and problem resolution.* New York: Norton.

Weber, J., & Fournier, D. (1985). Family support and a child's adjustment to death. *Family Relations, 34*(1), 43–49.

Weitz, R. (1991). *Life with AIDS*. New Brunswick, NJ: Rutgers University Press.

Werner-Beland, J. A. (Ed.). (1980). *Grief responses to long-term illness and disability.* Reston, VA: Reston.

Whall, A. L., & Fawcett, J. (1991). *Family theory development in nursing: State of the science and art.* Philadelphia: Davis.

Yalom, I. D., & Greaves, C. (1977). Group therapy with the terminally ill. *American Journal of Psychiatry, 134,* 396–400.

Chapter 15

The Lived Experience of Suffering

John Daly

Suffering is an experience which is commonly encountered in everyday life (Eriksson, 1992; Starck & McGovern, 1992) and a phenomenon that frequently confronts nurses in practice. Though the phenomenon is "as old as human kind, its scientific study has only begun recently" (Duffy, 1992, p. 291). While numerous theoretical views of suffering may be found in the literature, in general such perspectives shed little light on the essence or "whatness" of suffering. More often than not these views only posit reasons for why one suffers. Where definitions for suffering have been advanced, shortcomings are apparent (Battenfield, 1984; Duffy, 1992). As Duffy (1992) notes, "The majority of definitions of suffering are too narrow and simplistic, conceptualizing suffering only as a degree of physical and/or psychological pain" (p. 299). The limitations of such definitions are understandable in light of the contemporary claim that suffering is a wholistic and complex phenomenon (Cassell, 1991; Duffy, 1992).

Suffering has not been adequately elucidated through scientific inquiry and consequently there is little in the research literature regarding the phenomenon. Studies of the phenomenon which have been conducted from a quantitative perspective show that suffering may or may not be related to pain (Cassell, 1991; Kahn & Steeves, 1986) or other abstract variables. Meaning is said to be a crucial determinant in this context (Kahn & Steeves, 1986). This author found in the literature no purely qualitative studies which investigated the meaning of suffering. Of the studies of suffering done to date none clearly specifies the meaning of the experience for people.

The extant literature, which is considerable, shows that suffering is a phenomenon which is poorly understood (Battenfield, 1984; Cassell, 1982; Copp, 1974, 1990a, 1990b; Duffy, 1992; Eriksson, 1992; Goldberg, 1986; Kahn & Steeves, 1986; Morse & Johnson, 1991; Starck & McGovern, 1992). A number of these perspectives are elaborated in chapter 4 of this book. The need for phenomenological studies to elucidate the essence of suffering is acknowledged in the literature (Duffy, 1992; Kahn & Steeves, 1986). This essence can only be uncovered by inquiry which seeks to illuminate the meaning of suffering. The study reported here, of the lived experience of suffering, sought to elucidate its structure by use of the Parse theory and research method (Parse, 1981, 1987). As knowledge of suffering is currently rooted in disciplines other than nursing (psychology, sociology, philosophy and anthropology), the findings of this study provide nursing science with fresh insights into suffering explicated within a theoretical framework. This contributes to the human science knowledge base of nursing and offers implications for practice and research.

NURSING PERSPECTIVE

Parse's (1981, 1987, 1992) theory of nursing, a human science perspective, was used as the theoretical grounding for this study. This theory provides a perspective on human becoming which is unique to the discipline of nursing. Parse's (1981, 1987, 1992) theory comprises principles which elucidate processes inherent in living. It has a significant focus on patterns of human living. From her perspective, humans are unitary, intentional, free-willed beings. Parse's theoretical principles reflect the three themes of her theory—meaning, rhythmicity, and cotranscendence (Parse, 1981, 1987, 1992). These principles describe complex processes which are basic to human becoming. Parse's first theoretical principle states: *Structuring meaning multidimensionally is cocreating reality through the languaging of valuing and imaging* (Parse, 1981, p. 42). This principle posits the human as cocreating meaning at many realms of the universe all-at-once; this is imbued with unique, cherished beliefs and values. The cocreated meaning unfolds in the human-universe process and is chosen and structured by the human. Parse's second theoretical principle is: *Cocreating rhythmical patterns of relating is living the paradoxical unity of revealing-concealing and enabling-limiting while connecting-separating* (Parse, 1981, p. 50). This principle explicates the paradox inherent in rhythmical patterns of relating (Parse, 1981) in the human-universe process. Humans live both sides of these rhythms all-at-once, though one side may be predominant in the moment (Parse, 1981, 1987). Parse's third theoretical principle states: *Cotranscending with the possibles is powering unique ways of originating in the process of transforming* (Parse, 1981, p. 55). This principle describes the process of moving beyond the now moment toward the not-yet, in the process of becoming. The process involves finding unique and valued ways of struggling in creating new possibles.

The theory of human becoming views the human as an open, unitary being and nursing as a basic science with a unique knowledge base. Moreover, the person is further conceptualized as recognized by "patterns of relating" and as a being "freely choosing meaning in situation" (Parse, 1992, p. 38). Parse (1981) defines health as a process of becoming uniquely lived by each individual. It is the human's lived experience, a non-linear entity that cannot be qualified as good or bad, more or less. It is not the opposite of disease or a state that the human being has, but rather a continuously changing process that the human cocreates. Health for the person reflects value priorities. From this perspective there are no standards of "normality" by which to assess the person. The person is the expert and ultimate authority on his or her own health.

To develop a perspective on the phenomenon for this study the researcher dwelled with the meaning of the lived experience of suffering to arrive at a definition. From the researcher's perspective, then, suffering is lived meaning, a way of being with a situation which is conveyed through the languaging of anguish. Suffering is an agonizing heaviness prompted through being with and apart from others, objects, and situations unfolding in an unburdening lightness (Daly, 1992). In this perspective suffering is the meaning given to the situation by the person who is living the experience of suffering. The meaning is shown through languaging valued images. Suffering unfolds in living the choices presented as different possibilities arise. In this way the person reveals and conceals all-at-once the who that he or she is. The suffering person is enabled and limited by the experience as he or she connects and separates with others all-at-once in the suffering moment. Suffering reflects pushing-resisting while the sufferer is powering to create new ways of becoming. This perspective was articulated prior to undertaking the investigation into the lived experience of suffering.

METHODOLOGY

The human becoming research methodology is conceptually congruent with the theory of human becoming (Oiler Boyd, 1990; Ray, 1990); it evolved from the principles of the theory in combination with rules for construction of methodology developed by Parse (1987). Moreover, it emanates from the ontological assumptions of the theory which are congruent with those of the human science perspective (Parse, 1981, 1987; Ray, 1990). Parse's research methodology represents an approach to the generation of knowledge which is unique to the discipline of nursing. Cody (1992a) states that "Parse's research methodology is phenomenological in the generic sense, but it flows from the theory of human becoming and is thus guided by a nursing perspective" (p. 28). Ray (1990) concurs, stating that "unlike presuppositionless phenomenology Parse's methodology is governed by its own paradigm and conditioned by the reflective theoretical man-living-health ontology and epistemology" (p. 44). This methodology comprises processes that "demonstrate that the inquiry is a 'kind of seeking' about human experience to constitute the structures of experience" (Ray, 1990, p. 44). Parse (1993) asserts that the purpose of research (using the Parse methodology) "is not to verify the theory or test it but, rather, the focus is on uncovering the essences of lived phenomena to gain further understanding of *universal* human experiences. This understanding evolves from connecting the descriptions given by people to the theory, thus making more explicit the essences of being human. The knowledge, as expanded through research, enriches the belief system of human becoming, which guides the nurse in practice" (p. 12). Parse's research methodology is described as follows, in relation to this research project.

Participant Selection

Parse (1987) advises that "participant selection is carefully done" (p. 175). A fundamental assumption with this method is "a person who agrees to participate in a study about a particular lived experience can give an authentic account of that experience when engaged in dialogue with the researcher" (Parse, 1987, p. 175). With this method persons who have lived the experience under investigation are invited to participate in the particular study. In terms of numbers of participants admitted to a particular study Parse (1987) states, "Two to ten participants are considered adequate in this method" (p. 175). An assumption here is that such a sample will probably achieve redundancy. Redundancy is an acceptable indicator of sample size sufficiency in qualitative research (Wilson, 1989).

Nine people were invited to participate in this study. They were recruited through distribution of a written invitation to which they responded by contacting the researcher directly by telephone to arrange an appropriate meeting time and place. The invitation was presented in a standard typed format on a single sheet of paper. It was titled "An invitation to participate in a study of the phenomenon of human suffering." All of the research participants in this study spoke English, though for two of the participants English was a second language. All participants admitted to the study were drawn from the general population, and they were asked to give an account of their experience of suffering. They chose what they wished to discuss with the researcher. Suffering had emerged in the lives of the participants for a variety of reasons. Each dialogical engagement took place in the home of the research participant, a relatively quiet and private setting. All research participants were informed that they were participating in a nursing research project which was being undertaken for a Doctor of Philosophy degree and that the study was investigating the lived experience of suffering. The principles of informed consent were observed, embraced, and implemented by the researcher. Research participants were apprised of the purpose of the study in considerable detail prior to their formal consent to participate. They were also advised of their rights as research participants, including the right to withdraw from the study at any time. Participants were asked to contact the researcher by telephone if they found that they had further questions regarding the project or if they experienced discomfort related to their involvement in the project. Informed consent was obtained for all participants in the study. None of the research participants contacted the researcher following dialogical engagement.

Dialogical Engagement

Parse specifies a unique approach to dialogue between the researcher and the research participant. This approach is described as "an intersubjective 'being with' in which the researcher and participant live the I-thou process as they move through an unstructured discussion about the lived experience" (Parse, 1987,

p. 176). In the I-thou engagement the researcher is truly present with the participant in dialogue as "the remembered, the now, and the not-yet unfold all at once" (Parse, 1987, p. 176). Dialogical engagement represents "a unique researcher-participant dialogue which is not an interview but rather a true presence" (Parse, 1992, p. 4). In dialogical engagement the researcher is with the research participant in a special way. This "being with" allows the researcher to "elicit a description from the participant about the entity being studied . . . . it is a unique way of 'becoming with' the participant and is not specified as an essential part of any other qualitative research methodology" (Parse, 1992, p. 42). Through dialogical engagement the researcher "uncovers the meaning of phenomena as humanly lived" (Parse, 1992, p. 41).

Consistent with Parse's (1987) recommendations, prior to engaging each research participant in dialogue, the researcher dwelled with the meaning of the lived experience of suffering. The researcher developed some dialogical directions for initiating and focusing discussion during the dialogical engagement. In this context the researcher does not develop a rigid set of questions to be put to the research participants during dialogical engagement, "but rather a sense of the ideas to be shared in centering the discussion on the entity as lived by the participants" (Parse, 1987, p. 176). The researcher in dialogical engagement aimed to focus on the phenomenon of inquiry "avoiding the introduction of new concepts and attempting to move with the flow of the participants' descriptions" (Cody, 1989, p. 27). Dialogical engagements began with the researcher posing the question "Would you tell me about your experience of suffering?" In this study all dialogical engagements were audiotaped. The dialogues were transcribed to a typed format to facilitate extraction-synthesis (Parse, 1987).

Extraction-Synthesis

In this phase of the research process the researcher proceeds by dwelling with the transcribed researcher-participant dialogue (or viewing the videotape if one is available). "Dwelling with" is engaging with the transcribed dialogue with deep concentration. The researcher dwells with the dialogue in a focused, centered and reflective way (Parse, 1987). "Dwelling with" is a constant in the extraction-synthesis process. Through this process the researcher extracts essences from the dialogue (Cody, 1989). Parse (1987) states that "the term extract was chosen to convey the meaning of the essence of a concentrate" (p. 176). Extracted essences are in the language of the research participant; they are expressed, therefore, at the concrete level of discourse. Once essences are extracted from a complete description, the researcher moves the essences to higher levels of abstraction. This process is carried out according to Parse's (1987, 1992) specifications. The extraction-synthesis process encompasses five major processes: (a) extracting essences (expressed in the participant's language), (b) synthesizing essences (this involves expressing the core idea of each extracted essence in the language of the researcher), (c) formulating a proposition for each participant, (d) extracting concepts from all formulated propositions, and (e) synthesizing a structure of the lived experience using core concepts (Parse, 1987). The structure evolved through this process answers the research question. Extraction-synthesis in this study was carried out in accordance with the methodology delineated by Parse (1987). Sample findings of this study for extraction-synthesis are presented in Table 15.1. Extraction-synthesis is followed by heuristic interpretation (Parse, 1987, 1992).

Heuristic Interpretation

Heuristic interpretation is a process of logical abstractions (Parse, 1987) that takes the study findings beyond the theory of human becoming through two processes, namely structural integration and conceptual interpretation. Here in sequential abstraction the language of the participants is moved logically to the language of Parse's theory and beyond. Structural integration is connecting the proposition and the emergent structure to the theory of human becoming (Parse, 1987). Conceptual

Table 15.1 Examples of Extraction-Synthesis Process With Related Propositions

Extracted Essences (Participant's Language)	*Synthesized Essences* (Researcher's Language)
PARTICIPANT 4	
In suffering, the participant had feelings of conflict, hurting, unbearable pain, strain, paranoia, and disharmony in relationships, being ill at ease, suicidal, and scared of the future. He believes that suffering is a lonely experience even if you are with supportive others.	Entanglement in utter anguish surfaces varied ways of engaging-disengaging.
Withdrawing in an imposed isolation, the participant turned toward self-destruction while battling himself to stop.	Self-estranging recoil prompts struggle for self-preservation.
The participant lost faith in the system and thought his situation was hopeless but he knew time would heal his situation and that there is always hope to carry on.	Disillusioning despair emerges with precious alternatives in enduring resilience.

Proposition. Suffering is entanglement in utter anguish surfacing varied ways of engaging-disengaging as self-estranging recoil prompts struggle for self-preservation while disillusioning despair emerges with precious alternatives in enduring resilience.

PARTICIPANT 7	
In suffering, the participant had feelings of being scared, unhappy, tortured, tormented, physical pain, shock, numbness, tiredness, and loss of control. She believes that suffering is fear of the unknown and death. She pushes it to the back of her mind and tries not to dwell on it too much, but does give it some thought.	Immersion in paralyzing anguish surfaces with engaging-disengaging contemplation.

Table 15.1 (Continued)

Extracted Essences (Participant's Language)	*Synthesized Essences* (Researcher's Language)
Though the participant did not want to deal with the suffering of her grandmother she faced the situation believing that she was sharing the suffering and would benefit from the experience.	Confronting the direful with the cherished during difficulties prompts enhancement.

Proposition. Suffering is immersion in paralyzing anguish surfacing with engaging-disenaging contemplation as confronting the direful with the cherished during difficulties prompts enhancement.

PARTICIPANT 8

For the participant suffering is being caught in a big pit with feelings of deep depression, sadness, pain, panic, hurt, emptiness, being scared, lonely, and nervous. She believes that having her usefulness taken from her is the biggest suffering though she has realized that she is still useful.	Entanglement with the deadening paralysis of anguish shifts views of self unfolding precious possibles.
Feeling insecure and unsettled, the participant was helped by the love and caring of others.	Nurturing ways of engaging-disengaging calm vulnerable agitation.
Though the participant does not understand why she must suffer she believed that it is a part of her challenge in life and that she must stay positive and fight it.	Incredulous bafflement unfolds resilient resignation.

Proposition. Suffering is entanglement with the deadening paralysis of anguish which shifts views of self unfolding precious possibles as nurturing ways of engaging-disengaging calm vulnerable agitation as incredulous bafflement unfolds resilient resignation.

interpretation involves specifying the structure of the lived experience using the concepts of the theory of human becoming and thereby developing a specific theoretical structure from the principles (Parse, 1987).

PRESENTATION OF DATA

Core Concepts

From the nine propositions which emerged in this study (see Table 15.2), three core concepts were extracted:

1. Paralyzing anguish with glimpses of precious possibilities.
2. Entanglements of engaging-disengaging.
3. Struggling in pursuit of fortification.

FINDINGS OF THE STUDY

The major finding of the study is the structure which is: the lived experience of suffering is *paralyzing anguish with glimpses of precious possibilities emerging with entanglements of engaging-disengaging while struggling in pursuit of fortification.*

The structure is moved from the language of the participants to the language of the theory of human becoming (Parse, 1987, 1992). Here the structure of the lived experience of suffering was initially raised one level of abstraction in the process of structural integration. This involves forging interpretive links with the theory of human becoming (see Table 15.3). The structure is linked conceptually with Parse's theory (Pilkington, 1993). At this level the lived experience of suffering is *an impotent wretchedness glancing the treasured enmeshed in the intimacy-solitude of resolute affirmation.* In conceptual interpretation the structure of the

Table 15.2   Emergent Propositions

Proposition, Participant 1

Suffering is sequestered anguish surfacing endurance with glimpses of desired possibilities while vacillating in engaging-disengaging gives rise to barriers that clash with desires as entanglement with disparate views resides amidst a struggle for release as personal insults prompt comfort-discomfort amidst self-reflections.

Proposition, Participant 2

Suffering is enforced segregation in anguished abandonment as sorrowful recoil arises with disillusionment in engaging-disengaging while alternatives prompt precious nurturing with fortitude as options unfold with the amusing and direful all-at-once.

Proposition, Participant 3

Suffering is anguished bafflement with paralyzing ambiguity as disengaging-engaging prompts endurance amidst diffidence in contemplating ways to move on while precious moments of contented confidence unfold with receptive assurance in the pursuit of fortification.

Proposition, Participant 4

Suffering is entanglement in utter anguish surfacing varied ways of engaging-disengaging as self-estranging recoil prompts struggle for self-preservation while disillusioning despair emerges with precious alternatives in enduring resilience.

Proposition, Participant 5

Suffering is paralyzing anguish surfacing with alternative views of the possible while fortification unfolds with engaging-disengaging all-at-once.

Proposition, Participant 6

Suffering is anguish that surfaces enhancement with expanding horizons as remembering the precious of what-was emerges while engaging-disengaging in moving with new ways of becoming as living with inevitable changes prompts focused movement.

Table 15.2   (Continued)

Proposition, Participant 7

Suffering is immersion in paralyzing anguish surfacing with engaging-disengaging contemplation as confronting the direful with the cherished during difficulties prompts enhancement.

Proposition, Participant 8

Suffering is entanglement with the deadening paralysis of anguish which shifts views of self unfolding precious possibles as nurturing ways of engaging-disengaging calm vulnerable agitation as incredulous bafflement unfolds resilient resignation.

Proposition, Participant 9

Suffering is the anguished ambiguity of dwelling with mutual woe prompting paralysis with the struggle to move as the comfort-discomfort of the undisclosed shifts engaging-disengaging while clinging to glimpses of the possibilities as anticipated anguish emerges with spiritual succour.

Table 15.3   Progressive Abstraction of Concepts With Heuristic Interpretation

CORE CONCEPT	*STRUCTURAL INTEGRATION*	*CONCEPTUAL INTERPRETATION*
Paralyzing anguish with glimpses of precious possibilities	→ Impotent wretchedness glancing the treasured	→ Valuing
Entanglements of engaging-disengaging	→ Enmeshed in the intimacy-solitude	→ Connecting-Separating
Struggling in pursuit of fortification	→ Resolute affirmation	→ Powering

lived experience of suffering was expressed using selected concepts of the theory of human becoming; this emerged as *valuing the connecting-separating of powering.*

DISCUSSION OF FINDINGS

The structure of the lived experience of suffering which emerged in this study illuminates the unitary nature of the phenomenon of suffering. Each core concept reflects extracts from the dialogues. The first core concept uncovered in this research study is *paralyzing anguish with glimpses of precious possibilities.* It is a salient pattern of the lived experience of suffering in relation to meaning. Each participant described the agony and immobility of suffering along with the cherished opportunities it presented. The concept of paralyzing anguish is reflected in the following examples from the transcribed dialogues.

Participant 2: "I think that it was excruciatingly painful . . . . I felt terribly empty, enormously angry . . . . and, and yet helpless in terms of how one might change that because I was stuck with it and I didn't want to take it out on my daughter."

Participant 7: "It's really . . . . it's really . . . . , it's unhappy. The situation I was in, your emotions just take control because usually we really keep ourselves in check almost as humans and . . . . then a situation comes up over which you have no control and you can't control that situation, you can't make that person better, you can't . . . . so your emotions just come . . . . just out of control and you are feeling all these things."

Participant 8: ". . . . but when I start thinking about my family and wanting to see my daughter married . . . . and see my grandchildren . . . . and R [husband] being on his own . . . . the depression sets in . . . . so I've got to be very aware . . . . but that is a . . . . a really . . . . it really . . . . hurts and that's a really big suffering. If you want to use the word suffering, as I've said I don't like the word suffering . . . . experience of illness and sickness . . . . but it's just that awful feeling that you are just so alone . . . . so alone in this big pit that you just can't seem to get out of."

In addition to conveying the paralyzing anguish of suffering many research participants acknowledged the positives they had in life. Precious possibilities existed simultaneously with paralyzing anguish. In combination with extreme anguish was the insight that suffering offered opportunities for growth and changes in cherished ways of being. For example, some participants believed that suffering was not necessarily a "bad thing"; one stated that "you can learn through it"; another said "it was a beneficial experience." Some participants indicated that they would not change the paths their lives had taken—even with the suffering—if they could. Most asserted that they valued the experience and grew through it. One said, "[Suffering] means a great deal to me so that when I'm over it I feel as though I'm past the step and I'm able to cope with anything . . . . that's my general feeling . . . . is that I'm able to cope with anything after going through it." Another participant said, "It can be a positive thing . . . . suffering. You learn from it. It is not pleasant but you learn from all of your experiences, the good and the bad, and I learned a lot. I learned a lot about myself and I learned a lot about my family . . . . each of my children handled their father's death in a different way. All suffered in their own way . . . . in different ways, and it's like I say, it can be positive and it can be negative . . ." At the level of structural integration, *paralyzing anguish with glimpses of precious possibilities* was conceptualized as *impotent wretchedness glancing the treasured.* All participants conveyed a sense of impotent wretchedness in suffering while glancing the treasured all-at-once. The impotent wretchedness rendered participants immobile yet they valued new possibles. The concept of impotent wretchedness is linked to the concept of valuing from Parse's theory.

Valuing, from Parse's (1981, 1992) first theoretical principle, relates to choosing meaning in situation which is reflective of personal values. From the perspective of Parse's (1981, 1987, 1992) theory, suffering may be regarded as a chosen way of being. To choose suffering as a way of being with a situation does not mean that people reflectively choose to experience pain or anguish. It does, however, mean that people choose the meaning given to the experience. From Parse's perspective the person who is suffering is living choices which are personal beliefs and values. Valuing relates, in part, to choosing meaning in a situation as it involves the process of confirming cherished beliefs (Cody, 1992b) through "choosing from imaged options and owning the choices" (Parse, 1981, p. 45). Suffering may be construed as a cocreated chosen way of becoming incarnated through the human-universe process. All participants revealed unique aspects of suffering reflecting their personal beliefs, values, hopes, and dreams. While participants may have regarded suffering as an undesirable experience, many indicated that they believed the experience was valuable, that it was a positive thing. In addition, many participants believed that suffering is not something to be avoided, though it is undesirable, but an inescapable part of life and for some a worthwhile experience. Suffering for the participants was not something that occurred for them alone but clearly involved others. This is consistent with Parse's view of lived experiences being cocreated (Parse, 1981, 1987, 1992). Suffering is constitutive of personal reality, a fundamental aspect of being in suffering. These findings support Parse's view that valuing is fundamental in the cocreation of reality (Parse, 1981, 1987, 1992).

The second core concept abstracted from the nine emergent propositions of this study was *entanglements of engaging-disengaging*. All of the research participants spoke of their experiences of being with and apart from others in suffering and some noted that caring support was helpful and that this sustained them. The concept of "entanglements of engaging-disengaging" captures the simultaneous "engaging with" and "disengaging from others" that characterized the lived experience of suffering; this theme pervaded the participants' descriptions. The study participants experienced a strong sense of aloneness and immersion in suffering at times, even in the presence of others, the paradox implicit in this way of being. *Entanglements of engaging-disengaging* is being with and apart from others in suffering and from the experience of suffering. The presence and support of close others was desired and valued by many research participants and yet this was also eschewed, making for entangling webs in relationships. One participant who was grieving the loss of her husband described feeling lonely and cut off from him, yet she found ways to reconnect with him. The following examples from the dialogues illustrate this concept:

Participant 1: "I guess I felt very . . . . sad a lot of the time that those feelings of alienation and being different . . . . even if I was in a big group of people and sense of being alone too . . . . a loneliness so although on the outside I might appear to be just gregariously chatting to people, and to those who really didn't know me very well, I was just someone who was either quiet or laughing or joking or dancing. On the real . . . . the real self inside was very sad, like I could even be close to tears in that sort of . . . . just company. It might be at a party or a dance or a dinner but inside I felt completely churned up and sad and an enormous overpowering feeling of despair even bordering on panic at times and . . . . a sense of being completely alone and that there was absolutely no one who could help me and not being able to pinpoint the reason why I felt that way but just feeling completely devastated really."

Participant 4: "To me it feels being ill at ease . . . . sometime the unbearable physical pains I have gone through . . . . maybe being suicidal I've thought of that . . . . it makes you feel very lonely even if you have a supportive family . . . . type of a hopelessness that if you carry on it doesn't . . . . one day seems to be one year long. Through my past experiences I know time will heal a lot so if you hang on and hang on . . . . there is always hope. During that dark period it is very lonely and very dark indeed."

Participant 6:   ". . . . then when he died I had to uproot myself. We were living in a big house, we were renting a big house . . . . I had no intention of staying there. It was marvelous . . . . for the purpose . . . . because I nursed him until three hours before he died. So I had to uproot myself and find a house to live in and move . . . . physically move, and OK I had a lot of help. But that . . . . it was a terribly busy time and in some ways it was good even though all our ties with the things we had done together were cut, in some ways it was moving and having to do all these things. It was after I had moved, and everything was right and I had gone back to work, or actually, before I had gone back to work, I came in here one day and I sat down and I thought OK well I am settled now, where is he, why doesn't he come back? I had this terribly strong feeling that he should walk through that door. I was, you know, I was right now so he could come back. But I got over that."

The core concept of entanglements of engaging-disengaging was structurally integrated with the theory of human becoming (Parse, 1992) as *enmeshed in the intimacy-solitude*. This concept captures the paradox in relating recognized by Parse (1981, 1987, 1992), as moving toward and apart from others simultaneously in suffering. The participants felt trapped in a complex web of relationships where they valued being close sometimes and not others. Intimacy was sought and valued, yet solitude was sought and valued all-at-once. There was a mixture of feelings enmeshed in the ambiguity of wanting to be with and alone all-at-once. At the level of conceptual interpretation this is expressed as *connecting-separating*, a concept from Parse's (1981, 1987, 1992) second theoretical principle. This is a paradoxical rhythm; both sides of the rhythm are present simultaneously according to Parse (1981, 1987, 1992) and unfold multidimensionally. Parse's (1981) second theoretical principle, "cocreating rhythmical patterns of relating is living the paradoxical unity of revealing-concealing, enabling-limiting and connecting-separating" (p. 50), posits paradoxical patterns of relating inherent in living. The participants' descriptions of their experiences of suffering were punctuated with connecting-separating as a paradoxical pattern of relating.

The third extracted core concept emerging from this study is *struggling in pursuit of fortification*. All participants sought ways to move through their suffering. A significant theme here was struggling to find ways to be with the anguish of their life situation. Paradox was evident as many participants felt they could "not control" their life situation in suffering but did find ways to do so. Struggle and pursuit of fortification may be conceptualized as being in "rhythmic interplay" with paralyzing anguish with glimpses of precious possibilities. The interplay is the all-at-once struggle for fortification while moving through the paralyzing anguish glimpsing other possibilities. Struggling in pursuit of fortification demonstrates mobilizing to actualize values and move beyond the struggle of suffering by affirming self. This suggests that suffering involves affirming personal existence through becoming, in the face of what may be regarded as adverse and difficult circumstances. The following examples from the dialogues illustrate the concept of "struggling in pursuit of fortification" in the language of the participants:

Participant 3: "Frustration and not being in control . . . . that sort of loop . . . . and a feeling of non-believing. I guess I've got a pretty good opinion of myself and my capabilities . . . . and the moment that something happens that shakes that belief in myself and my capabilities, I go into this state of . . . . wonderment. What the hell is going on here? Why? I have to analyze why it is going that way and hopefully if I get through that analysis I can get control back."

Participant 8: "I don't accept [suffering]; I just think I am going to . . . . I don't think about this . . . . If I start thinking about it I start to get panicky and nervous and upset . . . . I just try to fill my life . . . . I think I stay positive . . . . as the doctor said to me a few weeks back . . . . many doctors would have had you gone

twelve months ago and you are still here . . . . but I think really . . . . probably because I am as stubborn as a strong mule
and I am not giving in to this. When I was alone in the hospital
last week I was so low . . . . I just cried all night and when I do
get into depression I just can't seem to come out of it . . . . then I
just come out of it all of a sudden . . . . If I take quiet time out
or . . . . meditate, get my mind onto other things I seem to be
OK . . . ."

Participant 9:   "It's hard to explain . . . . really in feelings. It
makes me probably depressed and more worried about not being
able to do something about it . . . . That's very hard . . . . that
feels like you just want to get out and do something. You'd like to
get to somebody and give them a push to get on with it. Get some
help somehow. People who were looking after M [participant's
wife] were doing all they could and there was no better care we
knew of . . . . but you still feel that things are not going right and
not being done."

Struggling in pursuit of fortification was structurally integrated
with the theory of human becoming as *resolute affirmation*. Resolute affirmation is deliberate determination to assert being who
one is when confronted with the possibility of non-being. This
concept is linked to Parse's theoretical concept of powering. Powering is pushing-resisting toward the not-yet (Parse, 1981), a
process which involves tension and struggle for the human. It is
conceptualized as tension in the rhythm of being - non-being
(Parse, 1981). Parse asserts that non-being "refers not only to dying but to the risk of losing one's self through being rejected,
threatened, or not recognized in a manner consistent with expectations" (Parse, 1981, p. 57). Parse labels the rhythm of powering
as pushing-resisting (Parse, 1981). The concept of powering is
"incarnating one's intentions and actions in moving toward possibles" (Parse, 1981, p. 57). Resolute affirmation means that the
person in suffering is propelling onward with fortified possibles.
This involves flux in the drive to fortify being over non-being in a
life situation. Powering is the third theoretical concept in the

theoretical structure of suffering, as it is congruent with struggling in pursuit of fortification.

CONCLUSIONS

This study generated a structure of the lived experience of suffering as conceptualized within the human becoming theory (Parse, 1992). The term structure is used here as Parse's (1987) definition of the term: "Structure is the paradoxical living of the remembered, the now moment, and the not-yet all-at-once" (p. 175). The study has contributed to expansion of the theory of human becoming by uncovering a new structure which represents a lived experience of health. The findings of this study have shed light on the ascribed meaning of suffering using Parse's (1987, 1992) research methodology. The findings corroborate Parse's (1987) view of universal lived experiences of health. The phenomenon of suffering emerged in this study as a unitary event and a process of multidimensional unfolding. This unfolding is cocreated and coconstituted. These findings stand in contradistinction to normative perspectives on suffering espoused in the literature (Battenfield, 1984; Benedict, 1989; Kübler-Ross, 1969; Wilson, Blazer, & Nashold, 1976). These findings show that the lived experience of suffering is a complex experience which unfolds in living many levels of the universe all-at-once. It is not the linear sequential process that has been posited in the small number of empirical studies which have investigated the phenomenon. The structure of the lived experience of suffering elucidated in this study sheds light on the experiential dimensions of the unitary suffering experience, which has not been done before. The structure explicated the ascribed meaning of the suffering experience for the study participants, it highlighted the paradoxical patterns of relating in suffering, and it demonstrated that the person in suffering is struggling with cotranscending with the possibles. Moreover the study shows that values are of prime importance in determining the meaning of suffering.

This study has contributed to the expansion of Parse's theory of human becoming (Parse, 1992), adding a different definition of suffering to the nursing domain and enhancing the knowledge base of the discipline in general. The lived experience of suffering is specified using Parse's theoretical concepts, therefore contributing to the growth of nursing science. With regard to research, this study demonstrates further support for the use of Parse's perspective and research method (Parse, 1987, 1992). The study enhances the nursing knowledge base in relation to suffering and consequently demonstrates further the value of Parse's theory and research method for knowledge development in the discipline of nursing. Parse's method allows apprehension of the complex nature of lived experiences of health (Cody, 1992b; Mitchell, 1990). Clearly this study lends support to nursing theory-based research, which is shown to be a viable and valuable avenue for apprehending and explicating the phenomena of concern to nursing.

RECOMMENDATIONS

Several recommendations for further research can be abstracted from the findings of this study. Since the participants for this study were drawn from the general population, it may be useful to further investigate the phenomenon of suffering using specific groups in the population at large. Further light may be shed on the phenomenon of suffering by exploring its nature and ascribed meaning with people who are living in difficult life circumstances or with members of a particular cultural group or age range. Phenomena which are often confused with suffering, such as pain and loss per se, could also be investigated to evolve specific structures. This could assist in achieving greater clarity with regard to what makes these entities phenomenologically distinct. This study focused on the lived experience for the individual; a future study could investigate the lived experience of suffering for families or other groups. The sub-concepts of the structure which emerged in this study could also be investigated. A final recommendation here is investigation of the lived experience of struggling to affirm self in suffering. This study used audiotaping; a future study of suffering could use videotaping. Cody (1992b) has had considerable success with this approach, and Parse (1994) has also used this method.

Recommendations for practice include the use of the theory of human becoming in nursing practice with people who are living suffering. Parse (1987) believes that practice in a scientific discipline is guided by theory. The structure of the lived experience of suffering may be considered by the nurse when she or he is practicing with the person who is or may be suffering (Cody, 1989). This is done with the nurse in true presence with the other (Parse, 1987, 1992). Being aware of the structure changes the way the nurse is with the person in suffering; it increases understanding of the phenomenon. The structure which emerged in this study shows that the person in suffering may be experiencing paralyzing anguish while glimpsing precious possibilities with entanglements of engaging-disengaging while struggling in pursuit of fortification. The nurse can be with the suffering person in an authentic way, aware of the possible struggle of suffering, the importance of ascribed meaning and values for the person in suffering, the shifting rhythm in interpersonal relating, and the struggle of the person in trying to find ways of fortifying self while living with paralyzing anguish. The nurse can be with the person in suffering in loving and ethically appropriate ways as the person finds new ways of becoming.

REFERENCES

Battenfield, B. L. (1984). Suffering: A conceptual description and content analysis of an operational schema. *Image: The Journal of Nursing Scholarship, Vol. XVI*(2), 36–41.

Benedict, S. (1989). The suffering associated with lung cancer. *Cancer Nursing, 12*(1), 34–40.

Cassell, E. J. (1982). The nature of suffering and the goals of medicine. *New England Journal of Medicine, 306,* 639–645.

Cassell, E. J. (1991). *The nature of suffering and the goals of medicine.* New York: Oxford University Press.

Cody, W. K. (1989). *Grieving a personal loss: A preliminary investigation of Parse's man-living-health methodology.* Unpublished master's thesis, Hunter College, The City University of New York, New York.

Cody, W. K. (1992a). *The continental European human science tradition: The horizon for the development of nursing as a unique science.* Unpublished manuscript, The University of South Carolina, Columbia, SC.

Cody, W. K. (1992b). *The meaning of grieving for families living with AIDS* (Doctoral dissertation, The University of South Carolina) (University Microfilms International No. 9307924).

Copp, L. A. (1974). The spectrum of suffering. *American Journal of Nursing, 74,* 491–495.

Copp, L. A. (1990a). Treatment, torture, suffering and compassion. *Journal of Professional Nursing, 6,* 1–2.

Copp, L. A. (1990b). The nature and prevention of suffering. *Journal of Professional Nursing, 6,* 247–249.

Daly, J. (1992). *Suffering: A view from Parse's theory of human becoming.* Paper presented at the International Consortium of Parse Scholars Annual Theory Seminar, Killington, VT.

Duffy, M. E. (1992). A theoretical and empirical review of the concept of suffering. In P. Starck & J. P. McGovern (Eds.), *The hidden dimension of illness: Human suffering.* New York: National League for Nursing Press.

Eriksson, K. (1992). The alleviation of suffering: The idea of caring. *Scandinavian Journal of Caring Sciences, 6*(2), 119–123.

Goldberg, C. (1986). Concerning human suffering. *The Psychiatric Journal of the University of Ottawa, 11,* 97–104.

Kahn, D. L., & Steeves, R. H. (1986). The experience of suffering: Conceptual clarification and theoretical definition. *Journal of Advanced Nursing, 11,* 623–631.

Kübler-Ross, E. (1969). *On death and dying.* New York: Macmillan.

Mitchell, G. J. (1990). The lived experience of taking life day-by-day in later life: Research guided by Parse's emergent method. *Nursing Science Quarterly, 3,* 29–36.

Morse, J. M., & Johnson, J. L. (1991). Toward a theory of illness: The illness-constellation model. In J. M. Morse & J. L. Johnson (Eds.), *The illness experience: Dimensions of suffering.* Newbury Park, CA: Sage.

Oiler Boyd, C. (1990). Critical appraisal of developing nursing research methods. *Nursing Science Quarterly, 3,* 42–43.

Parse, R. R. (1981). Man-living-health: A theory of nursing. New York: Wiley.

Parse, R. R. (1987). Nursing science: Major paradigms, theories and critiques. Philadelphia: Saunders.

Parse, R. R. (1992). Human becoming: Parse's theory of nursing. *Nursing Science Quarterly, 5,* 35–42.

Parse, R. R. (1993). Response: Theory guides research and practice. *Nursing Science Quarterly, 6,* 12.

Parse, R. R. (1994). Quality of life: Sciencing and living the art of human becoming. *Nursing Science Quarterly, 7,* 16–21.

Pilkington, F. B. (1993). The lived experience of grieving the loss of an important other. *Nursing Science Quarterly, 6,* 130–139.

Ray, M. A. (1990). Critical reflective analysis of Parse's and Newman's research methodologies. *Nursing Science Quarterly, 3,* 44–46.

Starck, P. L., & McGovern, J. P. (Eds.). (1992). *The hidden dimension of illness: Human suffering.* New York: National League for Nursing.

Wilson, H. S. (1989). Nursing research. Menlo Park, CA: Addison-Wesley.

Wilson, W. P., Blazer, D. G., & Nashold, B. S. (1976). Observations on pain and suffering. *Psychosomatics, 17*(2), 73–76.

Chapter 16

Of Life Immense in Passion, Pulse, and Power: Dialoguing With Whitman and Parse— A Hermeneutic Study

William K. Cody

*I*n this hermeneutic study, selected poems from Walt Whitman's (1892/1983) *Leaves of Grass* were interpreted in light of Parse's (1981, 1992, 1994a) human becoming theory. *Leaves of Grass* is, by Whitman's own description, an uncompromising expression of his own "Personality" within the context of the "spirit and facts" of his time (Whitman, 1892/1983, p. 444). The human becoming theory articulates Parse's perspective of the *human-universe-health* process (Parse, 1992). Each author's work, then, relates to the question, *what does it mean to be human?* This, the central question of the human sciences, was also the research question posed in this study.

In the first section of this chapter, a brief overview of hermeneutics is presented, leading to a discussion of specific beliefs about interpretation and understanding that are consistent with Parse's theory. In the pages which follow, the poetry of Walt Whitman is introduced, and selections from *Leaves of Grass* which relate to the research question are presented. Interpretive commentary is interspersed among the verse. In the final pages of the chapter, an interpretation of the meaning of the text in relation to the question, what does it mean to be human?, is explicated and reflected upon.

DILTHEY, HUMAN SCIENCE, AND HERMENEUTICS

Until the mid-19th century, hermeneutics was principally concerned with the interpretation of Biblical texts, and it has played an important role in theology and the history of religion. Present-day understanding of classical texts from antiquity represents centuries of hermeneutic inquiry as well. Juridicial hermeneutics forms another major branch of the discipline. In the 19th century, several German scholars explicated hermeneutics as the principal mode of historical inquiry. Wilhelm Dilthey further suggested that hermeneutics could be regarded as the principal methodology of all the human sciences. For Dilthey, human studies were to be concerned with one central phenomenon, *life as it is humanly lived.* Although he posited the *lived experience* as the fundamental datum of human science, Dilthey (in contradistinction to the phenomenologists) believed that lived experience was too overwhelmingly personal to be rigorously studied through direct investigation. Instead, he proposed that the proper objects of study in the human sciences were *"expressions of life,"* literary works, works of art, social organizations, and cultures, through which, he said, an understanding of lived experience could be gained (Dilthey, 1988; Ermarth, 1978; Polkinghorne, 1983).

HEIDEGGER AND GADAMER:
HERMENEUTIC ONTOLOGY

Martin Heidegger (1927/1962) shifted hermeneutics from methodology into *ontology* in his study, *Being and Time,* in which he proposed that *understanding* was a fundamental form of human existence: "The kind of Being which Dasein [the human] has, as potentiality-for-Being, lies existentially in understanding" (p. 183). The dichotomy of subject and object (or subjective and objective knowledge) dissolves in this frame of reference. Being-in-the-world, Heidegger said, is a unitary phenomenon, in which one's having-been and potentiality-for-Being are disclosed as standing-out against the *horizonal unity of temporality* (pp. 383–418). This means that the human being has something like a horizon upon which past, present, and future are disclosed, and these comprise one's "world." Ontologically, the horizon of one's life (or Being) is unitary; however, the horizon as it appears in the moment ("Being-there") may be regarded as a horizon, and thus there are innumerable horizons in one's whole life experience.

The "hermeneutic circle," as described by Heidegger and elaborated by Gadamer, represents "understanding as the interplay of the movement of tradition and the movement of the interpreter" (Gadamer, 1989, p. 293). A *tradition* is a belief system which *lives* through *discourse*. A text, as something written and read, is a form of discourse. The image of a circle illustrates the "tension" in the interplay "between the . . . text's strangeness and familiarity to us. . . . *The true locus of hermeneutics is this in-between*" (p. 295), that is, the process, or *movement* of understanding. "It is enough to say that we understand in a *different* way, *if we understand at all*" (p. 297). Thus, the movement is best characterized not as a circle but a *spiral* and is called "the hermeneutic spiral" in this chapter.

Gadamer (1976, 1989) wrote of philosophical hermeneutics as a discipline concerned with the fundamental conditions of understanding (human existence) in all its modes. This is the hermeneutic tradition with which this study, rooted in nursing science, connects. This study is not concerned with "objective" knowledge of what the author meant (although every clue to his intent is significant) but rather with *what the text means for the interpreter*. Making this explicit merely reflects the epistemological significance of a hermeneutic ontology.

All human life unfolds in a context of meaning. "Upon careful reflection, a brief moment of experience holds seemingly endless information which lies throughout different strata of awareness" (Polkinghorne, 1983, p. 215). In the encounter with the unfamiliar a different experience surfaces as a possibility, a potential horizon. Understanding is the realization of that potential, and this is referred to as *the fusion of horizons*. With regard to interpreting a text, the fusion of horizons has been described as a "a dialectical interaction between the expectations of the interpreter and the meanings in the text. . . . Interpretation is a mediation or construction between each interpreter's own language and the language of the text" (Polkinghorne, 1983, p. 226). Language is the horizon of hermeneutic ontology (Gadamer, 1989).

THE HERMENEUTIC SITUATION FOR THE STUDY

Both Whitman and Parse, as groundbreakers and visionaries, were obliged to create the vocabularies through which to give voice to their visions. Each author drew on tradition and broke with tradition to found a *new* tradition. In this study, the researcher set out to coparticipate in a dialogue between the two traditions they originated. Gadamer (1989) has written, "Working out the hermeneutic situation means acquiring the right horizon of inquiry for the questions evoked by the encounter with tradition" (p. 302). This means clarifying and making explicit one's orientation toward the encounter.

The hermeneutic process has been described differently by various authors. Dilthey (1988) once proposed that understanding of a text was achieved through the reader's self-projection into the author's world. Heidegger (1962) and Gadamer (1989) believed that this was impossible and proposed that understanding emerging from one's *fore-knowing* or *"prejudice"* was the only understanding possible. This fore-knowing or prejudice is always with one but is not static; it is "worked out" in the encounter with the unfamiliar, here called the *hermeneutic spiral*. Gadamer and others have further described the *situatedness* which is the condition for all understanding. Every human being is embedded in a historico-cultural context within which one understands all that *is* in his or her world; yet that which is first encountered as unfamiliar presents a possibility of further understanding and becoming familiar. The very fact that one can connect with something other and unfamiliar attests to the openness of one's horizon, or situatedness (Gadamer, 1989, p. 295).

Bernstein (1983), drawing on Gadamer's work, discusses the dynamics of discourse in communities (not necessarily geographic in the modern world), in which encounters between the familiar and the unfamiliar continually unfold through a primal dialogue, or *dialectic*, which is fundamentally hermeneutic in nature. This is an intersubjective process through which human beings, confronted with different beliefs, understand the other, assimilate new ideas, and most importantly, understand themselves. One cannot rise above this dialectic process for an objective view; understanding surfaces through *participation* in it (Bernstein, 1983; Gadamer, 1989). Such understanding precedes, succeeds, and pervades objective knowledge. This is clearly seen in the process of reflectively deciding upon an action, which is never based solely on objective knowledge itself but is worked out through what is traditionally referred to as *phronesis*, practical/moral reasoning based in human values (Bernstein, 1983; Gadamer, 1989). In a similar vein, Gadamer (1989) and Langer (1967) have explored the interrelation of aesthetics, symbology, understanding, and knowledge, with particular attention to the *truths* which live through symbols and art and are neither accessible nor explicable through objectivist inquiry.

Ricoeur (1976) has discussed what he calls the *"productive distanciation"* between reader and text, which is "a dialectical trait," the "struggle between the otherness that transforms all spatial and temporal distance into cultural estrangement and the ownness by which all understanding aims at the extension of self-understanding" (p. 43). Distanciation, then, is the condition that makes appropriation of the meaning of the text possible. Ricoeur also explicated the dynamic interaction (first conceived in structural linguistics) between the language system *(langue)* and the speech event *(parole)*, which he extends to textual discourse. Discourse draws on the organized patterns of an extant language system, a system of encoded meanings, yet brings it to *life* and introduces new meanings—for example, through metaphors, which live in discursive events and are not found in dictionaries. There is, then, an ongoing dialectic between discourse as event and as meaning, and thus a perpetual *"surplus of meaning"* (Ricoeur, 1976). This echoes a common theme throughout the human science tradition, the inexhaustibility of meaning.

Through reflecting on these ideas from hermeneutics and hermeneutic ontology in light of the assumptions and principles of Parse's (1981, 1992, 1994a) theory, the researcher explicated the processes of *discoursing, interpreting, and understanding* from the perspective of Parse's theory of human becoming. This explication is presented in Table 16.1, which shows the congruence of the ontological beliefs of the human becoming theory and hermeneutics as a mode of inquiry. The major author from whom the researcher drew for his understanding of hermeneutics is Gadamer (1976, 1989), whose views are generally consistent with Parse's.

HERMENEUTICS AND NURSING AS A HUMAN SCIENCE

Hermeneutic inquiry has received only limited attention in nursing to date (Allen & Jensen, 1990; Reeder, 1988; Thompson, 1990), and there has been minimal scholarly discussion of the relation between hermeneutic ontology and the ontology of any extant theory of nursing. The predominant paradigm in nursing is rooted in an empirical-analytical tradition, in which the researcher's personal interpretation, in the main, is considered biased, unreliable, and of questionable validity. The consequence of this stance is to limit the range of human phenomena investigated, the research questions asked, and the depth in which the human is understood.

Table 16.1   Discoursing, Interpreting, and Understanding: Explication of the Human Becoming Perspective

Parses' Theory of Human Becoming	Connections With Hermeneutics
Assumption 1	
Human becoming is freely choosing personal meaning in situation in the intersubjective process of relating value priorities.	Understanding as a mode of Being (Heidegger, Gadamer)
Principle 1	
Structuring meaning multidimensionally is cocreating reality through the languaging of imaging and valuing.	Language as the horizon of hermeneutic ontology (Gadamer) Fore-knowing; prejudice (Heidegger, Gadamer) Artistic truths (Gadamer, Langer)

Explication 1   *Discoursing* is the interplay of shared and unshared meanings through which beliefs are appropriated and disappropriated. A text, as something written and read, is a form of discourse. Author and reader are *discoursing* whenever the text is read.

Assumption 2	
Human becoming is cocreating rhythmical patterns of relating in open process with the universe.	The hermeneutic circle (Heidegger, Gadamer)
Principle 2	
Cocreating rhythmical patterns of relating is living the paradoxical unity of revealing-concealing, enabling-limiting while connecting-separating.	Langue/parole; the surplus of meaning (Ricoeur) Situatedness (Gadamer) Productive distanciation (Ricoeur)

Explication 2   *Interpreting* is expanding the meaning moment through dwelling in situated openness with the disclosed and the hidden. Interpreting a text is constructing meanings with the text through the rhythmic movement between the language of the text and the language of the researcher.

Table 16.1   (Continued)

Assumption 3

Human becoming is cotranscending multidimensionally with the emerging possibles.	Horizonal unity of temporality (Heidegger)

Principle 3

Cotranscending with the possibles is powering unique ways of originating in the process of transforming.	The fusion of horizons (Gadamer)
	Dialectic (Gadamer, Bernstein)
	Phronesis (Gadamer, Bernstein)

Explication 3 — *Understanding* is choosing from possibilities a unique way of moving beyond the meaning moment. Understanding a text is interweaving the meaning of the text with the pattern of one's life in a chosen way.

Parse's theory of human becoming quoted from Parse (1992, p. 38); elements of hermeneutics taken from Bernstein (1983), Gadamer (1989), Heidegger (1962), Langer (1967), and Ricoeur (1976).

The simultaneity paradigm, however, birthed by Rogers (1970) and expanded and specified by Parse (1981, 1987), posits a new basis for understanding the phenomena of concern to nursing (actually, then, different phenomena) and invites exploration of different modes of inquiry. The use of hermeneutic inquiry is consistent with the beliefs underpinning the simultaneity paradigm: that the human-universe-health process is an evolving unity characterized by multidimensional patterns in which the human coparticipates through personal knowing and choosing (Parse, 1987).

The use of hermeneutic inquiry has even greater relevance to Parse's human becoming theory specifically, since Parse (1981) views nursing as a *human science* concerned with the human's qualitative health experience. Health is defined in the theory as a "process of becoming as experienced and described by the person"

(Parse, 1992, p. 36). Nursing inquiry from the human becoming perspective focuses on uncovering the meanings of lived experiences of health. Parse's (1987, 1990b) research methodology is intended for the phenomenological study of lived experiences. Parse's methodology is clearly a *hermeneutic*-phenomenological one, but it is not intended to facilitate engagement with a literary text. For this study, the researcher borrowed a page from Dilthey to investigate the meaning of a specified *expression of life*, namely Whitman's *Leaves of Grass.*

THE HORIZON OF INQUIRY: PARSE'S HUMAN BECOMING THEORY

This author's understanding of what it means to be human is rooted in the belief system of Parse's (1981, 1992) human becoming theory. He lives in this tradition. The central belief of the tradition is specified at the theoretical level of discourse: human becoming is "structuring meaning multidimensionally in cocreating rhythmical patterns of relating while cotranscending with the possibles" (Parse, 1981, p. 41). The human becoming theory has been elaborated and further specified by Parse (1987, 1990a, 1990b, 1992, 1993, 1994a) and others (for example, Cody, 1991; Jonas, 1992; Mitchell, 1990; Smith, 1990). For nurses who are living the tradition, the theory guides practice and inquiry.

Within the belief system of the human becoming theory are beliefs and concepts that are interconnected with the discursive traditions of human science as founded by Dilthey (1988), existential-phenomenology (Heidegger, 1962), and hermeneutic ontology (Gadamer, 1989). The preeminent concern with humanly lived experience shows the connection between Parse's work and Dilthey's human science tradition. The belief that structuring meaning is cocreating reality is related to Heidegger's view that understanding is a mode of Being. The belief that "the human is coexisting while coconstituting rhythmical patterns with the universe" (Parse, 1992, p. 38) is related to ideas about traditions, discourse, and dialectic discussed by Gadamer and Ricoeur.

But there are also crucial distinctions between Parse's perspective and those of the other authors. For example, the hermeneuts (some more than others) tend to differentiate "understanding" and "meaning" in a way that preserves the subject-object dichotomy, which is in conflict with Parse's principle of *structuring meaning multidimensionally* with its key philosophical concept of *cocreating*. For the most part the hermeneuts also continue to regard understanding and misunderstanding as opposites, despite their own assertions of the ontological significance of understanding itself. This is connected with Heidegger's view of "authentic" and "inauthentic" Being. Parse, in contrast, speaks of *"freely choosing personal meaning* [italics added] in situations in the intersubjective process of relating value priorities" (1992, p. 38). "Misunderstanding" as a construct is illogical from this frame of reference. These and other distinctions necessitated the explication of a hermeneutic process for interpreting and understanding discourse congruent with the human becoming belief system—the researcher's belief system (see Table 16.1). There would be no point at all to conducting hermeneutic inquiry if the processes of inquiry used were incongruent with the researcher's ontological beliefs.

A horizon of inquiry is *always open,* since, as Gadamer (1989, p. 304) stated, "The historical movement of human life consists in the fact that it is never absolutely bound to any one standpoint, and hence can never have a truly closed horizon." Thus, Whitman's work (though in a sense "fixed" in the text) is open to further interpretation; and the theory of human becoming, the nursing tradition in which this author lives, is open to further interpretation through discourse which connects it with other traditions. The goal of this particular interpretation is enhancement of the human becoming belief system, the horizon of inquiry for the study, through exploring Whitman's "answer" to the question, what does it mean to be human?

SIGNIFICANCE FOR NURSING SCIENCE

From the perspective of the theory of human becoming, the goal of nursing inquiry is to enhance understanding of lived experiences of health—multidimensional experiences of becoming with the universe. Whitman dedicated his life to the expression of what it meant for him to be a human being in his world. There is a fit between the researcher's goal of enhanced understanding of humanly lived experience and Whitman's purpose in chronicling his own life. Approaching Whitman's text from the perspective of Parse's theory, reflectively aware of his stated purpose, therefore has the potential to contribute to the expansion of nursing as a human science. Dialoguing with Whitman, through the medium of his poetry, and Parse, through the language and ideas in her theory, offers the possibility of expanding and specifying the theory through working out the "tension" in the interplay "between the . . . text's strangeness and familiarity" (Gadamer, 1989, p. 295).

THE TRAJECTORY OF THE STUDY

The hermeneutic processes used in this study were not formalized beforehand but were worked out along the way (see Table 16.1). The trajectory of the study is presented in Table 16.2. "The hermeneutic spiral" is not an extraordinary process but is inherent in life; it describes the way of all understanding. "The fusion of horizons" is simply the transformative moment in understanding (Gadamer, 1989, pp. 302–307).

In engaging with *Leaves of Grass*, the researcher read the entire text several times, with particular attention to sections of special interest, specifically those poems most relevant to the research question. Selected passages were marked for reference, and notes were made pertaining to various possible interpretations. Unfamiliar words were found in the dictionary and their

Table 16.2   The Trajectory of the Study

Major Process

Moving through the hermeneutic spiral: A continuous all-at-once process, the rhythms of which are the meaning moments.

Dimensions of the Process

Engaging: The researcher, who lives the belief system (tradition) of Parse's human becoming theory of nursing, initiated a dialogue with Whitman's poems, which were presented by the poet as an expression of his life. This connects across traditions with Dilthey's work on expressions of life.

Questioning: Whitman's stated purpose fit with the central question of human science, what does it mean to be human? Gadamer says, "The text asks the question." The question surfaced in the dialogue and the researcher chose to seek an answer with the text.

Configuring the inquiry: The researcher reflected on the tradition and language of Parse's nursing theory as the horizon for interpreting a literary expression of life. A critical examination of hermeneutic theories in light of Parse's nursing theory led to an explication of the processes of discoursing, interpreting, and understanding from the human becoming perspective.

Constructing meanings: This was the moment-to-moment moving between Whitman's language and the researcher's language, a process of questioning and answering and questioning anew. This is the essence of the hermeneutic process. Here the researcher's tradition and language (human becoming theory) were engaged directly in the struggle with Whitman's tradition and language. The literary traditions associated with Whitman's work are American romanticism (of which it is considered the apex) and American modernism (the origin).

Fusing horizons: This is assigning meaning to the text through appropriating and disappropriating beliefs. Truths emerging from the researcher-text dialectic were identified by the researcher.

Disseminating possibilities: The researcher set in text for publication his interpretation of Whitman's perspective, offering it as a possibility for the enhancement of nursing science. He proposes that hermeneutic inquiry surfaces truths of vital importance to the discipline of nursing.

definitions *apropos* to Whitman's era noted. Several secondary sources (Allen, 1955; Asselineau, 1960; Miller, 1957, 1964) were perused to enrich the researcher's knowledge base. The researcher's own *reading of the text*, however, was the predominant mode of this inquiry.

As to technique, the fundamental unit of interpretation, as Ricoeur (1976) has pointed out, is the *sentence*, which consists essentially of an identifier (noun) and a predicate (verb). A given sentence may be understood in two contexts, that of *la langue* and that of *la parole* (discussed previously); for interpretive clarity it must be understood in both contexts; thus, the reader must engage with the language system for the literal meaning and the text as a situated whole for the figurative meaning. Working out this process in coherence with the researcher's beliefs about human becoming (Parse, 1981, 1987, 1992), the event of reading is seen as the meaning moment: connecting all-at-once with the contexts available in the moment, the reader moves onward to a new understanding through appropriating-disappropriating the possible meanings as they arise. There can be no absolute certainty that the meaning appropriated is the meaning the author intended. *Fusing horizons* is choosing the meaning of the text from among the possible interpretations and making explicit the understanding reached through the hermeneutic process. Gadamer and Parse would agree that *understanding* in this sense goes beyond reflection alone. It is the way the meaning *lives* in the interpreter's life. It is a form of truth.

WALT WHITMAN

Walt Whitman is widely regarded as one of the greatest American poets. *Leaves of Grass*, his *magnum opus*, first published in 1855, is a book of poems on which he labored for nearly forty years. The work, unique both philosophically and stylistically, proclaimed reverence for the individual, celebration of everyday life, and personal communion with the universe, in boldly rambling free verse. Whitman worked on *Leaves of Grass* for the rest of his life. The final edition, the seventh, was published in 1892; his book had grown from 95 pages to over 400. This was the edition used in this study (Whitman, 1892/1983).

Whitman is considered to be the first poet to fully capture the "spirit" of America, with his proud emphasis on the common person and individualistic "Democracy." He is associated with romanticism and transcendentalism for his love of nature and his emphasis on spirit and intuition. He is known for his synthesis of these views in positing that the body and the soul are united in communion with nature. But the consensus of criticism is that his greatest contribution is in explicating *the self*. Largely in connection with the theme of the self, the frank intimacy of his poems, and his free-flowing style, he is considered the primary originator of American literary modernism (Allen, 1955; Asselineau, 1960; Miller, 1957, 1964).

Whitman (1892/1983) wrote that his aim in writing *Leaves of Grass* was "to articulate and faithfully express in literary or poetic form, and uncompromisingly, my own physical, emotional, moral, intellectual, and aesthetic Personality, in the midst of, and tallying, the momentous spirit and facts of its immediate days . . ." (p. 444). He also wrote, "I avowedly chant 'the great pride of man in himself,' and permit it to be more or less a *motif* of all my verse" (Whitman, 1892/1983, p. 453). Whitman regarded the body and soul as "identical" (p. 451) and repeatedly explored this theme in his poems. Another major theme for Whitman was the relationship between himself and his world, or, more accurately, his "kosmos" or universe. This is connected with his celebration of the "New World," a liberating and heretofore unknown realm in which human individuality and communion with one another and nature are equally celebrated. In the midst of his lifelong work, his world became embroiled with the Civil War. Whitman volunteered to minister to the wounded Union soldiers and wrote voluminously about his experiences with the war. These poems, however, do not "ask" the research question for this study so clearly as others, and, in light of space limitations, are not addressed herein. In reading *Leaves of Grass* one meets a poet who seeks to uncover his own way of being, in the "presence" of the reader, through vividly and eloquently describing his own world.

ENGAGING WITH WHITMAN'S POETRY

In *Leaves of Grass*, Whitman presents the reader with an elaborate tapestry, a detailed and deeply considered perspective of one man's life. It would be impossible to represent this monumental work (truly a whole life's work) adequately in this chapter. Selected short poems and sections of longer poems from the text are presented. The researcher's comments are interjected to draw out the interpretive connections to Parse's theory. The opening lines of *Leaves of Grass* read as follows:

From **"One's-Self I Sing"**

One's-Self I sing, a simple separate person,
Yet utter the word Democratic, the word En-Masse . . .
Of Life immense in passion, pulse, and power,
Cheerful, for freest action form'd under the laws divine,
The Modern Man I sing.

The title of this study is taken from this poem, in which one line concisely suggests Whitman's beliefs about *life—"immense in passion, pulse, and power."* The three qualities of "life" named in this line directly and vividly relate to Parse's three central themes, *meaning, rhythmicity, and transcendence* and their corresponding principles. Both authors posit the human as: passionate, never without meaning in life; moving with others and the universe in rhythmic, flowing patterns; and moving and acting with a fundamental freedom through the very power of one's existence as who one is.

The first score of poems in *Leaves of Grass* are collectively titled "Inscriptions" and serve to introduce the book. The following
poem is essentially a dedication of Whitman's work to the human
being.

"For Him I Sing"

For him I sing,
I raise the present on the past,
(As some perennial tree out of its roots, the present on the
    past,)
With time and space I him dilate and fuse the immortal laws,
To make himself by them the law unto himself.

The last two lines allude to Whitman's belief that the human being
need not succumb to the conventional notions of time and space,
nor abide with any law other than that of the self.

From "I Hear America Singing"

I hear America singing, the varied carols I hear,
Those of mechanics, each one singing his as it should be
        blithe and strong,
The carpenter singing his as he measures his plank or beam,
The mason singing his as he makes ready for work, or leaves
        off work,
The boatman singing what belongs to him in his boat . . .
The delicious singing of the mother, or of the young wife
        at work, or of the girl sewing or washing,
Each singing what belongs to him or her and to none
        else. . . .

Here Whitman is celebrating the diversity of human life. He affirms that the song each person sings is the expression of who

each one is. In every case the song is unique, and yet he hears and appreciates each among the myriad for what it is. This is one of his major themes. Parse, too, says that each person's way of being is unique, that "it is like a fingerprint in that it belongs to only one human being and while others coexist in the large journey of life, each lives his or her own way on the journey" (1990a, p. 139). She says that health is "a personal commitment," the living of values that cannot be prescribed or described by societal norms . . . [and] cannot be described as good or bad, more or less" (p. 137).

"Starting from Paumanok" is the first long poem in *Leaves of Grass.* Paumanok was Whitman's birthplace on Long Island. His rock-solid belief in his own life experience is proclaimed in every stanza.

From **"Starting from Paumanok"**

Starting from fish-shape Paumanok where I was born,
Well-begotten, and rais'd by a perfect mother,
After roaming many lands, lover of populous pavements. . . .
Aware of the fresh free giver the flowing Missouri, aware of
    mighty Niagara,
Aware of the buffalo herds grazing the plains . . .

Of earth, rocks, Fifth-month flowers experienced, stars, rain,
    snow, my amaze,
Having studied the mocking-bird's tones and the flight of the
    mountain-hawk . . .
Solitary, singing in the West, I strike up for a New World. . . .

Victory, union, faith, identity, time,
The indissoluble compacts, riches, mystery,
Eternal progress, the kosmos, and the modern reports.

This then is life,
Here is what has come to the surface after so many throes
    and convulsions. . . .

Whitman is further announcing his themes as he describes how his perspective arose within the whole of his life experience. For Whitman, life *is* "victory, union, faith, identity, time, / the indissoluble compacts, riches, mystery, / eternal progress, the kosmos, and the modern reports. . . ." Parse (1981, 1992) closely concurs with Whitman in that she describes living health as the multidimensional human-universe process replete with paradoxical struggles and joys inspired by one's personal beliefs, manifesting the interconnectedness of the individual with multiple realms of the universe all-at-once. Whitman believes he has reached a new understanding of life, something fundamentally closer to truth than the historically received views. He writes, "Here is what has come to the surface after so many throes and convulsions. . . ." He continues—

. . . I sat studying at the feet of the great masters,
Now if eligible O that the great masters might return and
    study me.

In the name of these States shall I scorn the antique?
Why there are the children of the antique to justify it.

These lines presage the idea, articulated by Parse (1981), that the human coexists with contemporaries, predecessors, and successors all-at-once, while also acknowledging the historicity of human existence. Parse says that the human cocreates predecessors (Whitman's "the great masters") as they cocreate the human in the now (Whitman's "the children of the antique") all-at-once.

Dead poets, philosophs, priests,
Martyrs, artists, inventors, governments long since,
Language-shapers on other shores,
Nations once powerful, now reduced, withdrawn, or desolate,
I dare not proceed till I respectfully credit what you have left
    wafted hither,

I have perused it, own it is admirable, (moving awhile among
    it,)
Think nothing can ever be greater, nothing can ever deserve
    more than it deserves,
Regarding it all intently a long while, then dismissing it,
I stand in my place with my own day here.

Here Whitman deferentially salutes the great shapers of thought
and movers of history, even though they be "dead" or "desolate"
now, "nothing can ever deserve more" than what they have "left
wafted hither." Nonetheless, Whitman resolutely claims his *own*
place and day "here." Parse (1981) says that "an experience of a
situation, while cocreated with others, belongs to one human being only" (p. 30) and that one's "personal reality incarnates all
that a person is, has been, and will become all-at-once" (p. 42).
"Starting from Paumanok," with the reference to Whitman's
birthplace, suggests that the poem in a sense tells his life story.
Whitman's journey through life extends backward and forward in
time and whisks him across continents and oceans in a heartbeat.
Parse says that human beings choose from options "from the various realms of the universe" and "what is *real* for each individual
is structured by that individual" (1992, p. 37). Further, in cotranscending with the possibles, "threads of what *was* and *is* [italics
added] weave with the new and can be recognized in the fabric of
one's life" (p. 39). These words echo the following lines as Whitman continues—

I will make the true poem of riches. . . .
And I will show that there is no imperfection in the present,
    and can be none in the future,
And I will show that whatever happens to anybody it may be
    turn'd to beautiful results,
And I will show that nothing can happen more beautiful than
    death,
And I will thread a thread through my poems that time and
    events are compact,

> And that all the things of the universe are perfect miracles,
>   each as profound as any.

The following lines of the poem reflect Whitman's great urge to express the fundamental unity which he believed connected all things.

> I will not make poems with reference to parts,
> But I will make poems, songs, thoughts, with reference to
>   ensemble,
> And I will not sing with reference to a day, but with
>   reference to all days,
> And I will not make a poem nor the least part of a poem but
>   has reference to the soul,
> Because having look'd at the objects of the universe, I find
>   there is no one nor any particle of one but has
>   reference to the soul. . . .
>
> Was somebody asking to see the soul?
> See, your own shape and countenance, persons, substances,
>   beasts, the trees, the running rivers, the rocks and
>   sands. . . .
> Behold, the body includes and is the meaning, the main
>   concern, and includes and is the soul. . . .

Several major themes are threaded through the foregoing lines. Whitman speaks of the perfect wholeness of the universe, without divisions among body, soul, and cosmos. Parse says that "humans are open beings in mutual process with the universe," and indeed, "the construct human becoming refers to the human-universe-health process" (1992, p. 41). Both authors portray human existence as having qualities of openness and timelessness, even as this expansive life is incarnated, in the body, for Whitman, and in the human-universe process for Parse. In the next stanza Whitman hails and calls out to numerous lands and people.

. . . Land of the ocean shores! land of sierras and peaks!
Land of boatmen and sailors! fishermen's land!
Inextricable lands! the clutch'd together! the passionate ones!
The side by side! the elder and younger brothers! the bony-
    limb'd!
The great women's land! the feminine! the experienced sisters
    and the inexperienced sisters!
Far-breath'd land! Arctic braced! Mexican breez'd! the
    diverse! the compact!
. . . O all and each well-loved by me! my intrepid nations! O
    I at any rate include you all with perfect love!
I cannot be discharged from you! not from one any sooner
    than another!

These lines reveal Whitman's conviction that he belonged to all that held meaning for him and that all that held meaning for him belonged to him. Whitman and his world are in essence described as inseparable. *The diverse and the compact* (taken together) is a recurring reference in Whitman's poems. Here he says to all the people and lands of the earth, "O I at any rate include you all with perfect love! / I cannot be discharged from you!" suggesting that these are in some sense in him, and he in them. Parse says the human is "not alone in any dimension of becoming" (1981, p. 20); synergistically and multidimensionally cotranscending with the possibles "powers and compounds the creation of individual patterns of relating" (p. 33). This idea connects to Whitman's poem here in that, while the title refers back to his birthplace, beginning with the first lines Whitman's verse encompasses towns, cities, continents, stars . . . and lovingly embraces every person on the far-ranging journey. He urges his companion (the reader) to join him in the ceaseless rush toward the new.

. . . With me with firm holding, yet haste, haste on. . . .

Bearded, sun-burnt, gray-neck'd, forbidding, I have arrived,
To be wrestled with as I pass for the solid prizes of the
    universe,
For such I afford whoever can persevere to win them. . . .

Expanding and swift, henceforth,
Elements, breeds, adjustments, turbulent, quick and audacious,
A world primal again, vistas of glory incessant and branching,
A new race dominating previous ones and grander far, with
      new contests,
New politics, new literatures and religions, new inventions
      and arts.

These, my voice announcing—I will sleep no more but arise,
You oceans that have been calm within me! how I feel you,
      fathomless, stirring, preparing unprecedented waves
      and storms. . . .

O a word to clear one's path ahead endlessly! . . . .

O to haste firm holding—to haste, haste on with me.

                    *   *   *

"Song of Myself" is one of Whitman's more famous and complex
poems. Its subject is his best known theme, which he once referred to as "the miracle of *identity*." The poem is 50 pages long;
the following excerpts were selected in relation to the central
theme of the poem and the research question for the study.

From **"Song of Myself"**

I celebrate myself, and sing myself,
And what I assume you shall assume,
For every atom belonging to me as good belongs to you.

I loafe and invite my soul,
I lean and loafe at my ease observing a spear of summer grass.
My tongue, every atom of my blood, form'd from this soil,
      this air,
Born here of parents born here from parents the same, and
      their parents the same,
I, now thirty-seven years old in perfect health begin,
Hoping to cease not till death.

Creeds and schools in abeyance,
Retiring back a while sufficed at what they are, but never
     forgotten,
I harbor for good or bad, I permit to speak at every hazard,
Nature without check with original energy. . . .

. . . The smoke of my own breath,
Echoes, ripples, buzz'd whispers, love-root, silk-thread,
     crotch and vine,
My respiration and inspiration, the beating of my heart, the
     passing of blood and air through my lungs,
The sniff of green leaves and dry leaves, and of the shore and
     dark-color'd sea-rocks, and of hay in the barn,
The sound of the belch'd words of my voice loos'd to the eddies
     of the wind. . . .
The play of shine and shade on the trees as the supple boughs
     wag,
The flight alone or in the rush of the streets, or along the
     fields and hill-sides,
The feeling of health, the full-noon trill, the song of me rising
     from bed and meeting the sun . . . .

In the context of the poem as a whole, when Whitman says he was "born here from parents born here and their parents the same," he seems to be talking about *the world,* as all human beings are born into a world. He also writes, "I, now 37 years old in perfect health . . ." although Whitman's "health," if construed in the conventional sense, was never what would ordinarily be called good (Allen, 1955). Yet he continued to write about his good, "robust," or even "perfect" health after he had suffered a stroke and hemiparalysis (though in 1891, a year before his death, he did concede a few lines about his "ills and exhaustions"). Clearly Whitman is working with an unconventional notion of "health." Parse says health *"is just the way the human is!"* (1990, p. 137). Whitman's use of the word, some 140 years ago, is surprisingly consistent with Parse's. Whitman's description of his communion with nature provides a vivid and loving portrayal of what Parse

(1992) calls the human-universe-health process, as he repeatedly emphasizes his interconnectedness with the universe (nature, the world, the cosmos) and its profoundly personal meaning in his life.

The next lines from "Song of Myself" reveal Whitman's beliefs about human knowledge and understanding:

> . ., . Stop this day and night with me and you shall possess
>   the origin of all poems,
> You shall possess the good of the earth and sun, (there are
>   millions of suns left,). . . .
> You shall no longer take things at second or third hand,
>   nor look through the eyes of the dead,
>   nor feed on the spectres in books,
> You shall not look through my eyes either, nor take things
>   from me,
> You shall listen to all sides and filter them from your self. . . .

Whitman continuously plays off the tension between his fiercely held views about the nature of the self's relation with the world and his insistence that the reader must nonetheless "filter" and decide every issue for her- or himself; indeed, he declares both passionately. Parse says the human cocreates becoming with the universe through freely choosing in situation (1992, p. 36) and refers to the human as "coauthor" of health, which is the set of choices the person in a situation makes from many realms of the universe (1990, p. 137). "Song of Myself" continues—

> I have heard what the talkers were talking, the talk of the
>   beginning and the end,
> But I do not talk of the beginning or the end.
>
> There was never any more inception than there is now,
> Nor any more youth or age then there is now,
> And will never be any more perfection than there is now,
> Nor any more heaven or hell than there is now.

Clear and sweet is my soul, and clear and sweet is all that is
    not my soul.
Lack one lacks both, and the unseen is proved by the seen,
Till that becomes unseen and receives proof in its turn . . .

This selection reflects Whitman's view of time, or more accurately, timelessness, with all eras throughout the millennia seam-
lessly interconnected and open to his presence (indeed he
declares, "I was there") yet moving ever onward. In the last three
lines above there is also a glimpse of the paradoxical themes
threaded throughout the poems.

I pass death with the dying and birth with the new-wash'd
    babe, and am not contain'd between my hat and boots,
And peruse manifold objects, no two alike and every one good,
The earth good and the stars good, and their adjuncts all
    good. . . .

In me the caresser of life wherever moving, backward as well
    as forward sluing . . . not a person or object missing,
Absorbing all to myself and for this song.

These lines are reflective of the unitary nature of the human-
universe-health process that Parse speaks of in all her works. She
says that the "birthings and dyings" of day-to-day living are created as one "chooses the meanings of a situation and, through this
choosing, the possibilities that [one] can become" (1981, p. 27).
    Whitman further says that the "body" and the "soul" are iden-
tical, that they are one; and yet he writes voluminously of his communion with all that makes up his world and says that he is "not
contained between his hat and his boots." Whitman describes
many such paradoxes without explanation. In this way, his work,
as an expression of life, gives evidence of the "paradoxical unity"
in lived experiences of human-universe interrelating of which
Parse (1981, 1992) speaks. When he writes of "absorbing all to
myself and for this song," he affirms that his entire experience of
his world goes to make up the "who" that he is. Long portions of

"Song of Myself" are *literally* about other people. Whitman sings of "the pure contralto," "the carpenter," "the deacons," "the farmer," "the lunatic," "the machinist," "the squaw," "the young sister," and dozens more, briefly saluting each in their environs and activities. Whitman's "self" is richly and diversely populated, and he embraces all those who reside there with him. Parse says that the human coexists with others at many different realms of the universe and that "structuring meaning multidimensionally is cocreating reality" (1981, p. 42). Being human, for Parse, is coexisting while experiencing life as a unique individual. The meaning of the individual's experiences, though these are cocreated with others at many realms of the universe, is uniquely structured by that individual, cocreating reality (Parse, 1992, p. 37). Each individual cocreates reality with infinite numbers of others as well.

Whitman further proclaims the connectedness of the individual, humanity, and the cosmos as immanent in life itself, immediate, complete, and open to everyone.

> I resist any thing better than my own diversity,
> Breathe the air but leave plenty after me,
> And am not stuck up, and am in my place . . .
>
> These are really the thoughts of all men in all ages and
>   lands, they are not original with me,
> If they are not yours as much as mine they are nothing, or
>   next to nothing,
> If they are not the riddle and the untying of the riddle they are
>   nothing,
> If they are not just as close as they are distant they are
>   nothing.
> This is the grass that grows wherever the land is and the water
>   is,
> This the common air that bathes the globe.

The next stanza actually seems to ask the question, what is a human being?

Who goes there? hankering, gross, mystical, nude;
How is it I extract strength from the beef I eat?
What is a man anyhow? what am I? what are you?

And the next line seems to answer—

All I mark as my own you shall offset it with your own,
Else it were time lost listening to me. . . .

Having pried through the strata, analyzed to a hair, counsel'd
    with doctors and calculated close,
I find no sweeter fat than sticks to my own bones.

Standing before the reader as a human being, Whitman chants
the following description in his "Song of Myself":

In all people I see myself, none more and not one a barley-corn
    less,
And the good or bad I say of myself I say of them.

I know I am solid and sound,
To me the converging objects of the universe perpetually flow,
All are written to me, and I must get what the writing means.

. . . I exist as I am, that is enough,
If no other in the world be aware I sit content,
And if each and all be aware I sit content.

One world is aware and by far the largest to me, and that is
    myself,
And whether I come to my own to-day or in ten thousand or
    ten million years,
I can cheerfully take it now, or with equal cheerfulness I can
    wait. . . .
I laugh at what you call dissolution,
And I know the amplitude of time. . . .

Space and Time! now I see it is true, what I guess'd at,
What I guess'd when I loaf'd on the grass,
What I guess'd while I lay alone in my bed,
And again as I walk'd the beach under the paling stars of the
       morning. . . .

I skirt sierras, my palms cover continents,
I am afoot with my vision. . . .

I do not know what is untried and afterward,
But I know it will in its turn prove sufficient, and cannot
       fail. . . .

What is known I strip away,
I launch all men and women forward with me into the
       Unknown. . . .

I am an acme of things accomplish'd, and I an encloser of
       things to be. . . .

All forces have been steadily employ'd to complete and delight
       me,
Now on this spot I stand with my robust soul. . . .

Every condition promulges [makes known] not only itself,
       it promulges what grows after and out of itself,
And the dark hush promulges as much as any. . . .

I know I have the best of time and space, and was never
       measured and never will be measured.

Whitman declares that each person must interpret the world for
her- or himself, "else it were time lost listening to me." He insists
that his own beliefs, come as they have to him through the ages,
across space and time, are simply "enough." To exist as one is: no
advice or calculation can improve upon it. The "converging objects of the universe perpetually flow" to him, and he says, "All
are written to me, and I must get what the writing means." For
Whitman there is no sharp division between the self and the

world, if any division at all. One's *self* is a world, and "a world" that transcends space and time. For Whitman, to be human is to engage with the cosmos in the "push" of all that is, forever moving onward toward the "Unknown." One's self is the incarnation of history and possibility. To be human is to relate with the whole universe as an incarnate being. And while he extols the vastness and diversity of the cosmos, he affirms that he has "the best of time and space," his own, and the best by virtue of being his own. Although Whitman exalts himself in a singularly majestic way, he clearly suggests that such a passionate belief in the self is available to anyone. Parse's view is consistent with Whitman's when she says that the human is the incarnation of the is, was, and will be (Parse, 1992, p. 38), continuously cotranscending multidimensionally with the possibles, and that all humans know their own way, the way that is best for them. Whitman continues—

. . . I have no chair, no church, no philosophy,
I lead no man to a dinner-table, library, exchange,
But each man and each woman of you I lead upon a knoll,
My left hand hooking you round the waist,
My right hand pointing to landscapes of continents and the
      public road.

Not I, not any one else can travel that road for you,
You must travel it for yourself. . . .

You are also asking me questions and I hear you,
I answer that I cannot answer, you must find out for yourself.

I have said that the soul is not more than the body,
And I have said that the body is not more than the soul,
And nothing, not God, is greater to one than one's self is. . . .

*   *   *

Another well-known poem, "Song of the Open Road," enlarges on the theme foreshadowed in the preceding line: "Not I, not any one

else can travel that road for you, / You must travel it for yourself. . . ." Here Whitman also builds upon the theme of the self by
integrating it with the concept of human freedom.

From **"Song of the Open Road"**

Afoot and light-hearted I take to the open road,
Healthy, free, the world before me,
The long brown path before me leading wherever I choose.

Henceforth I ask not good fortune, I myself am good fortune,
Henceforth I whimper no more, postpone no more, need
      nothing,
Done with indoor complaints, libraries, querulous criticisms,
Strong and content I travel the open road. . . .

(Still here I carry my old delicious burdens,
I carry them, men and women, I carry them with me wherever
      I go,
I swear it is impossible for me to get rid of them,
I am fill'd with them, and I will fill them in return.). . . .

Allons! to that which is endless as it was beginningless,
To undergo much, tramps of days, rests of nights . . .
To see nothing anywhere but what you may reach it and pass it,

To conceive no time, however distant, but what you may reach
      it and pass it,
To look up or down no road but it stretches and waits for
      you . . .
To see no being, not God's or any, but you also go thither . . .
To take the best of the farmer's farm and the rich man's
      elegant villa, and the chaste blessings of the
      well-married couple, and the fruits of orchards and
      flowers of gardens . . .
To carry buildings and streets with you afterward wherever
      you go. . . .

To take your lovers on the road with you, for all that you leave
  them behind you,
To know the universe itself as a road, as many roads, as roads
  for traveling souls. . . .

Of the progress of the souls of men and women along the
  grand roads of the universe, all other progress is the
  needed emblem and sustenance.
Forever alive, forever forward,
Stately, solemn, sad, withdrawn, baffled, mad, turbulent,
  feeble, dissatisfied.
Desperate, proud, fond, sick, accepted by men, rejected by
  men,
They go! they go! I know that they go, but I know not where
  they go
But I know that they go toward the best—toward something
  great. . . .

"Song of the Open Road" is perhaps the purest expression of the
theme the researcher came to think of simply as the *onward, onward* theme. It is expressed repeatedly in *Leaves of Grass*, for example, in "Song of Myself," in the line, "I launch all men and
women forward with me into the Unknown. . . ." and in the last
line of "Starting from Paumanok," which beseeches the reader
". . . to haste, haste on with me." Whitman's concept of the "open
road" is surely analogous to Parse's belief in the openness of human becoming, continuously "cotranscending with the unfolding
possibilities" (Parse, 1992, p. 38). But like Whitman's "old delicious burdens," one carries one's experiences with one wherever
one goes ("To carry buildings and streets with you . . ."), and the
continuation of one's journey is the continuous cocreating of patterns of living. The open road is that of the possibilities open to
any human being, and from which each must choose.

  Whitman's invitation to travel the road with him is not a plea
to share his belief system down to the last particular, but to embrace the openness of possibility that is already there in being

human: "To know the universe itself as a road, as many roads, as roads for traveling souls. . . ." He rejects the supposed limitations of those who are "sad," "withdrawn," "mad," "feeble," "desperate," "sick," or "rejected by men," and declares these, like everyone, to be "Forever alive, forever [progressing] forward," saying, "They go! they go! I know that they go, but I know not where they go / But I know that they go toward the best—toward something great. . . ." Whitman challenges any value system that presumes to judge the worth of any man or woman or their course in life. He proclaims each self as the embodiment of a world, carrying environs and "lovers" along wherever the self goes. And though he does not know "where" any particular self may choose to journey, he knows that it will be "great." This does not mean that everyone's destiny is to be "great" in the sense of power or fame, but that each one's destiny is great in that it is revered as belonging to a self, and no one other than the self can truly assess its direction or value. Parse closely concurs with this view. She writes:

> Each human lives a way, his or her *own* way, which is both alike and different from the "ways" of others. It is *like* that of others in that it is a personal way of being; each individual has a personal way of being. It is *different* from others in that it is one's own.
>
> (Parse, 1992, p. 40)

CODA

Dialoguing with Whitman and Parse led to the following interpretation (the researcher's perspective of Whitman's perspective), which answers the research question, what does it mean to be human? To be human means to be *oneself,* embodied and sensual yet "not contained between my hat and boots." The self is one's interrelationship with the "kosmos," free and unbounded by space and time; the self includes all that is in one's universe. The human communes irrepressibly with the various sensuous and awe-inspiring phenomena of nature, which is everywhere alive and in no way separate from the meaning the human gives to any aspect of it. The self is sacred, and this is the sacredness of the cosmos and of God. Reality is not limited to the objective world; indeed *truth* reaches well beyond that limited realm. Human awareness is coextensive with the universe, transcends the idea of death, and is accessible as such to everyone. Free individuals live in communion with one another in a world of continual discovery and innovation, yet they celebrate the "greatness" of the commonplace and each individual. Time is unrestrictive yet ever flowing; it is the interconnection and the "perfection" of everything in the universe, encompassing the known and the unknown in the forward movement toward possibilities. The human "travels the open road," choosing a personal life course, wherever it may lead. Health is contentment with the self as the who one is in the face of challenges and hardships. Death is beautiful, a natural continuation of life to be embraced with the same joy with which one celebrates life itself.

This interpretation emerged as the researcher explored and reflected on the meaning of being human as expressed by the poet Whitman and by the theorist Parse. Whitman's view of the human as a *self*, a uniquely experienced unity of the body-soul-universe, is "familiar," in Gadamer's sense, though it is not the same as Parse's view of the human as an open being cocreating becoming with the universe. Whitman's view of the self living in communion with all others is not unfamiliar. The idea of the human's freedom to travel "the open road," the universe open to possibilities, is very similar to Parse's view. Several of Whitman's themes are connected with other traditions (belief systems) and truths for him which the researcher can appreciate while not sharing in them—for example, his attitude toward body and soul. Living and writing long before Heidegger or Einstein were published, Whitman seems to have been striving to express something like the unity represented in the constructs "being-in-the-world" and "space-time." Yet the unity of body and soul seems for him a nebulous, shifting concept, as he proclaims their unity in one stanza and celebrates each separately in others—connecting the body with sensual pleasures and the soul with other souls and "eternity," thus playing out the very traditions from which he simultaneously departs. Similarly, the communion and human freedom he celebrates expansively throughout *Leaves of Grass* appear to be closely tied to American democracy, associated with the "New World" (though his concept of "Democracy" is far removed from the political status quo).

Parse (1981, 1992) gives voice to a more radically *unitary* view of the human-universe-health process and possibly a more fundamental *freedom* in human existence (at least a freedom that is not tied to a particular political system, though she, too, would denounce oppressive forms of government). In their views of *health*, the researcher finds Whitman and Parse to be basically in agreement. Health, for Whitman, is the way he is, consistently described as "good" or "perfect." Parse, who posits health as the experiential process of human becoming, certainly would not argue with Whitman's assertion. Both authors argue for the uniqueness, sanctity, and expansiveness of the self, never forgetting the interconnectedness of everything in the universe, and both point to the diversity of being-becoming as evidence of its essential unity. Both take an uncompromising stand against judging or directing other selves as they progress along "the open road," each in a unique way. Overall, there is greater consonance than dissonance between the two views.

CONCLUDING REFLECTIONS

Gadamer has said that language is the horizon of hermeneutic ontology. This means that *truths* are disclosed in discourse through interpretation and understanding. In this study, the researcher coparticipated in two traditions which were founded in and *live* through language. The belief system of Parse's theory was expanded through making explicit the interconnections, similarities, and differences in relation to Whitman's perspective, the expression of life projected into the text more than one hundred years ago. The striking similarities and the new possibilities of meaning to be found in reading the text from Parse's perspective illustrate the generativity of interpretation as described in the hermeneutic concepts of situatedness, fore-knowing, and the dialectic of distanciation and appropriation.

Traditions *live* in discourse. This study uncovered new realms of meaning in Whitman's work, while his eloquence brought to life in vivid detail the ideas about human becoming articulated in Parse's theory. *Leaves of Grass* stands as testimony to the inexhaustible meaningfulness of each human life, to the paradoxical unity of individuality-communality in coexisting with others, and to the freedom of the human to choose from possibilities whatever the circumstances. In short, as Whitman himself said, his book bears witness to life "immense in passion, pulse, and power."

The implications of this study for nursing as a human science are not really original with this author, but are manifold. Recalling Gadamer's (1989) discussion of artistic truths and his "dialogue" with Bernstein (1983) on phronesis, it can be said that there are truths about human beings that are not accessible through objective science. That which is most sacred to human beings is the prime example; the sacred is unintelligible through objectivist methods (Langer, 1967). At the same time, the overall tradition of nursing is to be actively concerned with whole human beings and their health comprehensively. The hermeneutic endeavor is not complete until the implications for *praxis* are worked out (Gadamer, 1989).

What kind of science, then, will guide nurses in service to humanity? Nurses have traditionally been "doers." The movement of nursing into higher education and research thus far has resulted largely in the more sophisticated study and use of techniques for illness care derived from objective science. Even the hermeneutic tradition has been conscripted to serve in the pursuit of greater "know-how" (Benner, 1984). Increasingly, however, nurse scholars are moving away from this fix-it model of nursing science to view nursing truly as a human science (Mitchell & Cody, 1992).

Viewing nursing as a human science radically transforms the "horizon of inquiry," moving it away from greater "know-how" (Benner, 1984) toward understanding (Parse, 1981, 1987, 1992).

Whitman has shown that the lived experience of a single person, upon reflection, reveals a panorama of a thousand universes. One might pose the question Dilthey once asked of personal experience: "Can I base a science on this?" One that is forever *in medias res,* forever seeking truth amidst infinite possibilities? Whitman's poetry suggests that the answer lies in "the miracle of identity," the self. And Parse might respond, "Yes, *the person knows.*"

The truths that are sought in nursing as a human science are not to be found in the laboratory nor to be reached through path analysis. The theory base for nursing science can only be rooted in a true understanding of what it means to be human. This does not mean one truth, but many truths. These truths are within every human being and are expressed through the values each one lives. The way *the nurse* understands these truths is the way he or she understands *self* as a nurse and is expressed through the values he or she lives in practice (Parse, 1987).

An example may be given with the researcher's personal understanding of *death* as described by Whitman. The researcher is a nurse who is often with persons who are living their dying. Whitman's view of the beauty of death was not as "familiar" to the researcher as his theme of the beauty of each self, a belief the researcher already shared. But, as a nurse guided by Parse's theory, who approaches persons in practice to be with them in true, loving presence, with the goal of quality of life as experienced by the person, this nurse researcher now sees clearly what was previously a prereflective glimmering: that he does believe in the beauty of death—the potential beauty of death; that believing in this possibility is *essential* for practice with those who are living their dying. This is a *truth* which changes the way the researcher as a nurse is with persons in practice.

Thus, the theory base that guides practice must be rooted fundamentally in human values and express those human values explicitly in the language of the science. Perhaps it is true for nursing science what the visionary Whitman (1855, p. vii) wrote in the very first publication of *Leaves of Grass:*

"In the beauty of poems are the tuft and final applause of science."

REFERENCES

Allen, G. W. (1955). *The solitary singer.* New York: Macmillan.

Allen, M. N., & Jensen, L. (1990). Hermeneutical inquiry: Meaning and scope. *Western Journal of Nursing Research, 12,* 241–253.

Asselineau, R. (1960). *The evolution of Walt Whitman: The development of a personality.* Cambridge: Harvard University Press.

Benner, P. L. (1984). *From novice to expert: Excellence and power in clinical nursing practice.* Menlo Park, CA: Addison-Wesley.

Bernstein, R. J. (1983). *Beyond objectivism and relativism: Science, hermeneutics, and praxis.* Philadelphia: University of Pennsylvania Press.

Cody, W. K. (1991). Grieving a personal loss. *Nursing Science Quarterly, 4,* 62–68.

Dilthey, W. (1988). *Introduction to the human sciences* (R. J. Bentanzos, Trans.). Detroit: Wayne State University Press. (Original work published 1883)

Ermarth, M. (1978). *Wilhelm Dilthey: The critique of historical reason.* Chicago: The University of Chicago Press.

Gadamer, H-G. (1976). *Philosophical hermeneutics* (D. E. Linge, Trans. & Ed.). Berkeley: University of California Press.

Gadamer, H-G. (1989). *Truth and method* (2nd rev. ed.). (Translation revised by J. Weinsheimer & D. G. Marshall). New York: Crossroad. (Original work published 1960)

Heidegger, M. (1962). *Being and time* (J. Macquarrie & E. Robinson, Trans.). San Francisco: Harper & Row. (Original work published 1927)

Jonas, C. (1992). The meaning of being an elder in Nepal. *Nursing Science Quarterly, 5,* 171–175.

Langer, S. (1967). *Philosophy in a new key: A study in the symbolism of reason, rite, and art* (3rd ed.). Cambridge, MA: Harvard University Press.

Miller, J. E. (1957). *A critical guide to Leaves of Grass.* Chicago: University of Chicago Press.

Miller, J. E. (Ed.). (1964). *Whitman's "Song of Myself"; Origin, growth, and meaning.* New York: Dodd, Mead.

Mitchell, G. J. (1990). The lived experience of taking life day-by-day in later life: Research guided by Parse's emerging method. *Nursing Science Quarterly, 3,* 170–176.

Mitchell, G. J., & Cody, W. K. (1992). Nursing knowledge and human science: Ontological and epistemological considerations. *Nursing Science Quarterly, 5,* 54–61.

Parse, R. R. (1981). *Man-living-health: A theory of nursing.* New York: Wiley.

Parse, R. R. (1987). Man-living-health theory of nursing. In R. R. Parse, *Nursing science: Major paradigms, theories, and critiques* (pp. 159–180). Philadelphia: Saunders.

Parse, R. R. (1990a). Health: A personal commitment. *Nursing Science Quarterly, 3,* 136–140.

Parse, R. R. (1990b). Parse's research methodology with an illustration of the lived experience of hope. *Nursing Science Quarterly, 3,* 9–17.

Parse, R. R. (1992). Human becoming: Parse's theory of nursing. *Nursing Science Quarterly, 5,* 35–42.

Parse, R. R. (1993). The experience of laughter: A phenomenological study. *Nursing Science Quarterly, 6,* 39–43.

Parse, R. R. (1994a). *Human becoming: A theory of nursing.* Manuscript submitted for publication.

Parse, R. R. (1994b). Laughing and health: A study using Parse's research method. *Nursing Science Quarterly, 7,* 55–64.

Polkinghorne, D. (1983). *Methodology for the human sciences: Systems of inquiry.* Albany: State University of New York Press.

Reeder, F. (1988). Hermeneutics. In B. Sarter (Ed.), *Paths to knowledge: Innovative methods for nursing* (pp. 193–238). New York: National League for Nursing Press.

Ricoeur, P. (1976). *Interpretation theory: Discourse and the surplus of meaning.* Fort Worth: Texas Christian University Press.

Rogers, M. E. (1970). *An introduction to the theoretical basis of nursing.* Philadelphia: Davis.

Smith, M. C. (1990). Struggling through a difficult time for unemployed persons. *Nursing Science Quarterly, 3,* 18–28.

Thompson, J. L. (1990). Hermeneutic inquiry. In L. E. Moody (Ed.), *Advancing nursing science through research.* (Vol. 2) (pp. 223–280). Newbury Park, CA: Sage.

Whitman, W. (1855). *Leaves of Grass.* New York: Author [facsimile of 1st ed.].

Whitman, W. (1983). *Leaves of Grass.* New York: Bantam. (Original [7th ed.] published in 1892)

Chapter 17

Evaluation of the Human Becoming Theory in Practice With Adults and Children

Marc D. A. Santopinto
Marlaine C. Smith

As nurses begin to develop practice methods from the foundations of nursing conceptual models and grand theories, there is a concomitant need to evaluate these theory-based practices. Making a significant improvement in nursing practice has always been a purported value of nursing theory. The challenge of the 21st century will be to investigate this claim more fully (Smith, 1991). There are few studies in the literature informing us through evaluation research about the difference that nursing theory makes when used as a foundation for practice (Fawcett, 1989; DeGroot, 1988; Silva, 1986). However, those few studies that have been completed have documented that important and valued changes in client, nurse, and cost outcomes have occurred following the introduction of a nursing model that guides nursing practice (Hoch, 1987; Mattice, 1991). Further investigations of indicators of change that occur with theory application are essential to support the value of theory-based nursing practice. The purpose of this chapter is to summarize the process and findings of an evaluation research study examining the implementation of theory-based practice, in particular Parse's (1981, 1987, 1992), in an acute-care setting.

BACKGROUND

Theory-based practice was a proposed standard of nursing practice for Canadian nurses (Canadian Nurses Association, 1986; College of Nurses of Ontario, 1990). As a result, nurses and administrators were challenged to select nursing theoretical frameworks to guide practice. While theoretic diversity is evident and accepted in the discipline, administrators were faced with providing a setting for nursing practice that would foster a more conscious and systematic integration of nursing theory in practice. Some administrators opted for instituting a particular model of theory-based practice within their organizations. Entire hospitals or long-term care facilities have structured nursing practices based on particular nursing theories. The adoption of a single theoretical framework to guide practice within a nursing division offers distinct advantages. A common vision of human beings, health, and nursing may ease documentation of care, streamline decision making, and facilitate communication. Only an explicit theoretical framework can offer the scope, integration and depth required of such a guiding vision. Nurses might then select their setting for practice based on the theoretical framework congruent with their values and beliefs.

This project was conceived out of a perceived need for change in nursing practice at the hospital in which it was eventually initiated. A survey of nurses' attitudes and morale was conducted at the hospital. Results revealed significant levels of disenchantment with traditional nursing practice. Many of these nurses felt that current patterns of nursing care failed to reflect their professional, intellectual, and personal expectations. Feelings of diminished self-worth, anger, and alienation from peers and superordinates were also relevant findings. A substantial number of respondents indicated an intent to abandon nursing as a career. Nurses cited the lack of opportunity to interact meaningfully with others and lack of structures to support therapeutic relationships with clients at the bedside. The inevitable sequelae of this malaise imperiled staff retention and exacerbated declining recruitment during what was, at the time, a looming national shortage of nurses.

One nurse administrator responded to the concerns uncovered in the survey by conducting qualitative research on the way nursing was conceptualized by staff nurses. The administrator decided to engage nursing staff in the selection of a nursing theory that might become the foundation for nursing practice at the hospital. Based on the belief that a common theoretical nursing perspective would enhance the quality of the work environment and enrich the quality of patients' health experiences, the administration opted for this bold organizational commitment. The nurse administrator spoke with nurses about their values and beliefs and, based on their responses, decided that Parse's (1981, 1987) theory of human becoming was congruent with many of the core values reflected in the staff's responses. The researchers for this study were then contacted because of their previous evaluation work with Parse's theory-based practice. Following consultations, the researchers were contracted to complete a 6-month evaluation study of the implementation of Parse's theory in practice.

PREVIOUS STUDIES

Several evaluation studies of Parse's theory had already been completed at the time of initiation of this study. The first study took place in an acute-care setting in a Florida hospital (Parse, 1988). The purpose of this qualitative evaluation study was to evaluate changes in nurses' beliefs and actions and patients' health experiences with the use of Parse's theory and Mayeroff's (1971) concepts of caring as a base for nursing practice. Data were collected prior to and 3 months post-implementation of the practice models. Four data sets were explored: (a) nursing documentation on patient records, (b) interviews with patients, (c) questionnaires completed by nurses related to their beliefs, and (d) narrative descriptions of characteristics and qualities of each nurse written by immediate supervisors. These data sources were accessed on three participating units: one implementing the Parse model, the second, the Mayeroff framework, and the third with no deliberate changes in practice patterns.

There were subtle qualitative differences noted in nursing values and the practice patterns of a few nurses on the Parse unit. Based on this study there were three suggestions: (a) increase the length of time for the implementation phase of any study evaluating the implementation of theory-based practice to at least 6 months; (b) enhance teaching and supervision of implementation of the theory-based practice model for the entire implementation phase of the study; and (c) garner more active administrative support for any theory-based practice project. The research design utilized in this study seemed useful in eliciting the answers to the research questions.

The second study was conducted by one of the researchers in a long-term psychiatric facility in Canada (Santopinto, 1989). The design was similar to the Parse (1988) study, except the researcher was also a clinical specialist leading implementation of the theory-based practice model on one unit. The pre-post interval for data collection was again 12 weeks long. In this study more substantive qualitative differences were noted in the patients' perceptions, the nurses' values, and nursing documentation on the study unit. An independent evaluator completed all data collection. Of particular note were the profound changes in the patients documented by videotaping of group sessions with the clinical specialist over the 12-week project. These elderly men, all labeled for many decades with psychiatric diagnoses and considered "hopeless cases" by many, showed very different patterns of being together in the group convened by the clinical specialist guided by Parse's theory. Prior to this time some of these clients had rarely spoken or revealed personal thoughts to others.

A third study was a pre- post-implementation evaluation study in another Canadian hospital (Mattice, 1991). Again, the clinical nurse specialist guided the implementation of Parse's theory-based practice model on the selected unit. This study again supported qualitative changes in the beliefs of nurses (reflected in their documentation, statements, and actual practice) and patient perceptions of nursing. During its 8-month implementation period economic advantages were noted in lower turnover rates and absenteeism.

A review of these early studies yielded important findings that served as a foundation for the development of the present study. First, the painful struggles of nurses engaged in a process of changing their practice was clearly evident; anguish and anger seemed an inevitable component of the change process. It seemed clear that qualitative changes in the selected indicators were more evident if the implementation phase was longer. Nurses needed to learn the theory and the practice method, and time was needed to accomplish this. Experience with these studies suggested that teaching and leading the implementation of theory-based practice required the full-time focus of a practice scholar over at least a 7- to 8-month period. Finally, it seemed evident that in future research studies it was important to: (a) engage and involve stakeholders throughout the process of the evaluation; (b) expand the evaluation of Parse's theory-based practice to practice settings with children (or patients who were other than verbally articulate); (c) explore the use of visual media to capture pattern change; and (d) examine perceptions of change in nursing practice from perspectives of other hospital personnel. The study that is reported in this chapter was designed to incorporate these recommendations.

PURPOSE

The purposes of this study were: (a) to discern changes in client-family health experiences, nurses' attitudes, beliefs, and practice patterns, and the organizational culture that might accompany the implementation of Parse's theory in an acute care setting, and (b) to generate data for informed administrative decision making related to implementing the model on a hospital-wide basis. The research question was: How does the initiation and implementation of Parse's theory-based practice model change client-family health experiences, nurses' attitudes, beliefs, and practice patterns, and the organizational culture?

DESIGN AND METHODOLOGY

The Evaluation Framework

Evaluation may be approached differently depending on one's perspectives on the process. Guba and Lincoln's (1989) constructivist paradigm was chosen as the model for this study. The constructivist paradigm addresses the participative relationship of evaluator with stakeholders in evaluation. The stakeholders are more fully involved in the creation of the evaluation plan as they co-construct the study as well as serve as "data sources." The constructivist paradigm incorporates a hermeneutic-dialectic process in which the researchers interpret data and illuminate the tensions within the data for further interpretation by the study participants. This openness allows for more in-depth reflection by both stakeholders and participants.

Design

A qualitative descriptive design incorporating data generation points prior to project implementation and 30 weeks following project implementation was used for the study. Process data

such as researcher's journals, meeting minutes, and participants' comments were collected throughout the study. An evaluator, not associated with the study, collected interview data
from nurses, administrators, patients, and families and reviewed nursing documentation in the patient records. The evaluator was a doctorally-prepared nurse researcher skilled in use of
qualitative evaluation methodologies and with a practice background in working with children and adults. Engaging an external evaluator had the advantage of promoting greater trust and
honest communication; participants could anonymously share
their perspectives with someone who had no stake in the out-
come of the project.

Prior to implementation of the study, stakeholders were surveyed to uncover what they wanted to know from the evaluation.
These stakeholders included: nurses, hospital and nursing administrators, physicians, the patient ombudsman, ancillary
health personnel on the units, researchers, patients and families.
Their questions were incorporated into questionnaires and interview schedules.

Setting

The setting for this study was a 400-bed community teaching hospital in a mid-sized Canadian city. The hospital served an ethni-
cally diverse population. The staffs of three units (110 nurses)
volunteered to be pilot units for the study: two adjoining 20-bed
pediatric units and a 42-bed medical-surgical unit.

Participants and Methods of Data Generation

Six groups of participants were selected for inclusion in this
study. Participants were all stakeholders in the evaluation of
nursing theory-based practice on the units. Participants provided
perspectives that were relevant to evaluating the indicators of
change. These participants were surveyed and/or interviewed

both before the project began and 30 weeks following its implementation. These participant groups are listed below:

1. Staff Nurses. All staff nurses from the three study units were offered an opportunity to participate in the project. The project was explained to the nurses in staff meetings, and all questions were addressed by the on-site principal investigator. A staff nurse questionnaire (Table 17.1) was given to every nurse participant after completion of the consent form. The survey was completed prior to the beginning of the project and at 30 weeks following implementation. Some staff nurses were nominated by their peers as key informants, nurses who were knowledgeable about the culture and values of the unit. Those selected as key informants engaged in an in-depth dialogue with the external evaluator. One staff nurse was videotaped in an admission interview with a client before the project began and at 30 weeks into the project. An end-of-shift report was tape-recorded at those same two data collection points for review by the researchers.

2. Adult Client Participants. The evaluator selected ten clients from the adult surgical unit and invited them to talk with her about their perceptions of nursing care. The interviews followed a semi-structured interview schedule (Table 17.2).

3. Child Client Participants. The evaluator selected five children from each of the pediatric units. The evaluator recorded a dialogue with the children and his or her nurses, and if situationally appropriate, invited the children to engage in play related to their perceptions of nurses (Table 17.3).

4. Parent Participants. The evaluator recorded a dialogue with the significant other(s) of the child participants. This dialogue was guided by a set of questions (Table 17.3).

5. Nurse Manager Participants. The evaluator interviewed the nurse managers on each of the three study units. These interviews

Table 17.1 Questionnaire for Nurse Participants

Introduction:

Please answer the following questions in your own words. There are no right or wrong answers, so simply take your time and answer as frankly as you can.

1. What, for you, is the most unique and important thing about being a nurse?
2. What beliefs and values guide you as you approach a new patient?
3. What is the meaning of health for you as a nurse?
4. Name three things you generally seek to accomplish with each of your patients.
5. What, for you, is quality nursing care?
6. Describe what quality of life means for you. How does this relate to the care you give your patients?
7. Briefly describe the present quality of your work life.
8. What do you offer patients that is unique and different from what others (doctors, social workers, O.T.s, etc.) provide?
9. If asked for advice, what would you say to a friend who was thinking of becoming a nurse?
10. Give a few reasons for your last answer.
11. What are your thoughts and feelings about remaining a nurse?
12. What are your thoughts and feelings about working on this unit?
13. What kinds of things do you usually chart about your patients?
14. In your opinion, how do other health professionals view nurses' charting written on your unit?
15. How do other professions view nursing's contribution to patient care on your unit?
16. What do independent action and intellectual challenge mean to you in relation to nursing?

Table 17.2   Questions for Adult Client Participants

1. What does the nurse do when he or she is with you?
2. What does the nurse discuss with you?
3. How often does the nurse initiate a conversation about your feelings and concerns?
4. Can you give some examples of important discussions you had with your nurse?
5. Who here in the hospital other than your family seems most concerned about hearing your hopes and concerns?
6. How do nurses have an impact on the quality of your life?
7. What do you want from the nurses that you do not get?

Table 17.3   Questions for Child and Parent Participants

1. What does the nurse do when he or she is with you?
2. What does the nurse talk about with you?
3. How often does the nurse talk with you about your feelings?
4. Can you tell me about an important talk you once had with a nurse?
5. Who here in the hospital listens to what you have to say?
6. What does the nurse do to make things better for you?

For the purposes of this study, a child is any individual below the age of 16. The above questions are intended to guide an open dialogue between the evaluator and the child. The evaluator will adapt the guiding questions to the level of comprehension of the child. If situationally appropriate, the evaluator may:

(a) invite the child to draw a picture of a nurse and talk about the picture.
(b) invite the child to play with a nurse puppet and a boy or girl puppet.
(c) observe the child in interaction with self or others.

utilized ethnographic interview processes as the evaluator sought descriptions of nursing practice and the unit culture from the administrators. During interviews the evaluator invited interpretations of some of the tensions perceived.

6. *Other Stakeholders.* The researchers and evaluator conducted interviews with physicians, child health workers, the patient ombudsman, and key representatives from health professions such as social work, psychology, and physical therapy to determine their opinions about nursing practice. Again, these interviews were conducted using ethnographic interview processes. The evaluator and researchers sought descriptions of nursing practice, observations, and perceptions of patient and family experiences, and any perceived changes on the units.

The researchers used photography prior to implementation of theory-based practice and at 30 weeks into the project in an attempt to capture the culture or life of the unit through another medium. A photographer was engaged with instructions to take photographs that captured the climate of life on the unit. The photographer spent some time walking through the units and then photographed scenes (with permission of those being photographed).

Protection of the Rights of Participants

The proposal was reviewed and approved by the Research Committee of the hospital in which the study was conducted. All participants who had completed surveys or were interviewed or photographed provided written consent. The participants were assured that they would not be identified by name in reports related to the study, that non-participation would not affect their employment or quality of health care in any way, and that they could withdraw from the study at any time. This meant that they did not have to be interviewed or complete questionnaires; however, all staff nurses did participate in learning the practice model by virtue of their assignment on the pilot units. All tape-recorded interviews were transcribed and maintained in a locked cabinet until they were destroyed.

Teaching Theory-Based Practice

The teaching of Parse's practice methodology and opportunities for guided practice were provided from week to week under the direction of the principal investigator. Video clips, lectures, small group discussions and one-to-one supervised practice were the teaching-learning strategies employed with nurses on the pilot units. A newsletter called *Creativity in Practice* was edited and disseminated throughout the hospital by the principal investigator. One edition of that newsletter appears in Table 17.4. During the latter half of the project, large polychrome posters illustrating guidelines for practice were placed in prominent areas of the three pilot units. Guest lecturers, practicing nurses who were expert in Parse's practice method, were invited to speak to the staff nurses. Generally, the theory was taught from a practice perspective. Nurses were engaged in reflections on and discussions about their values and beliefs. For example, nurses would examine the meaning of focusing on the uniqueness of the person, rather than focusing on the diagnostic labels or diseases. Emphasis was placed on values of respect, relationship, and concern for dignity and freedom. Nurses discussed focusing on lived reality as described by the person, rather than on caregiver interpretations of it. The goal of nursing in this model is quality of life as perceived by the client. Participants explored ways of eliciting the meaning of experience from children who were not articulate. Finally, written feedback on the quality of each teaching venue was elicited from all project participants. This feedback was used to continually revise teaching strategies in accordance with the evaluation framework.

Procedures

The following is an outline that summarizes the elements of the process utilized in implementing this evaluation study in each of

Table 17.4   Newsletter Reprint

CREATIVITY IN PRACTICE

Editor: Marc Santopinto, RN, MScN / Consultant in Parse's Theory

Editorial

Nurses often say they don't have enough time to be with their patients. Each day is filled with admissions, umpteen meds to be delivered on time, and the call bell rings on and on. . . . How can the nurse be truly present with people when there is simply not enough time? The shortness of each day mirrors the shortness of life itself. Not enough time to be with our children while they are still young. Not enough time to get out of the house alone with one's spouse. How can one find the time to get a proper night's sleep? Time just for yourself. Time to exercise. Time to watch the sun set. Time to make new friends and be with old ones. Time to just sit and think. Time to really live the values you believe in.

The nurse guided by Parse's theory creates time just to be there with patients. The time we *create* is different from the time we *have*. The time we *have* is simply filled, while the time we *create* is chosen. Creating time allows us to stretch out to innovative ways of nursing in a rapidly changing world. The nurse guided by Parse's theory creates time to reshape personal value priorities. Like a mountain stream that sparkles in the afternoon sunshine, one's

values seem from the distance to be motionless and stable. But when one pauses to sip the waters, the stream of one's personal beliefs reveals the freshness of movement and constant renewal.

Sometimes, the nurse will be able to find no more than two or three minutes to spend with a patient. But two minutes of true presence can radically transform a patient's way of living health.

The nurse creates time to be truly present with others because "filling time" is no longer an acceptable option. Because creating time to be with a lonely human being may actually take less time than avoiding contact. And lastly, the nurse takes time to be with patients because, alas, life itself is so short. The time we have remaining is far too precious to waste on anything of less value.

Marc Santopinto, RN, MScN

The Parse Project:
A Status Report

The goals of the Parse project were to introduce 110 nurses to a new nursing approach over 30 weeks, and

Table 17.4   (Continued)

to describe changes in patients and nurses over this time period. Individual and small group teaching has been carried out by the project director and by expert nurses working under his direction. Over 60 nurses have participated in a concentrated three-hour workshop on Parse's approach to nursing. Anonymous written feedback from pilot unit nurses has shown substantial and growing support both for the theory and for the methods of teaching used.

The progress of the learning process on all three pilot units is consistent with the experience of nurses involved in earlier, comparable evaluation projects. Expenses related to the project are being managed by the project director well within budget, and all of the study objectives are being met on target.

The early weeks of the Parse project were hallmarked by turbulence associated with the change process. Similar patterns of uncertainty and anxiety have been revealed in previous evaluation studies. The Parse project is now entering a new phase. Posters, guided practice, and small group work are being used to push the project forward toward a favorable conclusion.

The study has already generated interest internationally. A preliminary report was presented at a scholarly conference sponsored by Discovery International, Inc. in Cincinnati, Ohio in March. A second invitation has been received to read a paper on this study at the National Nursing Theory Conference at the University of California at Los Angeles in September. Applications to present our findings at other scholarly conferences have been submitted for peer review.

Many nurses are discovering a changing scope of practice and patients are seeing the difference.

Do You Believe . . .

. . . that people have the right to make their own choices in life, together with their family and friends?

. . . that each human being's experience of the world is unique?

. . . that people make small and big life decisions based upon what they value?

. . . that human beings are responsible for all the outcomes of the choices they make?

. . . that if others are to understand you, they must respect what you value?

. . . that each human being has a unique way of being with the people and objects he or she loves?

. . . that people struggle back and forth between different options as they move toward life dreams?

. . . that nurses have a role that is different from that of physicians?

. . . that the center of nursing practice is human relationship?

Table 17.4 (Continued)

. . . that the way you are with a person can make a real and immediate difference to the quality of his or her life?

These are some of the beliefs and assumptions that Parse's theory is built upon. Nurses who hold these beliefs find guidance and support in Parse's practice method.

This approach is much more than simple respect for patients, caring, or listening to their concerns. Based upon the human sciences, Parse's approach to practice is specific, feasible, and can be learned. This way of practice was developed by nurses for nurses. It is unique to nursing. No other category of health care workers structure their practice in this way.

Credits: These guiding beliefs and assumptions have been adapted, with permission, from an unpublished manuscript prepared by Gail J. Mitchell.

Parse Charting

Charting should reflect those task- and safety-related issues that have been legally and ethically expected of nurses. Charting should also reflect the caring and healing relationship between nurse and person. If your charting fails to reflect this unique focus, you are not giving yourself credit for what you do.

A common myth is that charting based on Parse's theory must be lengthy. Theory-based charting can be extremely brief. The following guidelines will help you to write brief sentences that apply Parse's theory.

1. Add a sentence that reflects what the person says. Don't label, or explain the person's thoughts, words, or actions.

Example:
Mr. S. says he wants to spend time with family and friends.

2. Document what the person says is important in his life.

Example:
Mr. S. says he just wants to get out of this hospital now, but adds that he is not going to leave until they tell him what is wrong with his leg.

3. Document the person's struggle back and forth as he talks about the important people and things in his life.

Example:
Mr. S. says he dislikes children. He then went on to talk in detail about how much he is looking forward to spending the summer with his grandchildren.

4. Describe the person's hopes and dreams.

Example:
Mr. S. said that all he wants is to die. He then asked how long the physio treatments would last and asked if the nurses could visit him at home after he leaves.

Parse charting reflects the patient's unique world. It shows the

Table 17.4   (Continued)

whole person, not just a part, system, or problem. And it's in plain English—the patient's own words.

Living the Theory:
Common Q's & A's

Q. I am already practicing this way. Why do I need a theory to help me do what I am already doing?

A. I know that you care about your patients and listen to their concerns. But Parse's practice approach is much more than this. Learning the theory itself will deepen and clarify some of your guiding beliefs. Your practice will be enhanced.

Q. How is practice guided by Parse's theory different?

A. The nurse guided by Parse's theory does not reassure patients or give them advice on what to do or how to be. The nurse does not label (diagnose) or impose expectations upon the patient. This is not and cannot be a canned or standardized approach. Traditional nursing focuses upon task completion. The Parse nurse focuses upon human interrelationships. In place of problem-solving, we provide true presence.

Q. Tell me what true presence is.

A. True presence is going to wherever the person is in his or her daily struggle. The nurse stays with the to-and-fro of shifting options as the

dreams unfold. True presence is immediately recognized by patients as a different way of being cared for.

Q. What do patients say about practice guided by Parse's theory?

A. They are often surprised. They say it makes them feel special and valued. It changes the way they think of nurses.

Q. What do the nurses think about it all?

A. Nurses are surprised to see how patients change as they talk about the meaning of their life situations. Other nurses say that it feels like a burden is lifted when they no longer feel they have to change the way people think, talk, or act. Nurses have known for years that, ultimately, patients choose what they want to do, based upon their own beliefs and values. Now, guided by Parse's theory, nurses can provide true presence to people during that process.

Q. But we can't just let people decide about their own health care.

A. Why not? You know they will anyway. If the patient wants information related to disease process, he or she will ask for it. The Parse nurse does not hesitate to provide patients with the teaching or information they request. But the Parse nurse focuses on unfolding meaning as the person struggles with his own shifting options.

the three phases: Pre-Implementation Data Generation, Implementation, and Post-Implementation Data Generation.

Pre-Implementation Phase

- Decision is made to implement Parse's theory-based practice on three pilot nursing units.
- Pilot units volunteer, and three are selected.
- Researchers spend one week introducing staff to the study. Letters and posters inform staff of the project.
- Researchers interview stakeholders to identify what they want to know from the evaluation and ask for identification of other stakeholders.
- Questionnaires are administered to all nurses on the pilot units.
- Videotaping of a nursing admission interview is conducted.
- Audiotape of a change-of-shift report is collected.
- Evaluator joins research team and conducts interviews with key informants, clients, families, administrators.
- Evaluator reviews nursing documentation.
- Random photography of "life on the unit" is completed.

Implementation Phase

- Principal investigator and other experts on Parse's theory-based practice begin teaching small groups of nurses about the theory and practice method.
- *Creativity in Practice,* a newsletter, is developed and used as a vehicle to highlight important points about the theory and the project in general. It is distributed monthly throughout the hospital.
- Posters on each unit highlight nursing documentation, client profiles, and other issues that support points made in teaching sessions.

- Principal investigator makes rounds (when invited) to model the application of Parse's theory in practice.
- Process data are gathered through: collection of opinions, concerns, memos, and letters; researcher's log; patient evalations during the time of the implementation; and any policy/ governance changes that occurred during the time of implementation.

Post-Implementation Phase

- Both researchers are on-site to initiate the week of data generation.
- Nurse questionnaires are administered to all staff nurses on pilot units.
- Evaluator returns to conduct interviews with clients, families, nurse administrators, and other key informants.
- Evaluator reviews nursing documentation.
- Evaluator prepares a report on findings from documentation and observations.
- Videotaping of a nursing admission interview is conducted.
- Audiotape of a change-of-shift report is collected.
- Random photography of "life on the unit" is completed.
- Principal investigators continue to analyze data.
- Findings are presented to hospital forum.

Although information from other sources was accessed, findings from four major data sets will be the focus here: (a) **Nursing documentation**—the way nurses recorded their observations, impressions, and actions. The evaluator described patterns of language in the nurses' notes that referred to clients, important others, and descriptions of daily practice (see Table 17.5 for guidelines used in evaluating documentation); (b) **Client-family interviews**—interviews conducted by the evaluator

Table 17.5   Guidelines for Evaluation of Documentation

The evaluator will randomly select ten charts from each pilot unit and will discern and describe patterns of language within the nurses' notes. The evaluator will focus attention on how nurses refer to clients and important others, and upon how nurses describe daily practice.

---

according to the Interview Guide and any other ways (such as puppet-play and drawings) of eliciting children's perceptions of nurses and nursing practice; (c) **Nurse questionnaires**— responses to a 16-item open-ended questionnaire that was distributed to the nurses at the two data-generation points; and (d) **Key informant interviews**—identified administrators, nurses, and health professionals who were interviewed about their perceptions of nursing practice and client care on the pilot units. Interviews were conducted using ethnographic processes and were tape-recorded. (Supplemental data, such as videotaped admission interviews, end-of-shift reports, and photography were also generated; analysis of these data will not appear here.)

Analysis

Analysis of the four data sets was accomplished using a qualitative analysis-synthesis process (Parse, Coyne, & Smith, 1985). The researchers reviewed and reflected on the qualitative data to identify themes or major ideas that described patterns of changes in: nurses' attitudes and beliefs, key informants' perceptions of nursing practice and organizational culture; and client-family perceptions of nursing practice. In a similar fashion the evaluator analyzed the nursing documentation and presented her findings in a report to the researchers. Findings are presented as themes or narrative excerpts exemplifying a central idea.

FINDINGS FROM THE EVALUATION

Documentation

The evaluator reviewed ten charts from each unit prior to implementation and 30 weeks following implementation of the practice model on the three units. The evaluator noted no changes in general charting format. However, prior to implementation of Parse's theory-based practice model, the evaluator found no nursing documentation related to clients' wishes, hopes, and feelings. Thirty weeks following implementation, the nurses were describing clients' perspectives on their life and health. Data from the nurse questionnaires supported this difference in that 50 percent of the nurses believed that their charting had changed significantly during the project. The external evaluator also commented that at 30 weeks, ritualized phrases such as "good day," "resting comfortably," "no complaints this shift," and "slept well" were much less frequently used. These phrases gave way to more focused accounts of how patients described their life situations. Again this difference was confirmed in responses to the Staff Nurse Questionnaire. One nurse stated, "I [now] make attempts to include the person as a whole, rather than compartmentalizing their needs and fragmenting their care. In my charting, I try to bring forward the patients' or families' expressed wishes or goals, rather than just physical and mental needs." Another nurse said, "My charting has been affected [by the project]. I am clearly more conscious of documenting what the patient perceives as important."

In summary, the major changes noted in nursing documentation at 30 weeks following the implementation of Parse's theory-based practice model were: **greater inclusion of client's perspectives of feelings, wishes, and hopes; less use of**

ritualized phrases in charting; and more focused accounts of how patients described their life situations.

Interviews/Observations of Discussions
With Clients and Families

At the beginning of the project, clients stated that their conversations with nurses related to feelings and concerns were minimal. They described the nurses as taking blood pressures, helping with morning care routines, and attending to medically-related procedures such as intravenous fluid and medication administration. When asked to describe a significant conversation they had with a nurse, examples given related to disease processes and functional limitations related to disease entities. Clients or families were unable to identify an instance where the nurse had influenced their quality of life. When asked what they wanted from nurses, the most common answer was: "More individual consideration." One child played nurse with another hospitalized child on the unit. The child said, "I'm the nurse and I'm giving you a needle. Stay still!" The other child struggled despite repeated orders to "Stay still!!!"

At the post-implementation phase, subtle changes were noted in client and family responses to these same questions. Several older pediatric and adult surgical clients said that the nurses asked at least once every day about their feelings, opinions, and concerns. On the pediatric units, the evaluator noticed that fewer babies were being left to cry alone, and that more children were being held by nurses at the nursing station. At the post-implementation data collection the evaluator observed more nurses in conversation with clients at the bedside rather than at the nursing station.

In summary, although not all clients answered questions differently in the post-implementation interviews, several clients noted that they were asked routinely about their feelings and concerns. The evaluator's observations of patterns of activity on the pediatric units reflected more attention being paid to children.

Nurse Questionnaires

Pilot unit nurses were invited to complete questionnaires prior to implementation of Parse's theory and 30 weeks following implementation. Analysis of these data will be presented according to the questions asked.

At the end of the project, nurses were asked what had changed for them. Although some nurses noticed little, if any, change in their way of being a nurse, by far the majority of nurses commented thoughtfully on changes they noted in their practice. The following were typical responses to that question:

> "My attitude has changed. I am much more **aware of each individual's uniqueness.** My tolerance level is at an all-time high."

> "I [now] look at patients as a **whole** rather than separating their disease. I learn to create time to spend with a client, and to look at personal values. What is important to that individual, where they are right now, and **to be truly present**. . . . I've learned to describe what the person says is important to him at this point, rather than just routinely documenting."

> "I . . . have a renewed awareness of the patient as an individual having his own unique experience. I try not to interview the patient looking for answers to my [own] problem list. I ask him how things are going . . . so I can discover **what is important to him.** Then I ask what I need to know. Now I know that it is not . . . particularly helpful to reassure a worried patient. If I just listen to him and he talks about it, he will feel better. I always hated reassuring patients because it felt like a lie I was supposed to tell."

The nurses' perceptions of health changed from the beginning to the end of the project. When asked to answer the question "What is health?" prior to implementation of Parse's theory, nurses talked about well-being, absence of illness, and the ability to function. The post-implementation questionnaires revealed that, instead of viewing health as a set of norms, nurses considered health to be living according to what was important to the person. Examples of responses follow:

> "Health is not just the absence of disease or a state of well-being. It means the way I view my own health based upon my **own values and beliefs.** I would hope I have the right to make my own choices."

> "Health means to me what it means to my patient and his family."

> "Health means asking the patient, **'What's important to you?'** initially when he is first admitted to the ward before asking our usual set of questions."

Prior to the implementation of the project, respondents were asked to define quality nursing care. Four themes were identified within those responses: coping under time constraints, completing tasks on time, being both effective and caring, and working well with others. At the 30th week, there were qualitative differences in the definitions of quality nursing care. Prior to the project, nurses tended to describe quality nursing care as an idealized state rarely achieved. At the conclusion, they were beginning to describe new ways of relating which they were daily creating. Examples of these differences follow:

> "I do not just try to finish my daily task(s) . . . I also try to provide true presence. **I focus now on the human interrelationship.** . . . What is important to my patient today? What is he feeling? How (have) things been going for him?"

> "Providing care according to the needs of the patient. **Respecting their needs** without deciding for them the changes or adaptations. Respecting the choices each patient makes toward his goals and dreams."

Another item in the questionnaire asked nurses to comment on the uniqueness of nursing practice. In the pre-implementation phase nurses stated that they helped people in illness, took care of patients' bio-psycho-social needs, had flexible work hours to meet their own needs, and had medical knowledge and technical ability to make people more healthy. Responses in the post-implementation phase were different:

> "It is mainly true presence with my patients."
>
> "I feel I give patients more than just facts. When I have the time, I take time out to find out what's important to them."
>
> "I don't have to diagnose; that is not my job. I see the client as a whole being and I can help the individual cope a little better with his or her disease knowing they have the right to make the choices they value as important to them."

The quality of the nurses' work lives was explored in the questionnaire. Before the project the following themes were extracted from the responses: bitter disenchantment together with moments of fulfillment; feeling rushed and unsafe while seeking satisfaction; living with short-staffing and little respect. Following 30 weeks of the project, responses were very different, indicating improved quality of work life. Exemplar responses follow:

> "I enjoy the relationships I have with my patients. I may suggest (alternatives) that patients and families have **without forcing them or labeling them** as 'unable to cope' or 'unable to adapt to stress.' I try to serve as a caregiver who allows others to have their own beliefs and goals of their own, and try to serve as a support for my patients toward their goals."
>
> "I am satisfied with my work life and deem it good quality. I respect people I work with and my clients but realize that they have the **right to make their own choices in life** with family and friends. Being with clients [can] truly make a difference to their quality of life."

Analysis of the responses to the Questionnaire for Nurse Participants before and after implementation of the study suggested differences in nurses' perceptions of human beings, health, and quality nursing practice. Responses indicated that many nurses were practicing differently based on Parse's theory-based practice method.

Key Informant Interviews

Key informants consisted of 18 nurses, nurse managers, and members of other health care disciplines who had daily contact with the three pilot units. Key informants were "nominated" by stakeholders in the hospital. Often nomination was initiated by the investigators' asking, "Do you know of anybody who holds a different opinion?" Key informants were interviewed prior to implementation and 30 weeks following implementation. They were able to describe what had happened, from their perspective, over the entire project. Their narratives provided frank and explicit descriptions of life on the pilot units.

In the data collected at the conclusion of the study there were shifts in the way nurses looked at themselves and their work. The first theme to emerge was **new images of self.** Some exemplars of this theme were:

> "When you practice this new way, you just feel so much better about yourself, because you touched a soul. You were really there for him."
>
> "The self-esteem of the nurses has increased definitely."

Many of the nurses talked about **improved morale** on the unit at the end of the study:

> "In the last three weeks there has been a big change in morale."
>
> "Our helping, friendly relationships are better."
>
> "For myself, I have a greater sense of accomplishment. This has been a challenging, trying and rewarding time. The project has been good, and I've learned a lot."

The evaluator noted changes related to the collective morale on the units and the individual morale of the nurses interviewed. The evaluator stated, "The morale seems better. Nurses aren't talking behind each other's backs."

Another theme to emerge at the end of the project was **new patterns of working with others.** Examples of this theme follow:

> "Now the nurses are more supportive of one another. When a child [recently] died, the nurses who took care of that baby were encouraged by their peers to leave the unit and share quiet time alone, to deal with their feelings. And the other nurses cared for them. They brought them coffee. I'm not sure this would have occurred six months ago. Now, the nurses are more tuned-in to the needs of other people."

> "[The nurses] seem friendlier now. They seem to work out their disagreements among themselves."

> "There's more a sense of unity [now]. We help each other out. So we have more quality time to spend with patients and their families."

Affirming personal power was another theme that emerged. Exemplars follow:

> "After the study, [there is] less bitching and acting like victims. The project awakened a will to go to meetings in the belief that we can actually foster change."

> "Before, nurses would take their concerns to the higher-ups. Now, they are more likely to deal with the person directly, like going directly to the doctor in charge."

> "Staff are advocating in the interests of their patients. People are standing up to the doctors, and saying [when] things are inappropriate."

> "Nurses are advocating more, taking a stand. There's more pride. But, the doctors don't see them any differently."

"Before Parse, we were asleep. Now we are awake. Nothing will ever be the same."

The theme of **seeking knowledge** came out of the key informant interviews at the conclusion of the study. One nurse put it this way:

"If you counted them up, you'd be surprised at the number of nurses who have recently decided to do university courses. Before the study, they were just here for their shifts. They say they are going back to school to get out of nursing, but they are signing up for nursing courses."

"I want to further my education. I think it's the only way nursing will get better."

"I've seen an increase over the last 6 months in the number of interdisciplinary conferences [to discuss patient care]. These are always initiated by the pilot unit nurses."

Over the course of the project, nurses described the theme of **shifting values and beliefs.** Here are some examples gleaned from the key informants:

"Although patient care has (always) been a priority, the nurses' attitudes have changed. Before, they would have labeled a patient as 'difficult.' Now, they attempt to find out what is important to [the patient]."

"The nurses are taking more time to be with patients. Now they are not [just] looking at convenience or at habit, but at what is important to the child and parents."

"The theory affirmed for them that it's okay to not just focus on tasks. It's okay to make time just to be with the patient."

"Before the project, nurses looked more at the clinical perspective than at the patient's perspective. There is a real difference now. The nurses are more focused on what the patient wants."

"Before [the project], you tried to make people better by 'fixing' them. Now, I don't tell them what to do. Family-centered care has definitely been enhanced because the paternalistic attitudes have changed. There's a greater interest in looking at where families are coming from."

"We don't take a generalized approach to admitting people any more. Instead, we now try to look at each person as unique."

"A priority is still physical care and getting things done, but now we also focus on family needs."

"The patient is now seen as a total person, rather than a label. We try to understand their needs and problems. We try to give them our true presence."

"We now find more time to be with the patients. We ask the child: 'What is this feeling like for you?' . . . rather than just going in and giving treatment. We now spend more quality time with them."

"More and more, [the nurses] are seeing the uniqueness of people and respecting others' values and beliefs, instead of imposing their own views on the patient. Now they pick up the direction from the person . . . More and more nurses are buying into the idea that you have to understand and value the beliefs of patients and their families."

Another key theme at the conclusion of the study was **looking beyond the labels.** The data revealed a strong change in the nurses' attitudes toward different cultures and beliefs:

"There's more of a concentrated effort to make a different-looking family more comfortable."

"There's still some labeling of people, but when you don't label patients, you see them, and not [just] the nationality."

"I think that we are more understanding of people. We look beyond the diagnosis to the person himself."

The theme of **changing patterns of practice** emerged. Some examples follow illustrating the comfort-discomfort lived by pilot unit nurses as they attempted to put new values into action:

> "It's risky and uncomfortable. I see opportunities to use Parse's method, but I let them slip away. But I see some nurses using it, and they get all kinds of stuff from patients that before would have just been held back."

> "Some try it out in safe situations, for example, at home with their children. And they see a real difference that they value."

> "Some [nurses] know it real well and are trying to teach it to the rest of us. Other's aren't using it but see real value in it."

> "I feel like I'm learning [the theory] and fumbling along."

As evidenced in the data, there is a struggle to break away from old familiar ideas:

> "Once [we had a] difficult patient, and we tried to use it on him. It worked sometimes, but not always."

> "Through Parse's theory, we have learned the skill of giving ourselves in true presence."

> "It's something you can use to approach a difficult situation. I'm [no longer] afraid to say: 'How do you feel about this?' Now it's okay to ask that. I'm more sensitive now, and that's not unprofessional. Before, staff [used to] skirt around questions. Now, they . . . ask . . ."

Patterns of comfort - discomfort in changing patterns of practice were also played out in the group dynamics of the pilot unit teams:

> "[Once] I tried to practice it, and I was put down by the other nurses."

> "A lot of us do like it. Some don't. We concentrate on it."

"I see them practicing Parse (theory) now, even if only a few would admit it. They are definitely spending more time with parents and children. The theoretical language still scares them . . . but people are really applying the new beliefs. . . . There are so many cases where they are using the theory with agitated parents, and turning these situations right around."

Some nurses remarked on the incongruence of Parse's theory with familiar concepts such as reality orientation and nursing diagnosis, and they began to appreciate the different opportunities offered by theory-based practice:

"I was working with one man who was confused, but not really confused. He just wanted to talk about the life he had led before coming to the hospital. It's a very different way of talking with (people)."

"I used it with a man who was contemplating suicide. I offered my time to him. He told me how bad it was for him. I didn't try to change what he thought. I didn't try to make him feel better. I just went with him to where he was. At the end of the conversation, he started to describe all he had. To understand Parse, you have to live the experience, and then you understand what it's about. At the end of [our] conversation, he looked so different . . . I was really busy that night, and I went home thinking: Among all the things that I had done that night, that experience meant the most to me."

One nurse described a woman who had been labeled by others as "non communicative":

"What evolved in that conversation was incredible. She became responsive and started talking. We just sat there and she turned her back. I thought this was my cue to leave but when I asked 'What's important to you?' she began to tell . . . how much she missed home and wanted her mother. She began to cry. After the dialogue, she was very different. Even the nurses on the next shift that night saw her as changed."

The last theme to emerge from the key informant interviews was **patients see the difference.**

"Families [who have frequent admissions with us] have noticed differences. I was using Parse's (theory) with a family and the mother said: 'What happened [to the nurses here]? What's changed? Is everybody around here [now] like this? The place must be under new management.'"

"Patients and parents have expressed their surprise. They say: 'I have never been to a hospital like this. Everything here is so meaningful.'"

After an encounter with a nurse, a mother said:

"I have never seen a hospital where there is so much caring."

At the conclusion of the study one mother wrote:

"Coming from a small city, the personal care you extended certainly was [a surprise]. We had become accustomed to the large city [attitude] of 'treat them and release them.' It was a nice touch, and we were impressed."

Another mother who frequently visited the study units wrote:

"Everyone was very friendly and accommodating. A pleasant change from the struggle and fight experienced previously. There is enough stress when your child is in the hospital without the added hassle of making sure that special needs are met. I wasn't very happy with my child's last stay in the hospital. I was afraid to voice my concerns for fear that if he were admitted another time, the nurses would be resentful. Fortunately, that did not happen."

One key informant noted that nurses seemed more self-assured at the conclusion of the study, and added that there were now fewer complaints about nursing care.

The key informant interviews provided the most notable indications of change in nurses' attitudes, values, beliefs, and practice patterns. Key informants, such as administrators and other health personnel, noticed differences in nursing practice and patient care. The narrative descriptions provided rich descriptions of the differences that occurred with the implementation of Parse's theory-based practice model.

REFLECTIONS ON THE PROCESS

The first weeks of the study were marked by turbulence related to the change process. Applying strategies of Guba and Lincoln's (1989) constructivist approach to evaluation, the investigators attempted to determine stakeholders' concerns and fears. Pilot unit nurses said that they felt devalued by the introduction of nursing theory. They felt that the implementation of a new nursing model implied that their practice was being judged as substandard or inferior. They were hurt and angry. Hospital administrators felt the anger of senior physicians who viewed the introduction of theory-based nursing practice as a threat. Anger was directed toward the principal investigator in multiple forms.

Organizational upheaval unrelated to the project contributed to the turbulent environment. Two research unit nurse managers departed from the hospital in the third month of the study. Responding to this loss, both pediatric pilot units were hastily amalgamated under a single head nurse. At the 12th week of the project, major budget cutbacks were announced throughout the hospital. Bed closures and massive nursing layoffs appeared inevitable. The 30 weeks of the Parse project were accompanied by unprecedented organizational changes that finally led to the resignation of three senior administrative officers after the successful completion of the project. Despite all confounding factors, teaching of the practice method continued and researchers became accustomed to living under constant pressure.

CONCLUSIONS

The purpose of this evaluation study was to discern changes in client-family health experiences, nursing attitudes, beliefs and practices, and the organizational culture that accompany the implementation of Parse's theory-based practice in an acute-care setting and to provide data for informed administrative decision making related to implementing the model on a hospital-wide basis.

Findings of this study did support that there were qualitative changes in client-family health experiences. These changes were subtle and certainly not experienced by all clients and family members that were interviewed. But, these changes were noticed and appreciated by some clients and family members. Several clients and family members specifically noted that they were asked about their feelings, concerns, and wishes. This was not evident in the interviews that were conducted in the pre-implementation phase. Other family members and clients were moved to write letters or comment to the nurse administrators on the units. Researchers were challenged to obtain children's perspectives. We could not discern changes through the interviews with the children, but the evaluator commented in her report that the nurses were with the children more during the post-implementation phase.

When nurses learn Parse's theory-based practice method, they tend to integrate it slowly as they "try it out" with family members and begin to appreciate the difference that it makes. The practice method is something that nurses grow with; therefore, the changes that clients and families will notice after about 7 months of learning and practice are expected to be subtle. Nurses did share that during some moments they felt that it made a surprising difference in the health experience of clients. These accounts were shared in the interviews.

Analysis of questionnaires, interviews, and nursing documentation indicated changes in nurses' attitudes, beliefs, and practices. Nurses described the changes in the way they had come to view their clients. For example, they talked about valuing the uniqueness of each person without labeling clients. They stated that they saw beyond the disease to the person as a whole being. They acknowledged the client's right to choose his or her own way and affirmed that health was a personal integration and living of values. Nurses structured practice based on these conceptual shifts by asking clients and families what was important to them and then communicating this to others. They stated that they were present with the client, that is, intent on being with the client to honor the client's agenda, not to assert their own.

The definition of quality nursing practice shifted from a dominant task-orientation to a relationship-orientation. At the 30th week nurses stated that quality practice is respecting the client-family's choices more than adhering to the health care provider's protocols. This description of quality practice was liberating, in that responsibility for quality became a partnership rather than the nurse's sole responsibility. These profound changes were noted by many of the respondents.

Nurses felt better about themselves, supported each other more frequently, and subsequently there was subtle improvement in morale on the units at the 30th week of the study. There seemed to be a difference in acknowledging personal power and responsibility. Nurses began to appreciate their special contribution to the health care team, and with this appreciation came a sense of pride and courage. Changes in nursing practice were evolutionary. Nurses were uncomfortable, and making changes was both awkward and risky. Some tried out new ways of being with their families and friends. Certainly, not all nurses came to value the theory or practice method. Those nurses who did not value it demeaned those who wanted to make some changes. Nurses who valued the theoretic perspective slowly integrated changes. Some provided stories of clients who seemed transformed by this different way of being with others.

Changes in organizational culture were more difficult to discern. Some changes appeared in the values of the unit. For example, children were more visible in the nursing station, on the laps of nurses rather than alone in their rooms. More nurses articulated differences in the way they perceived their clients and some family members felt a difference in the climate of the units. Nurses felt that a caring ethic was more evident in the way they interacted with each other.

Findings of the evaluation study were reported to the hospital administration in a written report and to the entire hospital community in an open forum. There was evidence that supported the continuing implementation of Parse's theory-based practice model on the pilot units and hospital-wide. However, the hospital administration and nursing administration changed after the study, and with these dramatic changes, the continuity of the project was not maintained.

RECOMMENDATIONS

Recommendations for future studies emerged from the experiences during this study. First, the evaluation of a newly implemented theory-based practice model requires at least a 12-month interval between implementation and post-implementation data generation. Some changes were noted in nursing values and practice, client-family experience, and unit culture at the end of 30 weeks; more consistent changes might be identified after a longer time interval. The principal investigator suggested that at least 6 months should elapse before other interested units began the process. Finally, he recommended that the values of the theory be integrated into the nursing service philosophy and introduced during the hospital's orientation program.

With the turmoil that accompanied these changes, the learning curve was erratic. The process of transformation was characterized by a paradoxical dialectic of open exploration and fearful withdrawal. In another context, Bruns (1989) has ably described such non-linear struggle: It is not a matter of clarity or transparency. There are bursts of sudden insight against the background of a slow dawning. Often, the bursts of light would darken quickly back into bewilderment. One finds one's path, then loses it just as quickly, doubling back to begin the search anew. Every glimpse of light draws one back into the darkness of uncertainty and doubt. Rather than a steady state of clarification (Bruns, 1989), the nurses experienced a hesitant groping toward a dimly-lit clearing of understanding.

Nurses were moved to change through witnessing the difference that this practice could make to their clients; therefore, one-on-one work with an expert nurse in the practice was the most effective teaching-learning strategy. However, it was very difficult for one practice scholar to be responsible for teaching 110 nurses. A team of nurses skilled in the theory-based practice model and on-site during the study might provide the support needed for a project of this scope.

Implementing one theory-based practice model on a unit-wide basis should be done only after careful consideration. If diversity of nursing models/theories is evident in the discipline, this diversity must be honored. Those nurses who espouse a different philosophy need not feel obligated to practice according to the one selected for the unit. Perhaps units could organize around frameworks selected by the majority of unit nurses; those not wishing to practice on those units could transfer to another unit. Another approach would be to allow diversity of approaches on the unit and to evaluate the differences in practice of those nurses who have chosen the model of interest.

Further work is recommended in using multiple modalities to gather the evidence needed to evaluate change. The photography used in this study has potential if used over time rather than at pre- and post-data generation points only. Nurses might be asked to view photographs and interpret them. Videotaping and audiotaping of encounters with clients also has potential to uncover changes in practice patterns. The researchers were challenged to access children's perspectives on nursing practice. We used puppet play and drawings but found that children had their own agenda and were not motivated to draw or play when we invited them to do so. Financial analysis could examine the cost-effectiveness of a theory-based practice model. For example, outcomes of turnover and nurse absenteeism could be investigated.

This descriptive qualitative evaluation study provided beginning evidence that with the introduction of Parse's theory-based practice model there were qualitative differences in patient-family health experiences, nurses' attitudes, values and beliefs, and the organizational culture. This study was conducted on two pediatric units and a general surgical unit in a 400-bed community hospital. The process of implementing theory-based practice on the units was characterized by turbulence. Substantive changes in values related to honoring client uniqueness, wholeness, and freedom to choose were described by the nurses. Some patients and family members noted that generally the staff were more friendly, supportive, and caring than they had been in the past. Administrators and nurses noticed some improvement in morale and a greater appreciation for the distinctive contribution of nursing to the health care team. Additional evaluation studies are essential for the further development of nursing theory-based practice methods and the growth of nursing as a professional discipline.

REFERENCES

Bruns, G. L. (1989). *Heidegger's estrangements: Language truth and poetry in the later writings.* New Haven: Yale University Press.

Canadian Nurses Association. (1986). *A definition of nursing practice: Standards for nursing practice.* Ottawa: Author.

College of Nurses of Ontario. (1990). *Standards of nursing practice:* Toronto: Author.

DeGroot, H. A. (1988). Scientific inquiry in nursing: A model for a new age. *Advances in Nursing Science, 10*(3), 1–21.

Fawcett, J. (1989). *Analysis and evaluation of conceptual models of nursing.* Philadelphia: Davis.

Guba, E. G., & Lincoln, Y. S. (1989). *Fourth generation evaluation.* Newbury Park, CA: Sage.

Hoch, C. (1987). Assessing delivery of nursing care. *Journal of Gerontological Nursing, 13,* 10–17.

Mattice, M. (1991). Parse's theory of nursing in practice: A manager's perspective. *Canadian Journal of Nursing Administration, 4*(1), 13.

Mayeroff, M. (1971). *On caring.* New York: Harper & Row.

Parse, R. R. (1981). *Man-living-health: A theory of nursing.* New York: Wiley.

Parse, R. R. (1987). *Nursing science: Major paradigms, theories, and critiques.* Philadelphia: Saunders.

Parse, R. R. (1988, September). *Parse's theory in practice: An evaluation study.* Paper presented at the National Symposium of Nursing Research. San Francisco, CA.

Parse, R. R. (1992). Human becoming: Parse's theory of nursing. *Nursing Science Quarterly, 5,* 35–42.

Parse, R. R., Coyne, A. B., & Smith, M. J. (1985). *Nursing research: Qualitative methods.* Bowie, MD: Brady.

Santopinto, M. D. A. (1989). *An evaluation of Parse's theory in the chronic care setting: A descriptive pilot study.* Paper presented at the 19th Quadrennial Congress of the International Council of Nurses, Seoul, Korea.

Silva, M. C. (1986). Research testing nursing theory: State of the art. *Advances in Nursing Science, 9*(1), 1–11.

Smith, M. C. (1991). Evaluating nursing theory-based practice. *Nursing Science Quarterly, 4,* 98–99.

Chapter 18

Evaluation of the Human Becoming Theory in Family Practice

Christine M. Jonas

*N*ursing practice in family practice settings traditionally has been dominated by a problem-based, medically-oriented approach. Typically, nurses prepare patients for examination and assessment by the doctor. Involved in the preparation is the recording of a brief history that focuses on the patient's chief complaint. Nurses may perform a physical assessment while trying to reach the correct medical diagnosis. Following the formal physician assessment and diagnosis, nurses in family practice might perform delegated interventions or health teaching based on the identified problem. Although opportunities for independent nursing practice do exist, the medical issues take precedence and often nurses do not avail themselves of the unique realm of nursing knowledge to guide autonomous practice.

Many nurses are familiar with this traditional problem-based scenario, but what happens when nurses in family practice change their knowledge base from bio-psycho-social theory to nursing theory? More specifically, what happens when nurses in a family practice unit learn and practice nursing from Parse's (1981, 1987, 1992) theoretical base? Parse's (1981, 1992) theory, called human becoming, is different from, yet complementary to, medical practice. The purpose of this chapter is to report findings from a descriptive evaluation study of Parse's theory in a family practice setting. Findings flow from nine staff nurse participants and their nurse manager who learned the theory over a 10-month period. Patient questionnaires provide data for further investigation.

BACKGROUND OF THE STUDY

The theory of human becoming has been used to guide practice in the community (Butler & Snodgrass, 1991; Rasmusson, Jonas, & Mitchell, 1991), in acute care (Mattice, 1991; Mattice & Mitchell, 1991; Mitchell & Copplestone, 1990; Mitchell & Pilkington, 1990; Quiquero, Knights, & Meo, 1991), and in long-term care (Mavely & Mitchell, 1994; Mitchell, 1986). Formal evaluations of the theory in practice have occurred in various settings, including an acute care unit in the same hospital as the Family Practice Unit (FPU) being discussed here (see chapter 19). That study was conducted following a request by the unit manager to teach nurses how to be with clients in a Parse-guided way (Mattice, 1991).

Findings from Mitchell's evaluation study (see chapter 19) revealed the following six patterns of change among staff nurses: (a) changed perspective of patient from "problem" to patient as "person," (b) changed morale in nurses, (c) less judging and labeling of patients, (d) more talking and listening to patients, (e) respecting the patient's right to choose, and (f) enhancing the quality of the nurse-person relationship. From the manager's perspective, Parse's theory enhanced quality of care for patients and improved satisfaction for nurses (Mattice, 1991). Staff nurses reported that "Parse's theory has opened our eyes and our thinking to a more humanistic way of nursing" (Quiquero, Knights, & Meo, 1991, p. 16). The findings of Mitchell's study expanded interest in Parse's theory in other hospitals as well as other areas of the hospital where the evaluation study was implemented. Santopinto and Smith (see chapter 17) identified similar themes in their evaluation of Parse-guided practice with children and adults admitted to the hospital. Additionally, preliminary findings in a psychiatric facility affirm consistent themes about nurse morale, satisfaction, and changes in the nurse-person relationship that enhance quality of life for persons receiving care (D. Northrup, personal communication, January 27, 1994).

The project to evaluate Parse's theory of nursing in family practice was initiated by the unit manager who, along with the staff nurses, wanted to change from traditional biomedical nursing to nursing theory-based practice. The nurse manager from family practice requested that several nurse specialists speak to the nurses about the differences among various nursing theories. Nurses on the FPU discussed basic values, assumptions, expectations, and anticipated outcomes of different theories. They decided to try to learn and evaluate Parse's theory with the rationale that it focused on the nurse-person process and on enhancing quality of life from the person's own perspective.

The purpose of the project was to evaluate Parse's theory in a family practice setting by describing the changes that occurred in practice from the perspectives of the staff nurses, the nurse manager, and the people who attend family practice. The question guiding this project was "What changes occur in nursing practice when Parse's theory is initiated in family practice, from the perspectives of the nursing staff, nurse manager, and people who attend the family practice unit?"

PARSE'S THEORY OF NURSING

Parse's theory of nursing (1981, 1987, 1992) focuses on human becoming as an open process that happens moment to moment in relationship with others. The focus with Parse's theory is not physical, psychological, social, or spiritual problems identified through assessment and comparison with norms. Health and quality of life are viewed from the person's perspective for nurses guided by Parse's theory. The assumptions and values of human becoming are very different from the traditional assumptions and values that nurses practice. These differences have been explicated elsewhere (Parse, 1987), but the changes in a family practice setting for nurses and patients have not been specified in the literature.

Parse's theory of nursing is grounded in human science (Mitchell & Cody, 1992; Parse, 1981, 1992). The theory "has its roots, then, in the belief that humans participate with the universe in the cocreation of health" (Parse, 1992, p. 37). Humans are viewed as open, unitary beings who cocreate health in rhythmical patterns. Health is not viewed in terms of being good or bad but, rather, as the way one lives personal values. Consistent with the human science perspective, the "essence of Parse's theory is embedded in meanings, patterns of relationships and in hopes and dreams" (Parse, 1992, p. 37). The different view of human beings and health in Parse's theory guides nurses to be with persons in a different way. The nurse is not the expert armed with standardized care plans which are used to "fix" the patient's health problem, as in traditional nursing. Rather, the nurse lives true presence and moves with the person as meanings are illuminated and relationships lived in the changing process of human becoming.

METHOD AND DESIGN

A pre-post-qualitative-descriptive design was chosen to generate data about the usefulness of Parse's theory for guiding practice. Guba and Lincoln (1989) described four generations of evaluation frameworks. The current project was guided by the third generation approach, which included, along with description, judgment by project participants on the value and merit of Parse's theory in a family practice setting.

Smith (1991) offered three basic guidelines for evaluating nursing theory-based practice: consistency, clarity, and change. Consistencies must be evident among the evaluation approach, the participants' and researcher's worldviews, and the philosophical assumptions of the theory being evaluated. This means that a theory such as Parse's that specifies simultaneous human-world processes would not be evaluated with a research model that required or generated causal relationships. The design of this research project, qualitative-descriptive, is thus consistent with Parse's theory. Clarity of reporting the research process, including intentions and outcomes, is crucial to good evaluation research. Evaluation studies should report enough detail and description so that others can reach the same conclusion about the consequences of the change. The change itself must be described and explored in an open way that encourages answers to "so what has happened here?"

Setting and Participants

The setting for this project was a Family Practice Unit (FPU) affiliated with a teaching hospital in a large urban setting in Canada. There were four registered nurses, three nursing assistants, and two health care aides employed on the unit. Team nursing was the mode of nursing care delivery on the unit. The nurses had not been exposed to nursing theories prior to the project; however, nurses were exposed to Parse's theory and other nursing theories in the process of choosing a theory that fit with their values and beliefs. Further, staff nurses elsewhere in the same facility were speaking openly, such as over meals in the cafeteria, about the limitations and opportunities of Parse's theory in practice.

Data Collection

The data were collected before and after teaching Parse's theory of nursing to the staff. A 10-month period between pre-project evaluation and post-project evaluation was considered the minimum amount of time needed to determine the influence of a theory in practice. Pre-project evaluation included asking nurses and the nurse manager to write about *what was most important in their nursing practice, how satisfied they were with their nursing practice, and how they would like to see their practice change.* During the post-project phase, 10 months later, nursing staff were asked again to write answers to the above questions. Additionally, nurses were asked to participate in focused interviews about changes in practice after learning about Parse's theory. These interviews were audiotape-recorded and transcribed. People who attended the FPU as patients were asked to participate in the evaluation of nursing care. Those who agreed to participate were asked to offer comments on the quality of nursing care received from the nurses.

Protection of Participants' Rights

All participants' data were protected for confidentiality. Nurses were given the choice of participating with all aspects of the project—answering questions in writing, interviews, and implementation of the theory. Participation in the project was considered consent. People who attended the unit were given a letter explaining reasons for the evaluation of nursing care. Included in the letter was a set of questions about what nursing care was like in the unit. Persons attending the unit were informed that they were not obligated to participate nor would their care be affected by their choice. They were also informed in the letter that choosing to answer the questions was considered consent.

Teaching the Theory

Parse's theory was taught to the nurses in small group sessions twice a week for the 10-month period. Modeled after Mitchell's approach (see chapter 19), sessions began with discussions that centered on the underlying values and beliefs of the theory. Gradually, sessions encompassed the concepts and principles of the theory and the practice methodology. The nursing practice guided by Parse's theory was demonstrated with persons attending the FPU by the author, a nurse specialist. Other Parse nurses not involved in the project were asked to visit the unit and to discuss practice guided by Parse. Discussion groups continued twice a week to provide an opportunity for the nurses to express their thoughts, concerns, and other issues linked to learning practice guided by Parse's theory of nursing. Videotapes of nurse-person discussions were also made for teaching purposes. The nurses gradually became knowledgeable about Parse's theory, and with guidance from the nurse specialist they began to change their practice. During discussions nurses related practice situations where they lived true presence according to Parse's theory. Nurses described both satisfaction and struggle with learning a new way of being with people. Weekly discussions centered on clarification of theory-guided experiences as nurses moved to a more enhanced understanding of the theory.

Data Analysis

Analysis of the pre- and post-project data followed a qualitative analysis-synthesis process. Major findings emerged from the following sources of data: (a) written comments from the questionnaires completed by nurses both pre- and post-project; (b) transcribed interviews with staff nurses about the changes they experienced in practice; (c) written and verbal data recorded with the nurse manager about the changes; and (d) written comments from the people who experienced care at the FPU. Participant responses to questions pre- and post-project were recorded and compared. Data from the interviews were read and reread with the audiotape playing in order for the researcher to identify the common themes surfacing in the data. The raw data and themes which the researcher identified were sent to two outside reviewers. The expert reviewers refined and verified the themes.

FINDINGS

Pre- and Post-Project Written Answers

Findings from the pre- and post-project written answers to questions did not show a radical difference. Prior to learning Parse's theory nurses primarily discussed meeting patients' needs as most important. Generally, nurses felt "fairly well satisfied" with practice, although they wanted more time and less focus on task completion. Pre-project data also indicated that nurses wanted more referrals from other disciplines in their areas of expertise.

After learning and integrating the values and beliefs of Parse's theory, nurses said that it was most important for them to be with patients to learn about them. Nurses described a growth with Parse's theory and a change in their sense of professional purpose. Practice was described as "very satisfying" with Parse's guidelines, and nurses said they wanted to learn more about new ways of thinking about and being with persons in practice. Table 18.1 contains examples of nurses' responses given prior to and after learning about Parse's theory.

Post-Project Interview

Post-project semi-structured interviews were conducted with the family practice nurses. Analysis of these data revealed six themes. Themes are numbered by frequency of occurrence, and examples of supporting statements follow.

Theme 1   Nurses described enhanced satisfaction and meaningfulness in practice.

- "I think it has enriched my practice; it has made nursing more interesting."
- "It makes me feel good, confident that I am achieving something."
- "I find the theory exciting and challenging."

Theme 2   Nurses reported how they became focused on time to listen.

- "I think the most frustrating thing is [the] time element, of finding the time . . . [yet] you do not have to spend half an

Table 18.1   Nurse Responses to Pre- and Post-Project Questions

Question	Pre-Project Response	Post-Project Response
What is most important in your nursing practice?	"Knowing that most of my patients' needs are being met."	"I feel privileged to have the opportunity to grow and learn from my patients."
	"To show I care."	"Being with patients has enhanced the way I practice nursing."
	"Helping my patients to understand their needs."	"It means great satisfaction."
	"Helping patients to the best of my ability, whether it be through listening, doing dressings, or whatever."	"My patients are most important to me, and from them and their experiences, I have grown and matured."
How satisfied are you with your practice?	"Fairly well satisfied, but would like to see a more independent nursing practice."	"Very satisfied; I need to be continually challenged. Parse does this for me."
	"I'd like to do more nursing and spend more time with patients."	"Just beginning to realize the great potential."
	"Doing the best I can each day brings satisfaction of its own."	"A new view to my nursing practice which brings a lot more satisfaction to all aspects of my nursing career."
How would you like to see your practice change?	"I would like more referrals from other health care professionals in the area of my expertise."	"I would wish for more time to be with the patient."
	"I'd like to do more nursing and spend more time with patients."	"Feel more confident with the use of Parse's theory."
		"I'd like to marry my need to give information with the patient's choices, hopes, and dreams."

hour. I know you can 'be with' people for two minutes and get a lot of satisfaction out of it."

- "You don't have the exact amount of time that you might like but . . . you might have this one brief encounter with them, only a few minutes, but that might be all that you need."
- "Nurses are spending more time with the patients listening to them rather than thinking that you have to fix their problems and you don't have the time."

Theme 3   Nurses described a heightened awareness of the person's perspective.

- "It is so much nicer to have the patient's point of view than for you to be projecting your own ideas on the patient all the time."
- "I think the theory helps to make you focus on the patient. You have that warm feeling with them and that is the joy."
- "Before I had all the answers, at least I thought I did. But I'm listening more and I am starting to hear more of what persons are saying."

Theme 4   Nurses clarified new benefits of being with clients.

- "It is a great way of being with people and I certainly feel very positive about it."
- "With Parse's theory you have achieved something because you have been with people and what they are going through and what coming to the FPU means to them."
- "I feel really good, just being there for the person."

Theme 5   Nurses reported struggling with living the different beliefs of Parse's theory.

- "[I'm] trying to use the theory and trying to get out of the old system."

- "I find it tough really—but I understand enough of it and appreciate enough of it to know that it will work for me in whatever, however far I want to go with it . . . because it is really basically very simple."
- "We have been taught one way and after say 20 years of nursing to all of a sudden change to something brand new, it's going to take a while."

Theme 6 Nurses indicated changed relationships with co-workers that were more nurturing and understanding.

- "I think it has brought the nursing staff closer together by having our meeting together and sharing this knowledge and learning experience."
- "I think we are all on the one wavelength rather than each one doing their own thing."
- "We tend to listen to one another and that is important."

Changes for the Unit Manager

The unit manager addressed the same three questions as staff nurses about practice pre- and post-project. Pre-project data indicated that the manager saw nursing as assisting people to maximize their health potential through education and doing tasks. Most important was to be trusted by patients, to be seen as a resource. The manager did think that nurses in family practice were trying to "emulate physicians," and she hoped that nursing models might provide nurses with a different identity. Practice was described as somewhat satisfying, and, although she felt autonomous, there was a sense of lacking nursing knowledge and unique direction.

Post-project data from the manager's answers to the questions indicated that practice now meant making a difference to clients because of a special nurse-person relationship. The manager felt that she had changed from focusing on duties to focusing on process, on relationships with patients, staff, and other nurses. Most important to the manager after the 10 months of learning Parse's theory was to establish a network with others who could continue to support and teach the theory and "not judging." As for satisfaction, the manager said that she had changed dramatically. She said, "I am excited about the change and about facing a future of further growth." The nurse manager discussed three central points in her interview after the project. The points are listed below with some quotes that typify descriptive comments.

- **New understanding about the uniqueness of nursing practice.**

  "I think by bringing Parse on the unit we have a much stronger sense of what nursing is—that we don't have to be doctors; we now have something to hang our hat on. I now talk with more confidence and with more ability because I have some sort of framework with which to discuss nursing. I strongly believe in what nursing has to offer now and I could not even define it a year ago. Now I believe I have something to offer."

- **Enhanced growth and satisfaction.**

  "The theory has so much potential for personal and individual growth and for nursing practice. I did not see any room for growth in nursing, and since I have started learning about Parse's theory—the implication for nursing—it is a never-ending field. I can make a difference."

- **Practice transformed from a "fix-it" model to a nurturing model.**

  "In the family practice unit you end up being mini-physicians. Walk-ins come in and you try to figure out and diagnose, do the tasks and the duties. I just ended up running the team, doing what I had to do. I didn't see much real room for growth. Now my practice is about being with and supporting personal growth."

The unit manager addressed concerns about the commitment required to learn Parse's theory. After 10 months she stated, "We are still having some difficulty applying it and still trying to understand. We still feel insecure in our attempts to apply it. But we have the belief that it is something of value." Later in the same discussion the manager said: "The problem with the theory is you do not apply it. The model allows you to grow and develop and understand and I think the model does not dictate to you. It's very much one of participating in, a growth model." The manager also acknowledged the challenge of presenting opportunities for growth of staff but of not being able to force it. She went on: "People take their growth so far. Some nurses may not grow with the theory any further. So that needs attention, but I think it will always need attention. I can't imagine that you ever arrive. So that requires manpower and recognition of that, and that is one of the problems of implementing the model."

Patient Comments About Nursing Practice on the FPU

Comments from some of the people ($n = 6$) who attended the FPU were collected with questions about quality of care. The small number of respondents, coupled with the lack of any comparison data, diminishes opportunities to attach great importance to the findings from patients. Three people commented that the quality of care received from the nurses was excellent, and they felt the nurses were really interested in how they were doing. One person commented that trips to the FPU were less stressful and more comfortable because of the nurse. Another person who attended the unit stated that the nurse "makes a big difference by making me feel like a person instead of a number." Four of the six people who returned questionnaires said that they did not notice any difference in nursing care over the past year. Data from patients does point to the need for studies that explore the consequences of nursing care that is structured in different theoretical perspectives. For example, one might ask, do patients perceive any difference in nursing care that is performed by nurses using Orem's self-care deficit theory compared with nurses guided by Parse's theory?

DISCUSSION

The findings suggest an increase in nurse satisfaction and patient-focused care with the introduction of Parse's theory of nursing. The six major themes in this study reflected changes in nurses' values and beliefs about human beings, health, and nursing practice. Changes were similar to, yet different from, the patterns and themes identified in Mitchell's evaluation study which took place on a medical unit, (see chapter 19) and Wallace's (1993) study of nurses learning Parse's theory in a chronic care setting.

The first theme, "Nurses indicated enhanced satisfaction and meaningfulness in practice" and the sixth theme, "Nurses indicated changed relationships with co-workers that were more nurturing and understanding," were similar to the pattern of "changed morale in nurses" which surfaced in Mitchell's study (see chapter 19). Nursing theory-based practice carves out the uniqueness of nursing which can lead to enhanced satisfaction and meaningfulness in practice. Similarly, Wallace (1993) reported a theme that focused on nurses' reporting that Parse's theory renewed their beliefs in the real purpose of nursing. Enhanced satisfaction and meaningfulness in practice as a result of theory-based practice has been reported in the literature (Heggie, Schoenmehl, Chang, & Grieco, 1989; Mattice, 1991; Mitchell & Pilkington, 1990; Quiquero, Knights, & Meo, 1991; Taylor, 1988, 1989).

The second theme, "Nurses reported a more focused time to listen," was similar to Mitchell's pattern of "more talking and listening" (see chapter 19) and Wallace's (1993) discovery that nurses in chronic care listened to patients more when guided by

Parse's perspective. In each project the nurses changed their priorities in practice from completing tasks to listening and being with patients. Tasks were still completed, but they were no longer the purpose or central focus of practice. Nurses spoke about how often, before practicing Parse's theory, they would sit and listen to a person and have already listed in their minds what the person "should" do for her/his health. Once the nurses thought more about the person's perspective, they no longer felt comfortable saying what the person should or should not do. One nurse from the FPU stated that she "was always taught that we were the trained professionals and we had all the answers and they did not know anything, so it is a complete reversal."

The third theme, "Nurses described a heightened awareness of the person's perspective" was similar to Mitchell's patterns of "changed perspective of patient from 'problem' to 'person'," "respecting the patient's right to choose" and "less judging and labeling" (see chapter 19). Likewise, Wallace (1993) identified a theme that highlighted the ways nurses developed a prevailing respect for persons as unique human beings, a respect that had not been focused on before Parse's theory. In the literature, nurses are acknowledging the importance of the person's perspective and meanings of lived experiences (Quiquero, Knights, & Meo, 1991; Rasmusson, Jonas, & Mitchell, 1991; Wondolowski & Davis, 1988, 1991). In support of this focus, Allan and Hall (1988) stated that "the time is overdue to move away from the technological imperative and toward holistic models that have as their major focus a concern with people's lives" (p. 33).

Lastly, the theme, "Nurses clarified new benefits of being with clients" revealed a similarity to Mitchell's pattern of "enhancing the quality of the nurse-person relationships" (see chapter 19). Wallace (1993) indicated that nurses in her study intensified efforts to "allow" patients to make choices when guided by Parse's theory. Liehr (1989) states that "it becomes increasingly clear that the unique gift a nurse has to offer is to share self by being truly present with another" (p. 7). Further, from Parse's human becoming theory, "True presence is crucial for promoting health and enhancing quality of life with individuals and with families" (Liehr, 1989, p. 8).

One different theme in this project was "Nurses reported struggling with living the different beliefs of Parse's theory." Though it was not named as a theme by Mitchell, it was evident in discussion of the process of change the nurses had undergone (see chapter 19). Heggie et al. (1989) implemented Rogers' nursing science in an acute care setting and described the "change to a nursing model (as) a slow and sometimes painful process requiring considerable time" (p. 147). The process of change seen in 10 months was very positive. The support from administration was critical during this time. Heggie et al. (1989) also acknowledged the importance of support from administration, considering it "a vital element to the success of the project" (p. 147).

The nurse manager noted that with Parse's theory there was a new understanding about the uniqueness of nursing practice. The manager described a change in practice from a "fix-it" model toward a nurturing model of nursing which supported the valued time for "being with" persons who attend the FPU. Jacobs and Heuther (1978) claimed that "external forces will have less influence on nursing when it creates its own internal stimuli for change and redefinition based on knowledge and practice generated by nursing science" (p. 64). Lastly, at post-evaluation the manager observed enhanced growth and satisfaction among the staff.

Only a few questionnaires were completed by the people who attended the FPU prior to the project's completion. These people commented on how their quality of life was enhanced by the nurses and their presence. With only a few completed questionnaires, it would be difficult to know that client satisfaction was enhanced with Parse's theory. However, from what staff nurses reported about their practice, more time was spent listening to the people who attended the FPU, nursing satisfaction increased, and quality of care improved. Further studies which capture the experience of the person in the nurse-person relationship are required. Mitchell found that the majority of patients and families at post-project reported an enhanced quality of life because of the way nurses were with them (see chapter 19).

In the current study, however, the changes that occurred with Parse's theory are most evident in comments of the nurses and nurse manager. The questions for people who attend the FPU might continue as a quality assurance measure, but more study is needed to clarify differences in practice experiences when nurses are guided by different theoretical perspectives.

CONCLUSION

Parse's theory was considered a valuable guide to practice for nurses in the family practice setting. Nurses continue to develop and grow with Parse's theory-based practice because of the satisfaction and meaningfulness of being with others in a way that makes a difference to quality of life. Teaching sessions guided by a nurse specialist continued. The sessions were guided by "Parse Learning Modules" (Jonas, Pilkington, Lyon, & MacDonald, 1992) created by the Parse Education Task Force at St. Michael's Hospital, Toronto, Ontario, Canada. The purpose of this task force was to address the concern of a growing number of nurses interested in the theory and the limited human resources to teach the content. The modules reflect the teaching pattern that occurred on the first pilot unit (see chapter 19).

The current evaluation project of Parse's theory contributes to the growing body of literature that indicates nursing theory-based practice enhances nurses' satisfaction and quality of care. An analysis of all the projects evaluating Parse's theory is strongly recommended. If nursing is a scientific discipline, its practice must be guided with nursing theory. Parse (1990) claims that "nursing theory-based practice is the challenge for the '90s" (p. 53). Further research evaluating the changes with theory-based practice is required to clearly establish the unique contributions made to human health.

REFERENCES

Allan, J. D., & Hall, B. A., (1988). Challenging the focus on technology: A critique of the medical model in a changing health care system. *Advances in Nursing Science, 10*(3), 22–34.

Butler, M. J., & Snodgrass, F. G. (1991). Beyond abuse: Parse's theory in practice. *Nursing Science Quarterly, 4*, 76–82.

Guba, E., & Lincoln, Y. (1989). *Fourth generation evaluation.* Newbury Park, CA: Sage.

Heggie, J. R., Schoenmehl, P. A., Chang, M. K., & Grieco, C. (1989). Selection and implementation of Dr. Martha Rogers' nursing conceptual model in an acute care setting. *Clinical Nurse Specialist, 3*(3), 143–147.

Jacobs, M. K., & Heuther, S. E. (1978). Nursing science: The theory-practice linkage. *Advances in Nursing Science, 1*(1), 63–73.

Jonas, C. M., Pilkington, B., Lyon, P., & MacDonald, G. E. (1992). *Parse's theory of human becoming: Learning modules.* Toronto: St. Michael's Hospital.

Liehr, P. R. (1989). The core of true presence: A loving center. *Nursing Science Quarterly, 2*, 7–8.

Mattice, M. (1991). Parse's theory of nursing in practice: A manager's perspective. *Canadian Journal of Nursing Administration, 4*(1), 11–13.

Mattice, M., & Mitchell, G. J. (1991). Caring for confused elders. *The Canadian Nurse, 86*(11), 16–17.

Mavely, R., & Mitchell, G. J. (1994). Consider karaoke. *The Canadian Nurse, 90*(1), 22–24.

Mitchell, G. J. (1986). Utilizing Parse's theory of man-living-health in Mrs. M's neighborhood. *Perspectives, 10*(4), 5–7.

Mitchell, G. J., & Cody, W. K. (1992). Nursing knowledge and human science: Ontological and epistemological considerations. *Nursing Science Quarterly, 5,* 54–61.

Mitchell, G. J., & Copplestone, C. (1990). Applying Parse's theory to perioperative nursing: A nontraditional approach. *AORN Journal, 51*(3), 787–798.

Mitchell, G. J., & Pilkington, B. (1990). Theoretical approaches in nursing: A comparison of Roy and Parse. *Nursing Science Quarterly, 3,* 81–87.

Parse, R. R. (1981). *Man-living-health: A theory of nursing.* New York: Wiley.

Parse, R. R. (1987). *Nursing science: Major paradigms, theories, and critiques.* Philadelphia: Saunders.

Parse, R. R. (1990). Nursing theory-based practice: A challenge for the 90s. *Nursing Science Quarterly, 3,* 53.

Parse, R. R. (1992). Human becoming: Parse's theory of nursing. *Nursing Science Quarterly, 5,* 35-42.

Parse, R. R., Coyne, A. B., & Smith, M. J. (1985). *Nursing research: Qualitative methods.* Bowie, MD: Brady.

Quiquero, A., Knights, D., & Meo, O. (1991). Theory as a guide to practice: Staff nurses choose Parse's theory. *Canadian Journal of Nursing Administration, 4*(1), 14–16.

Rasmusson, D., Jonas, C. M., & Mitchell, G. J. (1991). The eye of the beholder: Parse's theory with homeless individuals. *Clinical Nurse Specialist, 5*(3), 139–143.

Smith, M. C. (1991). Evaluating nursing theory-based practice. *Nursing Science Quarterly, 4*(3), 98–99.

Taylor, S. G. (1988). Nursing theory and nursing process: Orem's theory in practice. *Nursing Science Quarterly, 1,* 111–119.

Taylor, S. G. (1989). An interpretation of family within Orem's general theory of nursing. *Nursing Science Quarterly, 2,* 131–137.

Wallace, S. (1993). *Nurses' learning about Parse's theory of nursing: An exploratory study.* Unpublished master's thesis, D'Youville University, Buffalo, NY.

Wondolowski, C., & Davis, D. K. (1988). The lived experience of aging in the oldest old: A phenomenological study. *The American Journal of Psychoanalysis, 48,* 261–270.

Wondolowski, C., & Davis, D. K. (1991). The lived experience of health in the oldest old: A phenomenological study. *Nursing Science Quarterly, 4,* 113–118.

Chapter 19

Evaluation of the Human Becoming Theory in Practice in an Acute Care Setting

Gail J. Mitchell

*T*he nursing profession is rapidly moving toward consolidation of a scientific base by which to guide practice, research, and education. The scientific base is organized in nursing theories. Different nursing theories are derived from distinct belief systems that structure knowledge about the human-health interrelationship. The healing opportunities in practice are thus largely determined by the guiding theoretical framework(s). The literature attests to the paucity of research investigating the outcomes of nursing theory implementation (DeGroot, 1988; Huckabay, 1991; Mayberry, 1991; McFarlane, 1980; Silva, 1986; Smith, 1991). It is a concern that closure on theory-based applications will occur before research that evaluates change in quality of care and nurse satisfaction. Therefore, rigorous scientific investigation of outcomes from theory application must be conducted to determine utility. The purpose of this research was to evaluate the changes that occur for nurses and clients during practice guided by Parse's theory of human becoming (1981, 1987, 1992, 1994).

PARSE'S THEORY OF HUMAN BECOMING

Parse's theory of human becoming offers a different structure for organizing knowledge and actions in nursing. The theory of human becoming is in no way similar to the problem-based approach that defines nurses as experts who assess human beings for problems that require professional intervention. From Parse's perspective, nursing is living true presence with others as they explicate meaning, synchronize rhythms, and move beyond in life. The goal of practice is enhancing quality of life from the perspective of those receiving nursing, as opposed to quality as defined by experts and societal norms. The nurse is not an expert on others' ways of living health. Rather, the nurse believes that individuals know and will choose what is best for themselves based on their personal values, relationships, hopes, and dreams. Parse proposes that human beings and the universe are irreducible. Persons are never isolated beings. All human beings live in a world with others who share a culture, language, and history, and yet, all human beings are free to choose their life projects. Instead of focusing on problems, the Parse nurse focuses on living true presence, on bearing witness as others live health and choose their own unique ways of becoming. Parse's theory directs attention to the lived experiences of human beings, and nurses respect every person's right to be and become the who they choose to be.

METHODS AND PURPOSES

Stevens (1984) suggests that whether a theory is integrated or not depends on its ability to make a meaningful difference to nurses in practice. And Hall (1993) suggests that if Parse's theory lives, it "will live on for its usefulness in setting standards and ethics for practice" (p. 10). The current research addresses the specific issue of meaningful usefulness. The objective of this study was to describe what happened to nurses' beliefs and actions and to clients' health experiences when Parse's theory was the base for practice. The research question was "What happens to nurses' beliefs and actions and clients' health experiences when Parse's theory is used as the base for practice?"

STUDY DESIGN

The research design was descriptive evaluation (Guba & Lincoln, 1989), with pre-project post-project data gathering. This design was the best choice, given the scope of planned change and limited resources and number of theory-based experts. The limitations of the one group, pre-test post-test design (Cook & Campbell, 1979) were outweighed by the potential benefits of descriptive evaluation that generates rich data in a contextual way. Moreover, the threats to causal inferences held little significance in this study since the planned change was directed at personal values and beliefs, as well as perceived quality of life and relationships. Values, beliefs, and quality of life as phenomena of interest are not amenable to objectification, operationalization, and manipulation. Smith (1991) drew attention to the importance of selecting evaluation methods that are consistent with the theory being evaluated. In this case, Parse's theory is consistent with qualitative description and inconsistent with objective measures and statistical analysis. Further, Smith (1991) stated, "Qualitative evaluation strategies are considered to be as legitimate as quantitative measurement, and the practitioner-researcher is responsive to the emerging findings throughout the process" (p. 98). The researcher's intent was to generate descriptions of change for nurses and clients as opposed to making causal inferences.

Setting

The medical unit evaluating Parse's theory housed 28 treatment beds and primarily admitted individuals with general medical and respiratory problems. The mode of nursing care on the unit was team or functional. There were 17 registered nurses, 8 registered nursing assistants, and 2 nursing assistants employed on the unit. Length of time in practice for nurse-subjects ranged from several months to more than 25 years. None of the nurses had been exposed to Parse's theory prior to the commencement of the project, and there was no change in staffing patterns during the evaluation project.

The unit manager requested that Parse's theory be evaluated on her unit. The decision followed analysis of congruence between Parse's theory, the philosophy of the Mission Statement of St. Michael's Hospital, and the goal of the nurses to improve the quality of care. Support of the unit manager was viewed as essential for instituting such radical change.

The data-gathering procedures as they occurred before and after 32 weeks of theory-based practice guided by Parse are shown in Table 19.1. The pre-evaluation was largely conducted by a nurse researcher from the United States who was not familiar with the hospital. Pre-evaluation was implemented with taped interviews with the unit manager and 14 patient-subjects, 20 chart audits, and 23 questionnaires from nurses about the content of discussions with patients, and their actions and priorities in practice. This same procedure was conducted 8 months later, and additionally, nurses were asked to answer the following: Please describe how your nursing practice has changed since the initiation of Parse's theory. Nurses were also requested to dialogue with the researcher on tape about changes in practice, changes perceived on the unit as a whole, charting with Parse's theory, and what they thought about keeping the theory as a guide for practice.

The protection for human subjects followed the ethical guidelines for confidentiality, disclosure of risks and benefits, right of refusal to participate, and parameters of participation. All patient, family, and nurse-subjects were asked to sign consent forms after their participation was explained and their questions answered.

Teaching Parse's Theory

Parse's theory was taught on the pilot unit for an 8-month period. Table 19.2 shows the progression of process and content. The first 2 months of teaching focused on the values and beliefs of Parse's

Table 19.1   Data-Gathering Procedures

Pre-Evaluation	Post-Evaluation
Taped interview with unit manager about strengths of nursing care on unit, concerns, charting, how care evaluated.*	Taped interview with unit manager to discuss changes, concerns, strengths, charting related to Parse's theory.*
Fourteen patients interviewed to determine perceived quality of nursing care and content of nurse-person discussions.*	Nine patients and three family members interviewed to determine perceived quality of nursing care and content of nurse-person discussions.*
Twenty charts reviewed to determine style and content of nursing documentation.*	Sixteen charts reviewed to determine style and content of nursing documentation.*
Twenty-three nurses completed questionnaires of open-ended questions about the content of discussions with patients, actions during specific patient situations, and priorities in practice.	Nineteen nurses completed questionnaires for pre-post comparison.
	Eighteen nurses submitted written account describing changes experienced with Parse's theory.
	Twenty-three nurses participated in taped interview with researcher about changes in practice and charting with Parse's theory.

*Conducted by outside evaluator.
Research conducted at St. Michael's Hospital, Toronto, Canada, by Gail J. Mitchell, 1990.

theory. This was a critical phase because it is not possible to "add" Parse's theory onto the traditional values and beliefs of the problem-based approach. In order to practice Parse's theory the very essence of what nurses value and believe about human beings and health is challenged. Consider the following, for instance. From Parse's perspective, human beings are unitary and cannot

Table 19.2   Teaching and Learning Parse's Theory

1 – 2 Months

Daily sessions on the unit with small groups of nurses. Sessions during this initial time period focused on:

- Comparing the values and beliefs of Parse's theory with the traditional beliefs of the problem-based, diagnostic model
- Challenging the belief that patients are different from other human beings, including nurses themselves
- Discussion of Parse's definitions of human beings and health in light of personal views and experiences
- Discussion of major themes of Parse's theory (meaning, rhythmicity, and transcendence) in relation to personal ways of living

2 – 4 Months

Daily sessions with small groups of nurses continued. One-to-one guidance began with nurses attempting to create new ways of being with persons in practice. Group sessions with individual patients in true presence with researcher, followed by discussion. Teaching focused on:

- Major concepts of Parse's theory in relation to human beings, health, and life experiences
- Parse's practice dimensions and processes
- Challenges related to changing ways of being with persons in practice
- Charting with Parse's theory

4 – 8 Months

Sessions on unit held twice a week. One-to-one sessions more common as researcher accompanied individual nurses during nurse-person discussions. Teaching and group discussions focused on:

- Ongoing struggle of living changing values and beliefs
- Surprise and pleasure with changed nurse-person relationships
- Theoretical principles of Parse's theory and related literature
- Overall changes on the unit for nurses and patients
- Emerging commitment to live Parse's theory in practice

be thought of as separate from the universe. There is no one true reality but many realities, some that can be known, many that cannot. The nurse does not know how others should live health, and health is linked not only to how one lives, but to paradox, quality of life, becoming-unfolding, and mystery. The new knowledge in Parse's theory compels belief, so the assumptions, values, and principles are gradually integrated to create a new knowledge base, a new horizon from which to view practice and research activities.

One of the first challenges to the traditional approach was directed at changing the assumption that patients are somehow different from other human beings, including nurses themselves. Nurses first thought about Parse's theory in relation to their own lives and ways of living health. For example, nurses spoke about how they made decisions in life based on what was important to them and their loved ones. After weighing pros and cons, considering benefits and losses, nurses and their family members made decisions based on what they believed was best for themselves. The nurses reflected on how they felt when others tried telling them how they should live, and they spoke about how they felt when others judged and labeled them for living the way they wanted. The nurses all concluded that they did not appreciate being judged, labeled, or told what to do by others.

Next, nurses considered what it was like to have a different set of standards or beliefs about persons who just happened to be patients. They thought about how they spent time in practice trying to get people to do things, or to make certain decisions, without any attempt to find out what the person or family thought might be best for themselves. Most difficult for nurses was letting go of the belief that there is some best way, some "right" way to live with an illness, to grieve, to feel sadness, to take care of self. Through this process of reflecting on personal values in relation to Parse's theory and the traditional problem-based approach, nurses slowly began to question inconsistencies and to choose the values they wanted to live in practice.

Between the second and fourth months nurses began to think about the concepts of Parse's theory in relation to practice and human health. The nurses accompanied the researcher in practice situations to witness a different way of relating with human beings. Parse's practice method was taught, and nurses began the process of changing ways of being with patients based on their emerging beliefs. Nurses were also introduced to charting the patient's personal health description, which included the individual's perceptions, meanings, views, concerns, hopes, fears, and dreams. The nurses charted what the person said and did rather than recording their own interpretations and opinions about what they thought was happening with patients.

During the last 4 months of the project nurses continued to integrate the beliefs of the human becoming theory. Teaching sessions focused on discussing the struggle of change, the challenges and benefits, the surprises and difficulties, and the changing nature of relationships with patients. Theoretical concepts and principles were further specified and linked with practice situations, and nurses discussed how Parse's theory was different and how patients and families viewed that difference.

PRESENTATION OF FINDINGS

Major findings will be discussed under the following headings: changes described by nurses, unit manager perceptions, patient/family perceptions of nursing care, and changes in charting.

Changes Described by Nurses

Post-project evaluation produced two sets of qualitative data from nurses for thematic analysis. The two sources, written responses and taped interviews, with their identified themes are shown in Table 19.3.

Eighteen nurse-subjects submitted written responses to a question which asked them to write about the way their practice

Table 19.3   Themes Extracted From Nurses' Written and Taped Accounts of Change With Parse's Theory

Written Responses	Taped Interviews
1. Thinking of patients as persons and having closer relationships.	1. Viewing Parse's theory as valuable for patients and nurses.
2. Seeing nursing practice as more professional and satisfying.	2. Spending more time talking, listening, and just being with patients.
3. Having more understanding by listening to the person's story; no longer judging and labeling patients.	3. Becoming more accepting, tolerant, patient, caring, and aware with patients.
4. Experiencing less pressure to make patients conform; involving patients in their own care and respecting their rights.	4. Having a changed attitude and understanding things from the patient's point of view instead of judging.
5. Struggling with the new; changing ways of thinking and acting in practice.	5. Feeling freed, relaxed, and more satisfied in practice.
	6. Going beyond the medical to viewing and knowing the patient as a human being.
	7. Respecting patients' wishes.
	8. Feeling threatened with change and struggling to keep control with patients.
	9. Feeling challenged and more professional as a nurse and being able to specify unique contribution.
	10. Experiencing growth and learning.

had changed since the initiation of Parse's theory. The most common theme was *thinking of patients as persons and having closer relationships.* Data which typified responses in this theme were as follows:

> We have to start helping the patients first before their illness. We have to start treating them as human beings, not only an illness. I feel Parse's theory has been able to show me how the person's concerns and hopes all come together and that their contributions make a big difference in getting well.

The second theme extracted from the written data was *seeing nursing practice as more professional and satisfying.* Nurses offered comments such as the following:

> When describing nursing to people it is difficult to discuss what makes nursing unique and different from medicine, a profession in its own right, rather than an adjunct to the profession of medicine. Since Parse's I now feel that I am a professional. I have developed a sense of pride in what I do, something I haven't felt for some time. I was questioning the value of nursing and seriously considering leaving nursing because I felt dissatisfied with my role as nurse and the lack of true contact with patients. The tasks of nursing do not give me a sense of satisfaction. I chose nursing because I felt it provided a way of making a difference in people's lives. Somewhere along the way, I got caught up in the task-oriented model and lost my ability to "be with" patients.

Another nurse offered this statement:

> Parse's theory gives us something to look at and value as nurses. It gives us a purpose and a new way to look at what we do and how we can improve our relationships with patients.

The third theme, *having more understanding by listening to the person's story; no longer judging and labeling patients,* is typified by the following:

I find I listen to the patients and talk with them, not at them. I talk about their illness, death, dying, everything that I used to avoid before Parse's theory.

Another nurse said:

The way I am with patients has changed. I listen and try to be truly present to them wherever they are. There is a lot less labeling of patients on the floor and nurses seem more respectful of patients' feelings. With patients who cannot communicate, I make an effort to be with their families in order to discover how things are for them.

Experiencing less pressure to make patients conform; involving patients in their own care and respecting their rights was the fourth theme. This was revealed in statements such as the following:

For me now I find nursing less stressful. I do not have to take on burdens for when patients make their own choices. I can say at the end of the day, I was there for the person and that's what really matters.

Another nurse offered:

My new practice has made me realize that just because a person is in the hospital, they should be able to make some choices.

The last theme, *struggling with the new; changing ways of thinking and acting in practice,* is typified by the following:

Certainly, using Parse's theory does not make my job easier in some ways. It requires energy, concentration and the ability to slow down and listen. Sometimes it raises dilemmas that I would not have been aware of before. Often these dilemmas occur because I disapprove or want to change a patient's feelings or actions. However, with some soul searching and serious thought, I am able to support the patient in his or her decisions.

Another nurse said:

> I feel uncomfortable at times trying to live Parse's theory. It requires a deeper level of giving of self and sometimes requires more emotional strength than normal.

Nurse-subjects were also asked to dialogue with the researcher on tape about the changes in their practice and on the unit. The ten most common themes are listed in Table 19.3. The most common theme, *viewing Parse's theory as valuable for patients and nurses,* was present in 19 of the 23 transcripts as indicated in the following:

> I think Parse's theory has been very useful, developed the human part of the profession. It is important to understand the medical problems but for us nurses I think it is important to understand people more.

Another nurse stated:

> I like how my charting has changed because I am putting down how the patients are feeling, not how I'm feeling about them.

Another nurse offered:

> I like Parse's because you get to find out more about the patient's situation and how they take things. And you ask more. Before if something seemed wrong with a person, I just left them alone. Now I talk to them and they tell me. I think the patients know we care more.

The second most common theme revolved around nurses saying they were *spending more time talking, listening, and just being with patients.* The following are typical of the 16 nurses contributing to this theme:

> We have time. I don't know why that seems to be different because before Parse's theory you still had the same amount of time we

have now but we never really seemed to talk to patients. We may have talked at them but not really with them. And we really didn't explore their personal thoughts and feelings before Parse's.

Another nurse stated:

Now it's like more nurses are sitting and talking to patients and you are getting the feeling of nurse and patient contact more now than before. Before we'd just go in and make the bed, give the bath, whip them up, and they'd sit in the chair the rest of the day. We'd go back to see if they were okay. But now I think nurses are talking more to patients, I know I am.

Fifteen nurses contributed statements to the third theme which related to their *becoming more accepting, tolerant, patient, caring, and aware with patients*. Comments such as the following were recorded:

I guess I feel more like I did when I first came out of school. Very much more aware of the patient and how important they are in their own care, and not getting so bogged down in the routines.

Another nurse offered:

With Parse's because you don't categorize, you don't have the limitations, therefore you are more open to the person.

Another said:

I think Parse's theory makes the focus on the patient. I am just more aware of the patient and how they feel about things.

The fourth theme was *having a changed attitude and understanding things from the patient's point of view instead of judging*. Of the 23 nurses, 15 offered comments such as the following:

With Mr. N, he said he feels very alone with his disease, that nobody knows but us and that is why he calls us because he can share, he can just be himself. Well, before Parse's I would have come to my own conclusions about why he couldn't tell his friends, but he had his own reasons for that. It turned out that it was because it might strip him of his dignity in death. Had I drawn my own conclusions, well . . . . I never would have found these things out.

Another nurse stated:

A lot of times before we ignored whatever the patient said. We always, what do you call it, judged right away.

And another said:

My attitude toward patients has changed. I find that I'm listening to their words more and I'm listening to get a better understanding of them as a person, and kind of in a new light.

Another nurse offered:

Before, we would have classified every street person as the same. You know, he's just another street person, there's no need to be nice to him because he's just going back to the street. But now, when you really sit down and talk to him, he's pleasant, like he's his own person. He's not just a street person anymore, he's a person.

More than half of the nurses spoke of *feeling freed, relaxed, and more satisfied in practice*. Typical comments were as follows:

I find now that I'm not telling others what I think they should do, I'm like freed, or there's just a weight lifted off my shoulders. Now I know I am with the patient instead of sometimes being angry or frustrated and apart from him. I feel I am where I should be as a nurse.

Another nurse said:

I find with Parse's theory it is really easy to go home at night, you are not stressed out. I don't worry. I find I am more relaxed now on the floor and I do get a lot of positive feedback from patients even though it is not always verbal.

Eleven nurse-subjects commented on *going beyond the medical to viewing and knowing the patient as a human being,* such as in the following:

I was the typical stereotype where you treat the illness and sometimes converse with the patient to relax them and make them comfortable. But with Parse's I see them as a whole and I see their ideas and their feelings and their goals as priority over what they are in the hospital for.

Another nurse stated:

I was skill-oriented, like that's what I was concentrating on. But sometimes, I guess I just forgot the person in the bed. Just go do this dressing and it was just a leg or whatever. But I think now you kind of have to look at the whole person and the dressing doesn't really matter. This way, I guess the whole person is healed rather than just the leg.

Theme number seven, *respecting patients' wishes,* was addressed by 10 of the 23 nurses as revealed in the following:

Nurses are really starting to think about, well what am I doing. Is this what the patient wants, or is this what I want, or is this just a hospital routine?

Another nurse offered:

Before if so and so didn't want to do something, I'd push or say, you have to do it. But now a person has more leeway, more space to have and vent their feelings.

And another said:

Personally, I feel we are more in touch with our patients and we are more patient-oriented. More into pleasing the patient rather than pleasing the nurse and what has to be done in the nurse's eyes. What has to be done in the patient's eyes comes first now.

Theme number eight was *feeling threatened with change and struggling to keep control with patients.* Seven nurses contributed to this theme in the following ways:

> I was really threatened with the talk about technicians doing the skills which we were taught were most important. And really threatened when the patients could choose, like when to have a bath.

Another nurse said:

> I find it hard to ask people about their feelings because I'm afraid I am imposing on them.

The ninth theme, *feeling challenged and more professional as a nurse and being able to specify unique contribution,* was present in 6 of the 23 taped interviews.

One nurse offered:

> I guess Parse's makes me feel like a professional rather than a worker. You feel like you have something to contribute, that sometimes you can make a difference. That you know you have information the doctors do not, and that it is necessary sometimes in order that they understand the patient better, or approach the patient differently.

Another nurse said:

> It has made me more human. And I feel that I'm more of a nurse than . . . I just feel I am better than I was.

Six nurses also contributed to the last theme, *experiencing growth and learning.* The following responses are typical of this theme:

We see an improvement in ourselves. That all of us have grown in this experience. That it is true we should be looking at the patient and going with the person and not to what we want.

Another nurse stated:

Parse's theory has taught me about nursing, not medicine, nursing. It is about feelings, it is about love, it is about honesty and it's about not looking at the patient's religion, or the color of their skin, you are a person and that's what nursing is all about.

Unit Manager Perceptions

The unit manager had been on the unit 4 years prior to the evaluation of Parse's theory. Pre-project she stated that nurses on her unit delivered "good" care and they demonstrated many caring behaviors toward patients. However, she felt practice could be improved and directed toward more human concerns. The manager also indicated that, pre-Parse, staff nurses typically sought her assistance with family "problems," especially social issues related to discharge planning. She said the nurses' charting habits were poor and records did not reflect what nurses were doing with clients.

Following 8 months of integrating Parse's theory in practice, the unit manager discussed important changes that had taken place in the areas of: patient reports of nursing actions, nurse perceptions of patients, nurse relationships with patients, nurse morale, nursing image and professional initiative, and personal satisfaction with change.

During the post-evaluation interview, the unit manager stated that patients frequently said that nurses were talking with them and treating them with dignity and respect. Patient complaints to the unit manager decreased from several per month to two in 6 months. Reports from physicians indicated that they, too, received reports from patients and family members about their perceptions of feeling really cared about by nurses on the Parse unit.

The unit manager noticed several changes which reflected how nurses' perceptions of patients changed with Parse's theory. She observed that nurses were not labeling patients and that individuals previously considered "difficult" to care for, such as persons with HIV or persons from the streets, were now considered with concern and respect. Nurses on the unit began challenging each other about judging and labeling patients, and nurses complained less about patients previously viewed as management problems. The unit manager believed that nurses were more respectful of patients when guided by Parse's theory. Nurses no longer viewed patients first as problems; rather, they were seeing them first as persons.

The unit manager reported that the major strengths of nurses practicing Parse's theory were that they were now really listening to patients and trying to participate in changes that patients wanted. She said the nurses were spending much less time in the nursing station talking to each other; she witnessed much more talking and listening to patients at the bedside.

The morale on the unit was changed when nurses integrated Parse's theory. According to the unit manager, nurses indicated that they felt more valued. Staff worked together differently and were more supportive and tolerant of each other. The unit manager said the nurses actually seemed to be happy when coming to work instead of dragging themselves in to a job. Nurses said they knew their relationships with patients were valued. Not all nurses changed ways of relating with each other, but overall the unit manager believed staff relationships demonstrated better understanding and were more supportive.

Nursing image and professional initiative were changed with Parse's theory. The unit manager reported nurses frequently spoke to other professionals about what the patients said they wanted for their lives. Nurses reported seeing the theory as valuable for patients and realizing that nursing practice was more than tasks. The unit manager said she heard nurses talking about being more sure of themselves and specifying what the uniqueness of nursing practice was in the overall care of the patient. The unit manager also reported that nurses were more interested in patients and requested time to improve themselves professionally in educational programs.

Problems referred to the unit manager changed over the course of the evaluation study. The unit manager stated that the problems referred to her at the time of the post-evaluation were more complex and more often involved ethical issues about choice, as opposed to resources for discharge. In Parse practice the patients were making more decisions about their own care, so nurses were not going to the unit manager for answers. The unit manager continued to have concerns about charting and care planning. The nurses were charting more information about the person and family, but they still did not consistently record how they were practicing.

Finally, the unit manager said that she "could not believe how much she had changed herself." She liked not telling patients what to do, and she had no idea her beliefs would change so dramatically. Her relationships with staff changed as she, too, integrated new ways of being with others. She described herself as happier and more self-confident. Practices of hiring and evaluating staff now included questions related to beliefs about Parse's worldview. Rather than having performance appraisals based solely on performance of tasks and attendance, for example, the unit manager evaluated how nurses were living Parse's theory in practice.

Patient/Family Perceptions of Nursing Care

During the pre-project data gathering, 14 patients were asked to describe the quality of nursing care encountered on the pilot unit. Post-project, nine patients and three family members were interviewed. Despite the small number of persons available for interview, descriptions indicated important changes consistent with other data sources.

The first question asked patients and family members to describe the quality of nursing care. In general, post-project descriptions were much more detailed and superlative, describing nurses as truly caring and understanding and indicating the importance of their taking time for talking and listening to the patient's preference. Patients and family members were asked what nurses talked to them about. Pre-project responses indicated nurses spoke little to patients about their personal situations. Post-project, the majority of patients and family members reported that nurses spoke to them about many things including physical needs, family, medical conditions, and how they were doing and feeling.

Another question explored with patient and family participants what differences the nurse made during the hospital experience. Again responses were more detailed post-project with changes noted in ways nurses made a difference by including music, talking, listening, and caring. There was no reference to these nurse actions in the pre-evaluation data. Participants were also asked what plans they had discussed with nurses about the future. Pre-project, 13 of the 14 patients said nurses had not discussed their plans with them. Post-project, 5 of 11 patients and family members reported they had discussed future plans with the nurse.

The last question asked patients and family members how their quality of life had changed since being on the unit with the nurses. Pre-project data indicated only one person reported a change in quality of life because of the way nurses were with him. In post-project evaluation, all patients and family members except two reported enhanced quality of life related to the nurses' being "kind, gentle, welcoming, willing to listen, willing to talk, and willing to do things the patients desired."

Changes in Charting

Pre-project, the style of charting by nurses was evaluated on 20 randomly selected charts. Specific characteristics were as follows. All charts contained a patient profile or admission assessment, which is a standardized form used throughout the hospital. The admission profile contained reason for admission, medications, allergies, physical assessment, vital signs, and a check-off psycho-social-spiritual assessment. Nurses charted in narrative format, and notes typically included: unusual incidents (falls); observed symptoms (shortness of breath, urine output adequate); patient complaints of pain and medications given; descriptions of how patients sleep, eat, walk, care for self; results of lab tests; physician consults/visits; nursing interventions (dressings, intravenous insertions, catheter care); preparations for tests and procedures; and insignificant observations supporting normality (sleeping, no complaints, condition stable, unchanged). Most nurses noted the presence of family or friends visiting but did not describe the nature of the patient's relationships or any concerns, thoughts, or feelings, expressed by family. Nurses sometimes recorded their interpretations of patient behavior. For example, "Mr. X appears sad." Direct quotes from patients describing their personal thoughts, feelings, concerns, or desires were rare. Only two direct quotes about the person's perspective were found in the nurses' notes. In general, pre-project the charting by nurses did not contain personal perspectives of persons or families, meaning of situations, plans, hopes, concerns, or desires. The focus of charting related to performance of tasks and procedures and descriptions of what patients were observed doing in relation to activities of daily living.

Post-project evaluation indicated that the charts still contained a patient profile and admission assessment, both required by hospital policy. And, nurses still recorded unusual incidents, observed symptoms, activities of daily living, complaints of pain, medications, and interventions. Notations about family and friends' visiting continued, as did nurse interpretations of patients, although interpretation was less pervasive. There was a dramatic increase in direct quotes from patients. For instance, "Mr. X said that he is unhappy today because his family was not able to visit." Nurses also used the patient's name in charting instead of "pt."

Also changed post-project was nurses' recording of patients' thoughts, feelings, hopes, dreams, and plans. Seven of the 16 charts reviewed post-evaluation contained written accounts from the person's perspective about what specific situations meant, feelings about relationships, hopes, and concerns. Six charts contained only the traditional charting typical of the pre-project charting style.

DISCUSSION OF THE FINDINGS

The research question in this study was "What happens to nurses beliefs and actions and patient health experiences when Parse's theory is used as the basis for practice?" Guba and Lincoln (1989) guide evaluators to look for patterns between different perspectives and recurring regularities from different data sources which increase the truth value and credibility of findings. This type of cross-checking revealed six recurring patterns, as indicated in Table 19.4.

The first pattern emerging from different data sources in this research was the *change in the nurses' perspective of patients from problems to patients as human beings*. The unit manager stated that she believed nurses were more respectful of patients and that

Table 19.4 Recurring Patterns Across All Data Sources

• Changed nurses' perspective of patient from problem to patient as human being

• Changed morale in nurses

• Less judging and labeling of patients

• More talking and listening to patients

• Respecting the patient's right to choose

• Enhancing quality of nurse-person relationship

---

the nurses no longer viewed patients as problems but as persons. The change in the nurses' charting was congruent with this new perspective of patients as persons, not problems. Post-project, nurses' notes contained multiple quotes from patients and descriptions of the individuals' personal meanings, relationships, fears, hopes, and dreams. Nurses also referred to persons by name when charting, rather than using the generic term, patient. Perhaps the most dramatic change was with the nurses' descriptions of how their perspectives changed. Fifteen of the 23 nurses interviewed spoke explicitly about seeing things from the patient's perspective and having more understanding of the person as a human being. Nurse responses on the questionnaire also reflected this changed perspective. Nurse-person discussions changed from focusing on problems and tests to focusing on the person and his or her experience, goals, plans, and concerns. Seeing patients as persons rather than problems was also the most common theme in the written evaluations of nurses.

Patient- and family-subjects also supported this changed pattern in the way they described how nurses were with them. Post-project reports from individuals described nurses as caring about them as persons, and individuals said they found the nurses to be understanding.

The second pattern of change in nurses' beliefs revolved around an *enhanced morale, satisfaction, and professional image.* The unit manager stated she perceived morale to be much better with Parse's theory. She said nurses spoke to her about feeling more sure of themselves and the uniqueness and value of their practice. The unit manager stated she was happier and more self-confident in her role as manager since Parse's theory was initiated.

Several patients reported nurses to be friendly and good-natured on the pre-project evaluation. Post-project, most of the patients and family members commented on the way the nurses worked together, how they had a collegiality, how they never got down, and how they helped and supported each other.

In the written responses, six nurse-subjects wrote specifically of how they felt more professional and proud. They wrote of knowing the unique contribution of nursing and of having a clear purpose with Parse's theory as their guide. These same thoughts were echoed during the taped interviews. One of the more interesting themes of the taped interviews with nurses related to morale and satisfaction—they reported feeling freed, less stressful, and more relaxed. Several nurses, as well as the unit manager, related this unburdening to their no longer being expected to tell patients what to do.

The third pattern reflecting a change in nurse actions supported in various data sources was that nurses were *judging and labeling patients much less when guided by Parse's theory*. The unit manager stated that she noticed the nurses were not only using labels less, they were challenging each other for making judgments instead of trying to understand from the patient's perspective.

One patient during pre-project evaluation reported that she thought nurses picked on some of the patients. There was no indication of such behavior in post-project evaluation, and the repeated references to the nurses' true caring, understanding, and family-like relationships with patients suggested acceptance. Not judging or labeling patients was also one of the themes in both the written responses and taped interviews of nurses describing changes in their practice with Parse's theory.

The next pattern of change in nursing actions revolved around nurses' *spending more time talking and listening to patients*. This pattern emerged from all data sources. The unit manager reported that nurses were really listening to patients and spending less time in the nursing station talking to each other and more time talking to patients. In post-project evaluation, in describing the quality of care received, there were seven references to the nurses' being attentive, talking, and listening. Patients and family members also said the nurses had influenced the quality of their lives by talking and listening to what they wanted and needed. There had been no reference to the nurses' talking and listening to patients in pre-project evaluation. The increased quotes and personal descriptions in the charts indicated nurses were talking and listening more to patients. Listening to the patient's perspective was contained in the themes from both the nurses' written responses and taped interviews.

The fifth pattern identified in the data which related to a change in nursing actions was *respecting the patient's right to choose*. The unit manager reported that patients were making more decisions about their own care and that nurses were clarifying patient choices to other health care professionals. Patient-subjects reported nurses were more willing to learn from them and to do what they wanted rather than their having to do what the nurses wanted. Not only was there no reference to this nursing action during the pre-project evaluation, one patient said at that time that the nurses had decreased the quality of her life by taking her to things she did not want to go to and by telling her what to do.

Respecting the patient's right to choose was a common theme in the nursing data. This change related to both nursing actions and the struggle to let go. Several nurses said that before Parse's theory, they forced or pushed patients to follow routines because that was the way it was supposed to be. Nurses in this study talked about patients' now having authority and control, which was sometimes hard for the nurses. Other nurses said Parse's theory helped them see that patients should not lose their rights at the hospital door, and they gained further awareness of the person's participation in health care.

The last pattern of change which emerged from all data sources related to patient health experiences. The pattern revolved around the *change in the perceived quality of the nurse-person relationship*. The unit manager reported that patients often spoke to her of how nurses treated them with dignity and respect. She also received comments from physicians that patients and family members were talking about the quality of nursing practice on the Parse unit. Complaints about care decreased dramatically during the pilot study. Physicians started requesting that patients on other floors who had been labeled as "difficult" be transferred to the Parse unit because they believed the nurses' approaches made a difference in how patients progressed.

Data from patients and family members changed from seeing the nurses as helpful, friendly, and good-natured, to seeing them as truly caring, understanding, gentle, attentive, and kind. Pre-project, the majority of patients said the nurses had no influence on their quality of life and one patient said quality went down because of nursing actions. Those who said nurses made a difference offered reasons related to what tasks nurses performed, such as giving pills and making beds, rather than because of the nurse-person relationship.

In post-project evaluation, the majority of patients and family members reported enhanced quality of life because of the way the nurses were with them. Patients said nurses conversed with them, made them feel welcome, joked, talked and listened to them, and cared about them. This change was consistent with the reports from 15 nurses about being more caring, attentive, and accepting with patients.

STRUGGLING THROUGH CHANGE

The struggle involved in this process of learning Parse's theory is worth exploring in more depth because it is not easy to change, especially to change values and beliefs. The time on the unit with the nurses was patterned by shifting rhythms of feeling enthusiasm and indifference, moving and stalling, being clear and being obscure, feeling pleasure and feeling pain, experiencing surprise and living the expected. For example, enthusiasm was evident when nurses during one week would be eager to attend sessions and excitedly talked about how much they were learning, and the next week these same nurses were indifferent about attending sessions and changing their practice. The pleasure was related to pride and satisfaction that came from being with persons in a different way, and the pain revolved around both the frustration of learning Parse's theory and letting go of old habits. Nurses were surprised when patients told them how important they were and when they saw the patient in a totally different way, and they sometimes slipped back to familiar patterns when things became difficult for them. The shifting of rhythms, although expected, was at times very difficult to endure for both the nurses and the researcher.

Perhaps the most frustrating aspect of guiding and bearing witness to the nurses' struggle was knowing that changing one's values and beliefs would take time and serious reflection, for it was also a choice, a personal process for which there were no pre-planned strategies. Witnessing the process of the nurses' changing and moving did reveal interesting patterns.

When unfamiliar ideas from Parse's theory were first introduced, nurses either rejected the thoughts outright or they restructured the ideas so they would be familiar with what was known. The rejection was shown in statements such as, "that is a ridiculous idea," "that will never work with the patients we have," and "we definitely do not have time for that." Changing the new ideas so they would seem more familiar was most often expressed as the belief that nurses already practiced Parse's theory and so there would be no need to change at all. This was viewed as the "same-thing phenomenon" (Mitchell, 1993) and was revealed in statements such as the following. "I already use Parse's theory," "this is the same as good communication" and "Parse's is the same as counseling." Many nurses spoke of the "rejection" and "same-thing phenomenon" at the same time revealing the paradox of seeing the theory as radically different and impossible, yet familiar and known. This paradoxical viewing reflects the complexity of Parse's theory, which is, all-at-once, simple and complex, concrete and abstract, understandable and elusive. It takes time to learn the theory because it encompasses all aspects of the human-health interrelationship and then relates this relationship to life patterns and theoretical concepts. A nurse needs to process this complexity over time, because grasping and integrating new knowledge does not happen in one moment but in many moments as old beliefs are analyzed and changed to the new.

LITERATURE RELATED TO THE FINDINGS

The findings from this study show how the nurses' perspectives changed from viewing the patient as a problem, to viewing the patient as a human being. This changed perspective has important implications for a discipline which is struggling to move beyond the biomedical, problem-based tradition to confirm nursing as a human science. In the literature there is an urgent call for nurses to focus on the person's perspective and meaning of health (Moch, 1989; Parse, 1981, 1992; Sarter, 1987; Woods et al., 1988). The traditional problem-based model has been criticized for encouraging the objective, reductionistic approach with human beings and their life experiences (Cull-Wilby & Pepin, 1987; Hall & Allan, 1986; Holmes, 1990; Wilson-Barnett, 1991). Parse's theory, which proposes that human beings are nonreducible unities, effectively changed the common practice of reducing human beings to their bio-psycho-social problems. It is not reasonable to ask nurses to assess and label human beings, as is expected in the nursing process, while at the same time expecting them to view individuals as complex wholes who are more than and different from their parts. Similarly, it is not acceptable to ask nurses to be caring, loving, and respectful of individual differences and rights, while simultaneously expecting objective assessments, judgmental comparisons, and successful manipulations. Nurses require new ways of thinking and practicing with persons, families, and groups, ways that are based in nursing theory.

Findings in this study revealed that nurses judged and labeled much less when guided by Parse's theory. Although assessing and labeling is an important component of traditional practice, it limits the nurse's ability to be with human beings. To assess and label is to stand apart from and to compare the other to some standard before passing a judgment that can be harmful to the person (Deegan, 1993; Mitchell, 1991). In Parse's theory there are no expectations for how others should live. There is no blueprint for how one should grieve, or for how family members should relate with each other, or for how to view a certain experience like having cancer, depression, Alzheimer's disease, or open heart surgery. Every person is unique, and the nurse guided by Parse's theory does not seek to "stand apart from" but to "be with."

It was mentioned previously that along with the struggle of letting go of control there was also a related unburdening. There is discussion in the literature about whether or not nurses can control human beings and their ways of thinking, feeling, and acting (see for example Allen, 1985; Carboni, 1991; Griffin, 1980; Mitchell, 1991; Mitchell & Cody, 1992; Moccia, 1988; Polifroni & Packard, 1993; Yeo, 1989). If controlling other human beings is an impossible and unethical goal, as some nurses suggest, then it makes sense that with the release from this expectation in practice, nurses would experience an unburdening. In Parse's theory, the nurse's focus is not to control, but to be with, to bear witness to the person's struggle of becoming. Being truly present without trying to control and fix is an achievable goal which may redefine nursing's unique purpose.

Reports of enhanced satisfaction and professional image as a consequence of nursing theory-based practice have been reported in the literature and are consistent with findings in this study (Jonas, 1993; Laurie-Shaw & Ives, 1988; Mastal, Hammond, & Roberts, 1982; Santopinto & Smith, chapter 17, this work).

The current research, however, was the first to describe the quality of the nurse-person relationship as perceived from the individuals receiving care. The changed perspective of the patient (from problem, to patient as human being), the decreased judging and labeling, and the increased respect for the patient's right to choose, all as a consequence of theory-based practice, have not been reported in the literature. These findings reflect the changed values and beliefs of nurses guided by Parse's nontraditional approach. Future research evaluating Parse's theory in other settings may further clarify and support the unique contribution of Parse's theory in practice.

Another unanticipated and important change on the Parse-guided unit was the way other health care professionals came to view the nurse's contribution to care planning. In multidisciplinary rounds nurses began presenting the person's personal views, plans, hopes, and dreams. It was not unusual for the person's story, as presented by the nurse, to be different from what other professionals had assessed. These differences frequently raised ethical issues and debates that came to be an important and valued part of patient care rounds. It was not unusual for a physician in discussing a particular patient to ask for the Parse perspective.

One of the consequences of the evaluation study that surprised everyone was the way staff nurses shared how they valued the theory. It was the staff nurses' talking about Parse's theory in cafeterias and committee meetings that led to an unanticipated request for additional education about the theory. The nursing administration at St. Michael's did not mandate that nurses learn Parse's theory. The fact that it remains as a guide to practice on the medical unit 4 years later and that staff nurses continue to request education is because Parse's theory made a meaningful difference for the nurses in practice and in their relationships with clients and families. This grassroots movement toward nursing theory-based practice is both exciting and inspiring for all nurses. Research evaluating Parse's theory needs to be replicated in other settings so that findings can be evaluated and critically analyzed. Other theories and approaches need to be evaluated as well so that nurses can choose the values and beliefs they want to live in practice and research. There also needs to be more involvement of persons receiving nursing care so that nurses know how individuals think and feel about the service nurses provide.

Nurses have a very important choice to make concerning the future direction of their discipline. Either nurses will commit their theories, research activities, and autonomous practice approaches to the human science tradition, or they will extend the biomedical, problem-based approach to all aspects of human life and ways of living. Parse's theory is one approach that clearly positions nursing as a human science and that views nurses as autonomous practitioners who coparticipate in the human-health process.

REFERENCES

Allen, D. G. (1985). Nursing research and social control: Alternate models of science that emphasize understanding and emancipation. *Image: Journal of Nursing Scholarship, 27*(2), 58–64.

Carboni, J. T. (1991). A Rogerian theoretical tapestry. *Nursing Science Quarterly, 4,* 130–136.

Cook, T. D., & Campbell, D. T. (1979). *Quasi-experimentation design & analysis issues for field settings.* Boston: Houghton Mifflin.

Cull-Wilby, B. L., & Pepin, J. L. (1987). Toward a coexistence of paradigms in nursing knowledge development. *Journal of Advanced Nursing, 12,* 515–521.

Deegan, P. E. (1993). Recovering our sense of value after being labeled. *Journal of Psychosocial Nursing, 31*(4), 7–11.

DeGroot, H. A. (1988). Scientific inquiry in nursing: A model for a new age. *Advances in Nursing Science, 10*(3), 1–21.

Griffin, A. P. (1980). Philosophy and nursing. *Journal of Advanced Nursing, 5*(3), 161–172.

Guba, E., & Lincoln, Y. (1989). *Fourth generation evaluation.* Newbury Park, CA: Sage.

Hall, B. A. (1993). The theory-research-practice triad. *Nursing Science Quarterly, 6,* 10–11.

Hall, B. A., & Allan, J. D. (1986). Sharpening nursing's focus by focusing on health. *Journal of Nursing and Health Care, 7,* 315–320.

Holmes, C. A. (1990). Alternatives to natural science foundations for nursing. *International Journal of Nursing Studies, 27,* 187–198.

Huckabay, L. M. D. (1991). The role of conceptual frameworks in nursing practice, administration, education, and research. *Nursing Administration Quarterly, 15*(3), 17–28.

Jonas, C. M. (1993). *Evaluating Parse's theory on nursing in family practice.* Unpublished manuscript. St. Michael's Hospital, Toronto, Canada.

Laurie-Shaw, B., & Ives, S. M. (1988). Implementing Orem's self-care deficit theory: Adopting a conceptual framework of nursing. *Canadian Journal of Nursing Administration, 1,* 16–19.

Mastal, M. F., Hammond, H., & Roberts, M. P. (1982). Theory into hospital practice: A pilot implementation. *The Journal of Nursing Administration, XII*(6), 9–15.

Mayberry, A. (1991). Merging nursing theories, models, and nursing practice: More than an administrative challenge. *Nursing Administration Quarterly, 15*(3), 44–53.

McFarlane, E. A. (1980). Nursing theory: The comparison of four theoretical proposals. *Journal of Advanced Nursing, 5*(1), 3–10.

Mitchell, G. J. (1991). Nursing diagnosis: An ethical analysis. *Image: Journal of Nursing Scholarship, 23*(2), 99–103.

Mitchell, G. J. (1993). The same-thing-yet-different phenomenon: A way of coming to know or not? *Nursing Science Quarterly, 6,* 61–62.

Mitchell, G. J., & Cody, W. K. (1992). Nursing knowledge and human science: Ontological and epistemological considerations. *Nursing Science Quarterly, 5,* 54–61.

Moccia, P. (1988). A critique of compromise: Beyond the methods debate. *Advances in Nursing Science, 19*(4), 1–9.

Moch, S. D. (1989). Health within illness: Conceptual evolution and practice possibilities. *Advances in Nursing Science, 11*(4), 23–31.

Parse, R. R. (1981). *Man-living-health: A theory of nursing.* New York: Wiley.

Parse, R. R. (1987). *Nursing science: Major paradigms, theories, and critiques.* Philadelphia: Saunders.

Parse, R. R. (1992). Human becoming: Parse's theory of nursing. *Nursing Science Quarterly, 5,* 35–42.

Parse, R. R. (1994). Parse's human becoming theory: Its research and practice implications. In M. E. Parker (Ed.), *Patterns of nursing theories in practice* (pp. 49–61). New York: National League for Nursing Press, Pub. No. 15-2548.

Polifroni, E. C., & Packard, S. (1993). Psychological determinism and the evolving nursing paradigm. *Nursing Science Quarterly, 6,* 63–68.

Sarter, B. (1987). Evolutionary idealism: A philosophical foundation for holistic nursing theory. *Advances in Nursing Science, 9*(2), 1–9.

Silva, M. C. (1986). Research testing nursing theory: State of the art. *Advances in Nursing Science, 9*(1), 1–11.

Smith, M. C. (1991). Evaluating nursing theory-based practice. *Nursing Science Quarterly, 4,* 98–99.

Stevens, B. (1984). *Nursing theory: Analysis, application, evaluation* (2nd ed.). Boston: Little, Brown.

Wilson-Barnett, J. (1991). The experiment - Is it worthwhile? *International Journal of Nursing Studies, 28*(1), 77–87.

Woods, N. F., Laffrey, S., Duffy, M., Lantz, M. J., Mitchell, E. S., Taylor, D., & Cowan, K. A. (1988). Being healthy: Women's images. *Advances in Nursing Science, 11*(1), 36–46.

Yeo, M. (1989). Integration of nursing theory and nursing ethics. *Advances in Nursing Science, 11,* 33–42.

Index

Absent presences, 22, 199
Acute care, evaluation study:
  charting changes, 386–389
  findings, 374–392
  methods of, 368
  nursing care, patient/family
    perceptions of, 385–386
  nursing literature, 394–396
  purpose of, 368
  setting, 369–370
  teaching Parse's theory, 370,
    373–374
  unit manager perceptions,
    383–385
Ageism, restriction and, 162–163,
  181–182
AIDS:
  bearing witness, 127–128
  case studies, 128–132, 209–218
  death, confronting, 122–123
  decision-making issues,
    126–127
  disclosure, 125–126
  grieving process:
    loss and, 124–125
    research study, 197–236
  impact of, 115–117
  incidence, 116
  losses, 124–125
  meaning of, 116–117
  social construction, 204
  struggle, 232

suffering, 123–124
theory-guided practice, 117–121
Ambiguity, possibilities emerging
  with, 218, 223–225
Anguish:
  agonizing heaviness, 50, 52–53,
    56, 246
  paralyzing, 246, 253, 255–257, 265
  suffering and, 50–53

Bearing witness:
  to AIDS patients, 127–128
  to aloneness with togetherness,
    218, 222–223, 230
  house-garden-wilderness
    metaphor, 67–68
  nurse's process, 119–120
  to nurses' struggle, 393
Behaviorist tradition, 30
Beliefs, shifting, 335–336
Bereavement, grieving process,
  201–203

Care planning, 37, 396
Caring-healing moment, 69
Certainty-uncertainty, 220, 224,
  228
Change:
  significance of, 202
  yielding to, 173–174
Charting, 323–324, 329, 386–389
Client's feelings, awareness of, 328